Generis
PUBLISHING

INTRODUCTION TO ELECTROENCEPHALOGRAPHY

B. A. Lobasyuk
L.B. Barcewicz

Title: **INTRODUCTION TO ELECTROENCEPHALOGRAPHY**

ISBN: 979-8-89966-538-7

Author: B. A. Lobasyuk, L.B. Barcewicz

Cover image: B.A. Lobasyuk

Publisher: Generis Publishing
Online orders: www.generis-publishing.com
Contact email: info@generis-publishing.com

Lobasyuk B.A., Barcewicz L.B.

INTRODUCTION TO ELECTROENCEPHALOGRAPHY

Odessa, 2026

Summary

The book comprehensively examines the theoretical, methodological, and clinical foundations of electroencephalography as one of the leading methods for studying the functional state of the brain. It outlines the diagnostic, prognostic, and monitoring value of EEG, as well as its application in neurosurgery, functional diagnostics, psychophysiology, neuroscience, experimental psychology, and cognitive research. The place of EEG among modern brain research methods and its integration with neuroimaging techniques are emphasized.

The historical development of the method is reviewed—from early investigations to the era of full digitalization, the introduction of quantitative analysis (qEEG), source localization, and the implementation of artificial intelligence. The main EEG rhythms (delta, theta, alpha, beta), their functional significance, and age-related dynamics are described. Modern concepts of EEG genesis are presented, including the role of cortical neurons, postsynaptic potentials, thalamocortical mechanisms, neuronal synchronization, and the network organization of brain activity.

The book details EEG recording conditions, functional tests, technical aspects, and methods of mathematical analysis, including time-domain, spectral (Fourier-based), time–frequency, correlation, and nonlinear approaches, as well as topographic data visualization.

Special attention is given to EEG characteristics under normal conditions (age-related changes, interhemispheric asymmetry, qEEG parameters) and their relationship to individual psychological traits.

The clinical section addresses EEG changes in alcohol dependence, schizophrenia, intellectual disability, Alzheimer's disease, Parkinsonism, affective and organic disorders, epilepsy, and pediatric conditions, including perinatal pathology and cerebral palsy.

Overall, the book serves as a systematic guide that integrates fundamental neurophysiological concepts, modern analytical methods, and clinical practice.

TABLE OF CONTENTS

Summary **7**

Introduction. The Significance of Electroencephalography in Clinical Practice **13**

1. Diagnostic Significance of EEG 13
2. Prognostic and Monitoring Value 13
3. Use of EEG in Neurosurgical Practice 14
4. EEG in Research and Functional Diagnostics 14
5. Advantages and Limitations of the Method 14
6. The Role of Electroencephalography in Psychophysiology and Neuroscience 15
7. EEG as a Tool for Studying Cognitive Processes 15
8. Study of Emotional and Psychophysiological States 16
9. EEG in Neuroscience and the Study of Brain Networks 16
10. Application of EEG in Experimental Psychology and Cognitive Research 16
11. Advantages and Limitations of EEG in Psychophysiology 17
12. The Place of Electroencephalography Among Brain Research Methods.. 17
13. Main Categories of Brain Research Methods 17
14. Limitations of EEG and the Need for Integration with Other Methods 19
15. Clinical Practice: 19
16. The Place of EEG Among Other Methods: Synergy and Uniqueness 20

Chapter 1. History of Electroencephalography **21**

1.1. Hans Berger. Introduction of the Electroencephalographic Method 29
1.2. Studies of Human Brain Electrical Activity (EEG) During Sleep 32
1.3. The Role of the Thalamocortical System and Electroencephalography... 33
1.4. The Modern Stage of Electroencephalography Development 34
1.4.1. Full Digitalization and Technical Advancement of EEG 35
1.4.2. Transition from Visual to Quantitative Analysis (qEEG) 35
1.4.3. Development of Source Localization and Spatial Analysis 35
1.4.4. Integration of EEG with Other Neuroimaging Methods 35

1.4.5. Expansion of Clinical and Functional-Diagnostic Applications............36
1.4.6. Development of EEG Research Applications..36
1.4.7. Implementation of Artificial Intelligence and Machine Learning.........36
Chapter 2. Electroencephalographic Rhythms 37
2.1. Delta Rhythm 38
2.2. Theta Rhythm...40
2.3. Alpha Rhythm 42
2.4. Beta Rhythm...45
Chapter 3. Genesis of the EEG...51
3.1. General Principles of EEG Formation 51
3.2. Role of Cortical Pyramidal Neurons...51
3.3. Postsynaptic Potentials as the Main Contribution 52
3.4. Synchronization of Neuronal Ensembles...52
3.5. Thalamocortical and Corticocortical Mechanisms 52
3.6. Role of Volume Conduction 53
3.7. Contemporary Network and Dynamic Concepts of EEG 53
3.7.1. Thalamocortical Theory (Classical)...54
3.7.2. Cortical Theory (Local Generators)...54
3.7.3. Active Inhibition Theory (Inhibition Hypothesis)................................55
3.7.4. Pacemaker Theory..55
3.7.5. Neuronal Ensemble and Synchronization Theory 56
3.7.6. Evolutionary–Adaptive Theory..56
3.7.7. Contemporary Consensus (Brief)..57
3.8. Lobasyuk B. A. Hypothesis on the Genesis of the EEG..........................57
3.9. Structures Forming EEG 59
3.10. Biophysics and Signal Propagation...62
Chapter 4. EEG Research Methods..65
4.1. Conditions for EEG Recording 65
4.1.1. Environmental Conditions 65
4.1.2. Subject Preparation 65
4.1.3. Technical Recording Conditions...66

4.1.4. Functional Tests (during standard EEG) 67
4.1.5. Special Recording Conditions 68
4.2. Practical EEG Research Methods 68
4.2.1. EEG Recording Methods 69
4.3. Functional Tests (Activation Methods) 69
4.4. Methods of Mathematical EEG Analysis 70
4.4.1. Time-Domain Analysis 70
4.4.2. Frequency-Domain Analysis 70
4.4.2.1. Fourier Transform 71
4.4.2.2. Periodometric Analysis 72
4.4.3. Time–Frequency Analysis 75
4.4.4. Correlation and Coherence Analysis 76
4.4.5. Nonlinear and Chaotic Analysis 78
4.4.6. Channel and Topographic Visualization 79
4.4.7. Methodological aspects 82
4.4.8. Main components of a modern electroencephalograph 82
4.4.9. EEG lead placement and recording 85
4.4.10. EEG segmentation 91
Chapter 5. EEG in the Normal State 97
5.1. EEG Development by Age Periods 97
5.2. Adult EEG 109
5.3. Quantitative Analysis (qEEG) Under Normal Conditions 111
5.4. Interhemispheric EEG Asymmetry 123
6. Influence of EEG rhythms on extraversion–introversion and SMIL test scores in left- and right-hemisphere-dominant individuals 137
7. EEG in Various Pathological Forms in Adults 147
7.1. The Effect of Ethanol on Electrogenesis 153
7.1.1. Study of the Effect of VER on ECoG Parameters 155
7.1.2. Changes in functional interhemispheric asymmetry (FIHA) indices of the ECoG following VER administration 157

7.1.3. Relationships Between ECoG Rhythm Amplitudes in the Left and Right Hemispheres Before and After VER Administration 158

7.1.4. EEG in Alcoholism 160

7.2. Electroencephalographic Changes in Schizophrenia 173

7.2.1. Quantitative EEG (qEEG) in Psychiatry 181

7.2.2. Study of EEG Features in Schizophrenia Using Computerized Electroencephalography 183

7.3. Analysis of Changes in Electrogenesis in Intellectual Disability Using Computer Electroencephalography 192

7.4. Major EEG Changes in Alzheimer's Disease 203

7.5. EEG in Parkinsonism 211

7.6. Affective Mental Disorders 228

7.7. EEG and Epilepsy 231

7.7.1. Modeling Epilepsy in Biological Models 231

7.7.1.1. Application Model of Multifocal Cortical Epilepsy 232

7.7.1.2. Development of a biological model of multifocal cortical epilepsy by intraperitoneal administration of BP and analysis of seizure activity evolution 235

7.7.2. Epilepsy Diagnosis in the Clinic 242

8. Pathology in Children 261

8.1. Preparation of the Child for EEG 262

8.2. Periodization of the Development of Electroencephalogenesis 264

8.3. Perinatal Pathology and EEG 265

8.4. Cerebral Palsy in Children 270

Литература 279

Literatura 313

Introduction.
The Significance of Electroencephalography in Clinical Practice

Electroencephalography (EEG) is an important tool of modern clinical medicine, providing direct recording of the electrical activity of the brain. The method is based on measuring fluctuations of brain potentials using electrodes placed on the surface of the scalp. EEG makes it possible to obtain objective data on the functional state of the cerebral cortex, identify pathological processes, monitor disease dynamics, and assess the effectiveness of treatment (Britton JW, Frey LC, Hopp JL, et al., 2016).

1. Diagnostic Significance of EEG

EEG is widely used for the diagnosis of various neurological disorders, primarily epilepsy. Specific patterns of electrical activity, such as spike–wave discharges or polyspikes, may indicate the presence of focal or generalized epileptic activity. In addition, EEG helps differentiate epileptic seizures from other conditions, such as syncopal episodes or psychogenic seizures, which is critically important for selecting appropriate therapy (Frauscher B, Rossetti AO, Beniczky S., 2024).

The method is also applied in the diagnosis of other disturbances of brain function, including encephalopathies of various etiologies (metabolic, toxic, infectious), acute and chronic cerebrovascular disorders, traumatic brain injuries, and neurodegenerative diseases. EEG can reveal diffuse or focal changes in electrical activity, allowing clinicians to determine the localization and nature of the pathological process.

2. Prognostic and Monitoring Value

EEG is actively used to monitor the condition of patients in intensive care and critical care units. Continuous or periodic monitoring of brain electrical activity makes it possible to assess the extent of cortical damage in severe trauma, stroke, or hypoxic–ischemic conditions. EEG is of particular importance in comatose states, as it allows assessment of coma depth, outcome prediction, and monitoring of the effectiveness of therapeutic interventions (Ivanova, O. M., & Ivanova, M. A., 2018; Dokukina, T. V., & Misyuk, N. N., 2013).

In pediatrics, EEG plays an important role in predicting neurobehavioral and cognitive impairments in children at risk of developmental delay or epileptic syndromes. Patterns of brain activity at early stages may serve as indicators of future problems and guide preventive or therapeutic measures.

3. Use of EEG in Neurosurgical Practice

EEG is also a valuable tool in the preparation for neurosurgical interventions. It helps localize epileptic foci in patients with pharmacoresistant epilepsy and determine optimal areas for surgical resection. In combination with neuroimaging methods (MRI, CT, PET), EEG enables more accurate surgical planning and improves treatment outcomes (Simon, M. V., 2022; Kuruvilla, A., & Flink, R., 2003; Flanary, J., et al., 2022; Redžepi, S., Burazerović, E., Redžepi, et al., 2025; Talairach, J., Bancaud, J., Szikla, G., et al., 1974).

4. EEG in Research and Functional Diagnostics

In addition to clinical applications, EEG is widely used in neurophysiological research. The method allows assessment of cognitive functions, levels of alertness, responses to stimuli, and the dynamics of brain activity under various psychoemotional states. Modern EEG analysis methods (e.g., spectral, coherence, and functional analysis) make it possible to detect changes in brain activity that are not accessible through other techniques (Zhang H., Zhou Q., Chen H., Hu X.-Q., Li W.-G., Bai Y., et al., 2023; Chaddad A., et al., 2023; Jadhav C. J., 2022; van der Stelt O., Belger A., 2007; Komkova Y. N., Sugrobova G. A., Bezrukikh M. M., 2023; Osorio F. A. C., et al., 2025).

5. Advantages and Limitations of the Method

EEG has several advantages: it is a non-invasive, safe, relatively inexpensive, and accessible method that provides real-time information about the functional state of the brain. However, it also has limitations, including low spatial resolution, sensitivity to artifacts (movement, blinking, muscle activity), and limited ability to accurately detect activity in certain deep brain structures. Therefore, EEG is often used in combination with other neuroimaging and neurophysiological methods.

Electroencephalography occupies a key position in modern clinical practice. It enables early diagnosis of neurological diseases, patient monitoring, surgical planning, and assessment of treatment effectiveness. Despite its limitations, EEG remains an indispensable tool for neurologists, neurosurgeons, and intensive care specialists, combining high informational value with safety and accessibility. The development of analytical methods and integration with modern technologies continue to expand the clinical and research applications of EEG, making it an important component of personalized medicine.

6. The Role of Electroencephalography in Psychophysiology and Neuroscience

Electroencephalography (EEG) is one of the fundamental methods for tudying brain function, playing a key role not only in clinical practice but also in psychophysiology and neuroscience. The method is based on recording the electrical activity of the cerebral cortex from the scalp and allows assessment of the dynamics of neuronal processes in real time. Due to its high temporal resolution, EEG provides unique data on information processing, cognitive activity, and emotional states.

7. EEG as a Tool for Studying Cognitive Processes

In psychophysiology, EEG is actively used to study cognitive functions such as attention, memory, perception, and learning. Different brain wave frequencies (delta, theta, alpha, beta, gamma) are associated with specific psychophysiological states:

Alpha rhythm (8–13 Hz) is usually associated with rest, relaxation, and reduced processing of external sensory information.

Beta rhythm (13–30 Hz) appears during active cognitive activity, focused attention, and problem solving.

Theta rhythm (4–8 Hz) often reflects processes of internal concentration, memory, and meditation.

Gamma rhythm (30–100 Hz) is associated with the integration of sensory information and high-level cognitive processing.

EEG enables researchers not only to record brain activity within these frequency bands but also to conduct advanced analyses of coherence and neural connectivity, providing insight into how different brain regions interact during specific tasks.

8. Study of Emotional and Psychophysiological States

EEG is an important tool for assessing emotional responses, stress levels, and emotional regulation. Research has shown that asymmetry of alpha activity in the frontal lobes may be associated with a predisposition to positive or negative emotions.

The method allows researchers to:

track responses to emotional stimuli, study physiological correlates of anxiety and depression, investigate the dynamics of brain activity during meditation, relaxation, and mindfulness training.

EEG is also widely used in biofeedback (neurofeedback), where individuals learn to become aware of and regulate their brain activity, thereby improving cognitive and emotional functioning.

9. EEG in Neuroscience and the Study of Brain Networks

In modern neuroscience, EEG is used to study functional brain connectivity, synchronization of neural networks, and the dynamics of information processing. Owing to its high temporal resolution, EEG makes it possible to capture instantaneous brain responses to external and internal stimuli, which is not feasible with methods that have low temporal precision, such as MRI.

Contemporary approaches, including spectral analysis, coherence, and functional connectivity analysis, make it possible to:

determine which brain regions are co-activated during the performance of cognitive tasks, investigate neural mechanisms of attention, memory, and learning, study pathological changes in brain activity associated with psychiatric and neurological disorders.

10. Application of EEG in Experimental Psychology and Cognitive Research

EEG enables experiments in which the dynamics of brain responses to sensory, cognitive, or emotional stimuli are recorded. Examples include studies of speech perception and visual processing, assessment of responses to complex cognitive tasks, investigation of decision-making and attentional processes, and examination of the neural mechanisms underlying learning and memory.

In addition, EEG is actively used in combination with other methods, such as functional magnetic resonance imaging (fMRI) and transcranial magnetic stimulation (TMS), allowing integration of data on the spatial and temporal organization of brain activity.

11. Advantages and Limitations of EEG in Psychophysiology

Advantages of EEG include high temporal resolution, enabling the recording of neural activity dynamics on the millisecond scale; non-invasiveness and safety; the possibility of multichannel recording and analysis of network interactions; and the relatively low cost and mobility of equipment for laboratory and clinical research.

Limitations include lower spatial resolution compared to MRI, sensitivity to artifacts (eye movements, blinking, muscle activity), and difficulties in studying deep brain structures without the use of additional methods.

EEG is an indispensable tool in psychophysiology and neuroscience, allowing researchers to investigate the dynamics of cognitive processes, emotional states, and functional interactions within neural networks. The method combines safety, high temporal resolution, and multichannel analytical capabilities, making it a key technique for both fundamental and applied brain research. Thanks to modern analytical approaches, EEG not only describes general patterns of brain activity but also reveals individual features of brain functioning, opening new possibilities for personalized cognitive and psychological diagnostics.

12. The Place of Electroencephalography Among Brain Research Methods

The study of the human brain is one of the most complex challenges in medicine and neuroscience. A wide range of methods is used for this purpose, each with its own advantages, limitations, and areas of application. Electroencephalography (EEG) occupies a special place among these methods due to its unique ability to directly record the electrical activity of the cerebral cortex with high temporal precision.

13. Main Categories of Brain Research Methods

Modern brain research methods can be broadly divided into three groups:

1. **Structural methods**, which allow assessment of brain anatomy:

- **Magnetic resonance imaging (MRI)** — provides high spatial resolution and enables detailed examination of brain anatomy and detection of pathological changes.

Computed tomography (CT) — a more accessible method used to diagnose trauma, hemorrhages, and tumors.

Functional methods, which record brain activity over time:

Functional MRI (fMRI) — evaluates blood flow changes associated with neural activity, offering high spatial resolution but relatively low temporal resolution.

PET and SPECT — assess metabolism and cerebral blood flow and are used in the diagnosis of neurodegenerative and tumor processes.

Magnetoencephalography (MEG) — records magnetic fields generated by neural activity with high temporal resolution.

2. **Electrophysiological methods**, based on the recording of neuronal electrical activity:

Electroencephalography (EEG) — records the summed potentials of cortical neurons through the skull, providing unparalleled temporal resolution.

Evoked potentials (EPs) — specialized forms of EEG responses elicited by sensory or cognitive stimuli.

2. Advantages of EEG Compared to Other Methods

EEG has several unique features that make it indispensable:

High temporal resolution — EEG records brain electrical activity with millisecond precision, making it ideal for studying dynamic processes such as sensory processing, cognitive responses, and epileptic seizures.

Direct recording of neural activity — unlike fMRI or PET, which measure indirect indicators (blood flow or metabolism), EEG reflects the immediate electrical oscillations of neurons.

Accessibility and safety — the method is non-invasive, does not involve ionizing radiation, and is relatively inexpensive and mobile.

Multichannel analysis capability — modern EEG systems can simultaneously record dozens or even hundreds of channels, enabling investigation of the spatial organization of brain activity.

14. Limitations of EEG and the Need for Integration with Other Methods

Despite its advantages, EEG has several limitations:

Low spatial resolution — it is more difficult to precisely localize the source of activity, especially in deep brain structures (e.g., the hippocampus or thalamus).

Sensitivity to artifacts — eye movements, blinking, muscle activity, and electrical noise can distort the signal.

Limited anatomical detail — EEG does not provide information about brain structure or vascular pathology.

Due to these limitations, EEG is often used in combination with other methods, such as:

fMRI for spatial localization of activity,

MEG for improved temporal and spatial accuracy,

MRI for constructing individualized head models in EEG analysis.

4. The Role of EEG in Clinical and Scientific Research*

15. Clinical Practice:

EEG is widely used for the diagnosis of epilepsy, encephalopathies, sleep disorders, comatose states, and for the assessment of brain activity in newborns. The possibility of long-term monitoring makes EEG indispensable in intensive care units and critical care settings.

Neuroscience and Psychophysiology:

EEG makes it possible to study cognitive processes, emotional states, functional brain networks, and responses to external stimuli. In combination with analytical methods such as spectral analysis and coherence, EEG reveals the dynamics of interactions between neural regions and patterns of brain activity.

Experimental Psychology and Neurocognitive Research:

EEG is used to investigate attention, memory, perception, decision-making, and learning. It is indispensable in studies of biofeedback (neurofeedback), cognitive training, and psychophysiological testing.

16. The Place of EEG Among Other Methods: Synergy and Uniqueness

EEG should not be regarded as a replacement for MRI or PET; rather, it is a complementary yet unique method. While structural techniques provide an accurate anatomical map and PET or fMRI demonstrate metabolism and blood flow, EEG captures neural activity in real time. This capability is critical for studying dynamic processes such as epileptic seizures, sensory processing, cognitive and emotional responses, and sleep–wake rhythms.

It is precisely the combination of EEG with other methods that enables a comprehensive understanding of brain function by integrating information about the structure, function, and dynamics of neural networks.

EEG occupies a special position among brain research methods due to its unique ability to directly record neuronal electrical activity with high temporal precision. It is indispensable both in clinical practice and in psychophysiology and neuroscience. Despite limitations in spatial localization, EEG integrates effectively with MRI, fMRI, PET, and MEG, providing comprehensive insight into the human brain. EEG continues to be a key tool for studying dynamic processes, functional networks, and the neurophysiological foundations of behavior and cognitive activity.

Chapter 1. History of Electroencephalography

The history of electrophysiology began with the study of the effects of electricity on the living organism. In the 18th century, physicists investigating electrical charges repeatedly encountered their irritating effects on biological tissues.

Electrical stimulation produced distinctive subjective sensations and various physiological effects, such as involuntary and convulsive muscle contractions and twitching. These phenomena attracted the attention of physicians and physiologists.

In the 18th century, the Italian physician **Luigi Galvani** was the first to discover bioelectricity—the ability of biological objects to generate electrical current. Galvani demonstrated this phenomenon using dissected frog legs.

Galvani reported his discovery in 1791. He observed that frog legs suspended on copper wires on his balcony contracted when they came into contact with zinc supports. He believed that the cause of the muscle contractions was "animal electricity" generated within the body of the animal itself, while the wire merely served to complete the electrical circuit. Galvani sent a copy of his work to **Alessandro Volta**, a professor of physics in Pavia (Northern Italy).

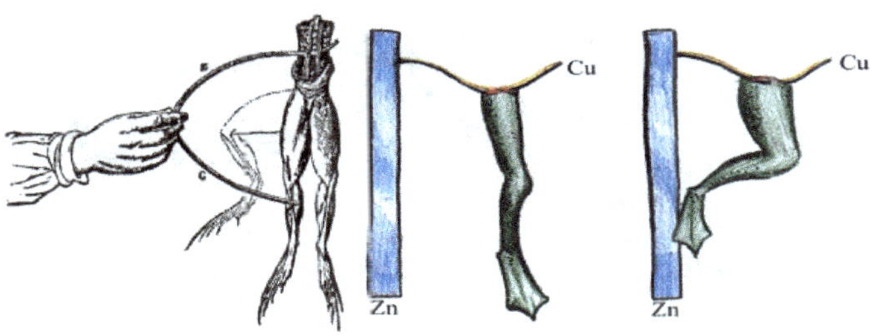

Figure 1. *Galvani's first experiment.*

Volta repeated Galvani's experiments, obtained the same results, and at first agreed with his conclusions, but later drew attention to the fact that "animal electricity" arises only when two different metals are present in the circuit. Volta showed that touching the tongue with two different metals connected to each other produces a sensation of taste.

Attempting to refute Galvani's thesis about the existence of "animal electricity," Volta suggested that a circuit containing two different metals in contact with a saline solution should be a source of continuous current—unlike an electrostatic machine, which produces only electrical discharges.

This proved to be the case. Volta published his work describing the first source of direct current (later called galvanic) in 1793. However, soon afterward Galvani demonstrated that "animal electricity" also exists in circuits that do not contain bimetallic contacts: he placed the nerve of a neuromuscular preparation onto a muscle so that one part of the nerve lay on an intact surface of the muscle and another part on a damaged one.

He was unable to continue his dispute with Volta. In 1796, Bologna came under French control, and Galvani, who refused to recognize the new government, was expelled from the university. He was forced to seek refuge with his brother, where he no longer engaged in scientific work until his death (1798). In 1800, Volta presented his discovery to Napoleon, for which he received a substantial reward. Thus, the dispute between two compatriots—different in political views, temperament, and education—gave impetus to the development of modern physics and biology.

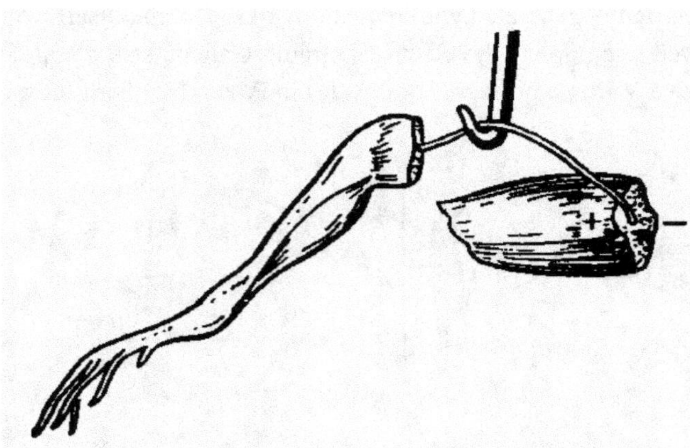

Figure 2. *Galvani's second experiment.*

Carlo Matteucci (1811–1868) showed in the 1830s–1840s that an electric current can always be detected in a muscle, flowing from its intact surface toward a transverse cut. He explained Galvani's second experiment by the outflow of negative charge along the nerve, acting as a conductor, from the interior of the muscle. Matteucci also showed that the electric current arising during tissue excitation is capable of stimulating another excitable tissue (the "secondary contraction" experiment).

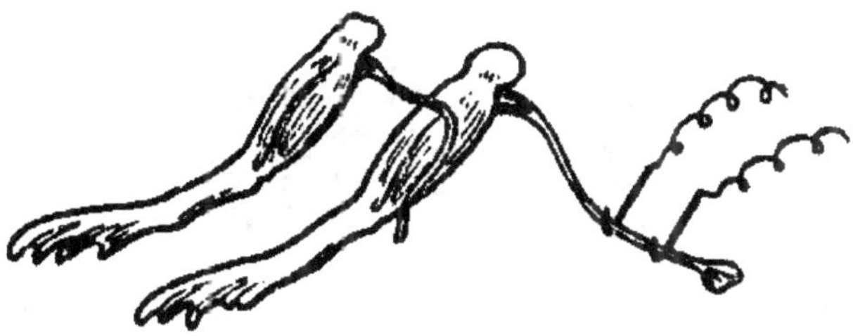

Figure 3. *Matteucci's experiment.*

"Action potential" or "nerve impulse."

The nerve impulse constitutes the material basis of the excitation process in the nervous system. For their research into the nature of the nerve impulse, the British scientists Alan Lloyd Hodgkin and Andrew Fielding Huxley were awarded the Nobel Prize in 1963.

How do our sense organs inform the brain about what is happening around us? And, in general, how do different parts of our body exchange information? Nature has devised two special communication systems for this purpose. The first, the humoral system (from the Latin *humor* — moisture, fluid), is based on diffusion or, in simpler organisms and in plants, on the transport of biologically active substances by the flow of fluid from the place where they are synthesized throughout the organism.

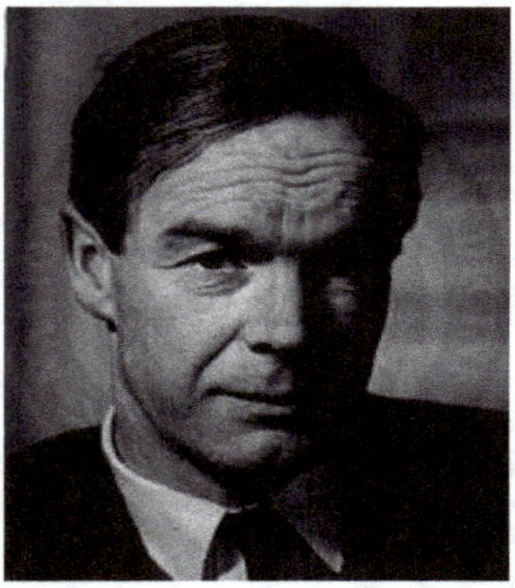

Figure 4. *Sir Alan Lloyd Hodgkin (5 February 1914, Banbury, England — 20 December 1998) was a British neurophysiologist and biophysicist, a laureate of the 1963 Nobel Prize in Physiology or Medicine (shared with John Eccles and Andrew Huxley) "for their discoveries concerning the ionic mechanisms involved in excitation and inhibition in the peripheral and central portions of the nerve cell."*

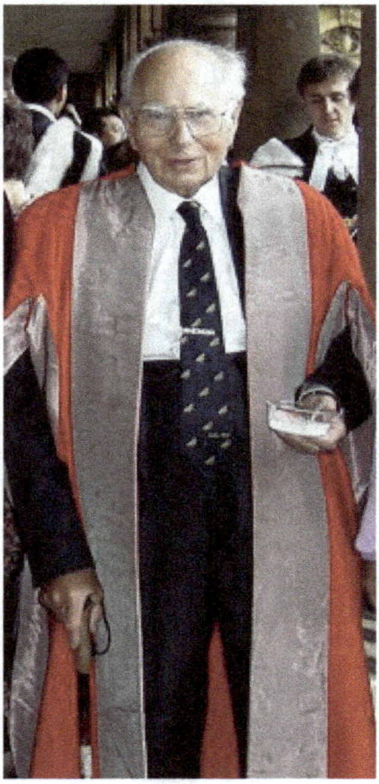

Figure 5. *Sir Andrew Fielding Huxley (22 November 1917, London — 30 May 2012) was an English neurophysiologist and biophysicist, a laureate of the 1963 Nobel Prize in Physiology or Medicine (shared with John Eccles and Alan Hodgkin) for their discoveries concerning the ionic mechanisms involved in excitation and inhibition in the peripheral and central portions of the nerve cell."*

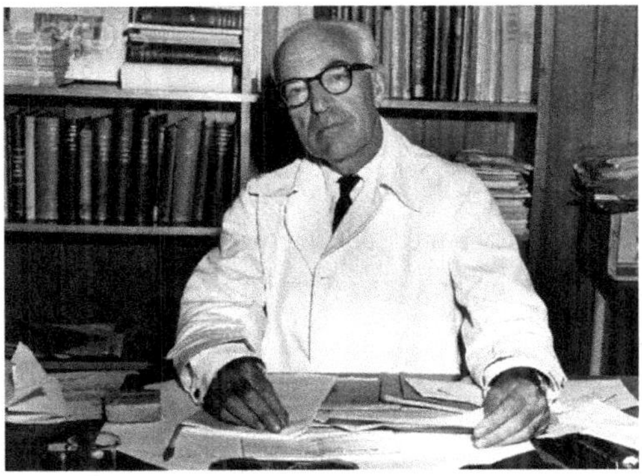

Figure 6. *Sir John Carew Eccles (27 January 1903, Melbourne, Australia — 2 May 1997, Locarno, Switzerland) was an Australian neurophysiologist and a laureate of the 1963 Nobel Prize in Physiology or Medicine. He served as President of the Australian Academy of Science from 1957 to 1961.*

The study of the electrical processes of the brain was initiated by D. du Bois-Reymond in 1849, who showed that the brain, like nerves and muscles, possesses electrogenic properties.

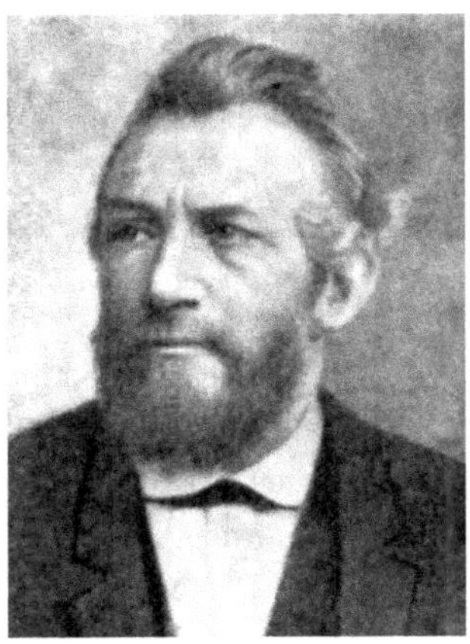

Figure 7. *Emil Heinrich du Bois-Reymond (7 November 1818, Berlin — 26 December 1896, Berlin) was a German physiologist of Swiss origin, a philosopher, and a foreign corresponding member of the St. Petersburg Academy of Sciences (1892).*

In the 19th century, the first physical instruments—string galvanometers—were developed, which made it possible to study weak electrical potentials from biological objects. In 1875, the English surgeon and physiologist Richard Caton reported for the first time at a meeting of the British Medical Association that he had succeeded in recording weak electrical currents from the brains of rabbits and monkeys. Thus, it was shown that the brain is a generator of electrical activity, i.e., brain biocurrents were discovered.

Professor I. Pravdich-Neminsky of Kazan University studied bioelectrical oscillations of the dog's brain under various conditions of the animal—at rest and during excitation. In essence, these were the first electroencephalograms.

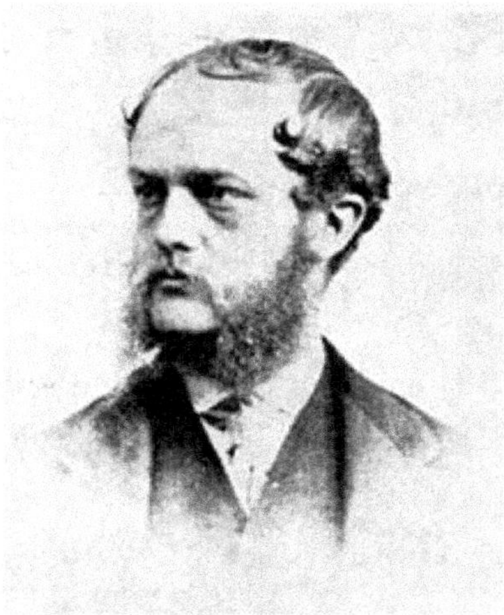

Figure 8. *Richard Caton (1842, Scarborough, Yorkshire — 2 January 1926) was an English physiologist and surgeon, a Fellow of the Royal Society of London.*

In 1882, I. M. Sechenov published the work *"Galvanic Phenomena in the Medulla Oblongata of the Frog,"* in which the existence of rhythmic activity was established for the first time. He called this activity spontaneous, since it arose without any apparent external causes. Sechenov showed that stimulation of peripheral nerves leads to suppression of spontaneous oscillations.

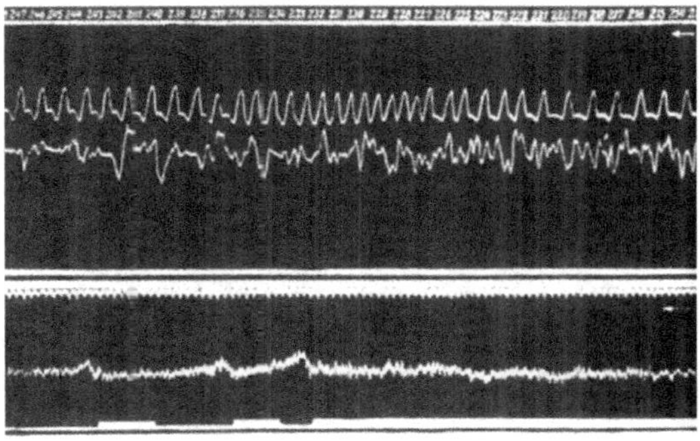

Figure 9. *The first published photograph of a dog's EEG.*

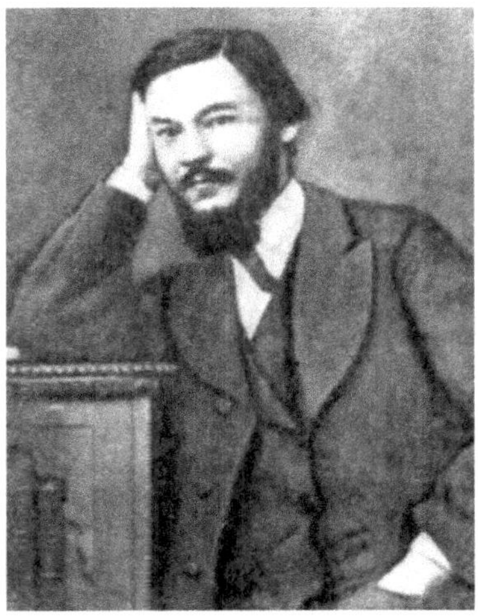

Figure 10. *Ivan Mikhailovich Sechenov (1 (13) August 1829 — 2 (15) November 1905) was a Russian physiologist and educator, publicist, rationalist thinker, founder of a physiological school, encyclopedic scholar, evolutionary biologist, psychologist, anthropologist, anatomist, histologist, pathologist, psychophysiologist, physical chemist, endocrinologist, ophthalmologist, hematologist, narcologist, hygienist, cultural studies scholar, instrument designer, and military engineer.*

In 1884, N. E. Vvedensky, in his work *"Studies on Nerve Centers,"* applied the telephone method to investigate the electrical activity of the frog's medulla oblongata and the cerebral cortex of rabbits and dogs. Vvedensky confirmed

Sechenov's main observations and showed that spontaneous activity can also be detected in the cerebral cortex of mammals.

In 1889, a major paper by the well-known Russian physiologist and student of Sechenov, B. F. Verigo, was published in the journal *Bulletin of Clinical and Forensic Psychiatry and Neuropathology*, in which he presented his observations on the electrical activity of the spinal cord and brain.

In 1929, the German physiologist and psychiatrist H. Berger recorded the bioelectrical potentials of the human brain, which are now called the electroencephalogram. In these studies, the main rhythm of human brain biocurrents was recorded for the first time—sinusoidal oscillations with a frequency of 8–12 cycles per second.

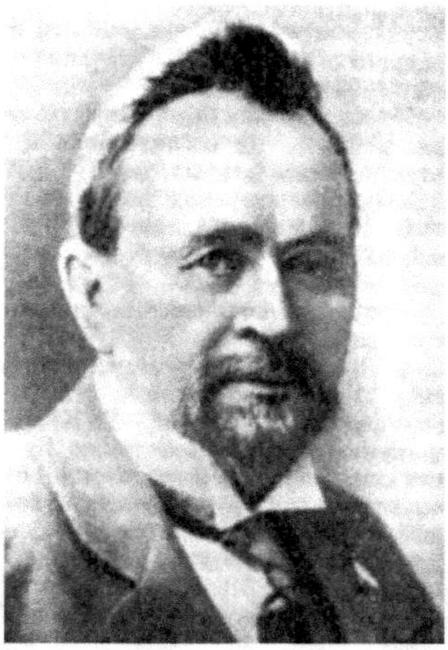

Figure 11. *Nikolay Yevgenyevich Vvedensky (16 (28) April 1852, Kochkovo village, Vologda Governorate — 16 September 1922, same place) was an outstanding physiologist, a student of I. M. Sechenov, and the founder of the study of general principles of excitability in the body's responsive systems.*

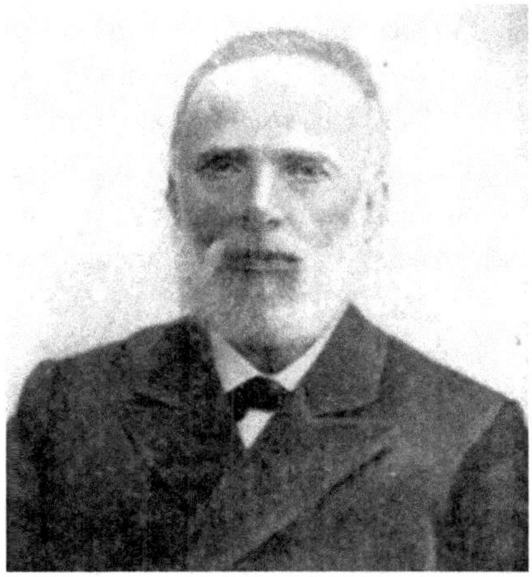

Figure 12. *Bronislav Fortunatovich Verigo (14 February 1860, Uzhvald estate, Dinaburg District, Vitebsk Governorate — 13 June 1925, Perm) was a Russian physiologist who was the first to establish the effect of oxygen on the blood's ability to bind carbon dioxide (the Verigo effect). He was also the author of works on electrophysiology.*

1.1. Hans Berger. Introduction of the Electroencephalographic Method

The German physiologist and psychiatrist Hans Berger (1929) recorded the bioelectrical potentials of the human brain, now called the electroencephalogram (EEG). In these studies, the main rhythm of human brain biocurrents was recorded for the first time—sinusoidal oscillations at a frequency of 8–12 cycles per second.

Electroencephalography (EEG) is a method for recording the electrical activity (biopotentials) of the brain through intact scalp tissues, allowing assessment of its physiological maturity, functional state, presence of focal lesions, generalized brain disorders, and their nature. Recording biopotentials directly from the exposed brain is called electrocorticography and is usually performed during neurosurgical operations.

EEG is sometimes compared to the "smoke of a locomotive" or the "noise of a car." Some consider EEG to be an "epiphenomenon" (a secondary, accompanying phenomenon that parallels the main process but is not necessarily causally linked to it).

Does this mean that EEG patterns cannot be a subject of scientific study?

The first recordings of electrical activity of the human cerebral cortex by H. Berger (1929) showed that the curve representing biopotentials is complex in pattern. If the elements of the electroencephalogram could be decoded, it would be possible to determine the state and specifics of processes occurring in the nervous system (Monakhov K.K., Bochkarev V.K., Nikiforov A.I., 1983). One of the most striking features of EEG is its spontaneous, autonomous character.

In his article *"Über das Elektrenkephalogramm des Menschen"* (On the Electroencephalogram of Man), German psychiatrist and neurophysiologist Hans Berger first described the method of recording electrical activity of the human brain from the surface of the skull and introduced the term *electroencephalogram* (EEG). This work became foundational in the history of electroencephalography—the method of measuring spontaneous electrical potentials of the brain using electrodes placed on the scalp, allowing the first continuous recording of human brain rhythms.

Berger conducted experiments for many years, initially on animals, but only in 1924 did he achieve reliable registration of brain electrical signals in humans using a galvanometer and amplifier. His 1929 publication presented the results of numerous experiments, including the description of regularly oscillating curves of electrical activity, which he later identified as distinct brain rhythms (alpha and beta rhythms—representing calm and active cortical states, respectively).

In his paper, Berger also discussed methodological aspects of recording (how to obtain signals), characteristics of the recordings, and possible physiological and psychophysiological interpretations of the curves obtained, including variations in activity under different states (consciousness/sleep, relaxation/activity). The EEG he presented laid the foundation for the systematic study of brain electrical activity and later found broad application in sleep research, epilepsy studies, cognitive process research, and clinical diagnostics.

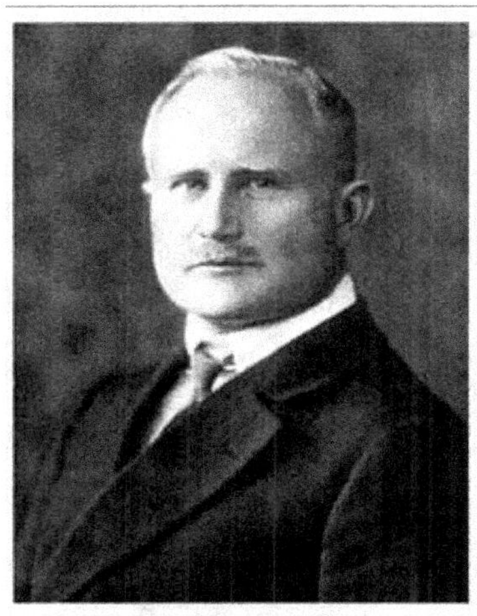

Figure 13. Hans Berger

Hans Berger (German: Hans Berger; May 21, 1873, Neuses near Coburg — June 1, 1941, Jena) was a German physiologist and psychiatrist, one of the founders of electroencephalography.

Hans Berger was born in the village of Neuses (Ger.) near the city of Coburg in Thuringia, Germany. He discovered the alpha rhythm of the human brain and was the creator of the electroencephalographic method for recording brain activity. He was a student of O. Binswanger. After completing his education and one year of military service, he worked from 1901 as a Privatdozent in Jena; from 1905 he was an associate professor, and from 1919 to 1938 he served as full professor and director of the Psychiatric Clinic of Jena University, which now bears his name. He also studied and described the chronic form of paranoia (1913).

This publication subsequently became the first in a series of works by Berger under the same title, in which he developed and expanded his observations on the measurement of electrical oscillations of the brain under normal and pathological conditions.

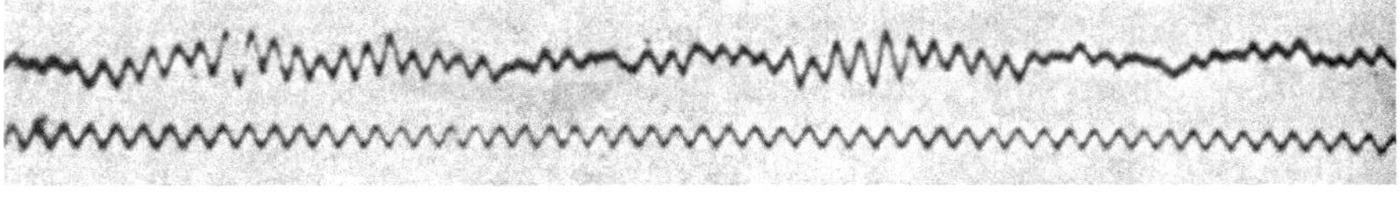

Figure 14. *The first human EEG recording was obtained by Hans Berger in 1925. Two electrodes were used: frontal and occipital.*

1.2. Studies of Human Brain Electrical Activity (EEG) During Sleep

In the article *"Cerebral states during sleep, as studied by human brain potentials"* (1937), Loomis A. L., Harvey E. N., and Hobart G. A. presented some of the first systematic studies of human brain electrical activity (EEG) during sleep, obtained using surface recordings of brain potentials. The authors employed amplifiers and automatic recording systems developed by themselves to continuously record EEG during sleep and wakefulness, which for the first time made it possible to describe the relationship between changes in brain electrical activity and different stages of sleep.

The study demonstrated that as the transition from wakefulness to sleep occurs, the EEG undergoes sequential qualitative changes. During the transition from wakefulness to sleep onset, a typical alpha rhythm is recorded, which disappears during deeper sleep. Subsequently, a sequence of states differing in amplitude and frequency spectrum of electrical activity appears; the authors designated these as distinct states (A–E).

Each of these states is characterized by specific EEG spectral features: state A — pronounced alpha rhythm, typical of quiet wakefulness or drowsiness; state B — reduced amplitude and rhythmicity, indicating the onset of sleep; states C–E — the emergence of slower, high-amplitude waves reflecting progressively deeper stages of sleep.

The authors also noted increasing difficulty in awakening subjects from the deeper states (D and E), indicating greater depth and stability of sleep. In addition, they suggested a relationship between certain EEG characteristics and dreaming, noting that low-amplitude, low-frequency EEG activity may be associated with richer internal experiences compared to deeper stages of sleep.

This work made a major contribution to the history of sleep research by laying the foundations for EEG-based sleep stage classification, which was later further developed and standardized by other researchers (e.g., Dement & Kleitman; Rechtschaffen & Kales).

1.3. The Role of the Thalamocortical System and Electroencephalography

The article by Steriade, McCormick, and Sejnowski (1993) is a review of the mechanisms underlying the generation, modulation, and physiological significance of oscillations in thalamocortical systems across different brain states—sleep and wakefulness. The authors emphasize that sleep and wakefulness are characterized by specific rhythmic patterns of brain electrical activity that arise from interactions between the thalamus and the cerebral cortex.

The paper discusses how low-frequency oscillations (characteristic of sleep) and fast rhythms (typical of wakefulness) emerge as a result of complex dynamics within thalamic and cortical neuronal networks. According to the authors, sleep is characterized by synchronized activity of billions of neurons, manifested as slow rhythms, whereas during awakening neuromodulatory systems are activated that suppress slow oscillations and induce fast rhythms and high brain reactivity.

The authors analyze data obtained at multiple levels—from molecular to network—using intracellular and extracellular recordings *in vivo* and *in vitro*, as well as computational modeling, allowing them to trace the mechanisms underlying transitions between oscillatory states. They demonstrate that thalamocortical oscillations result from intrinsic neuronal properties, their interconnections, and the action of neurotransmitter systems, and that these oscillations play a key role in regulating consciousness, attention, and information processing across different functional states of the brain.

The work highlights that synchronization within thalamocortical networks accompanies the transition from wakefulness to rest and subsequently to deep sleep, and also influences behavior and perception. Such integration of physiological data sheds light on fundamental principles of brain function and provides a basis for further research into the neurodynamics of sleep, consciousness, and cognitive states.

In the article *"Low-frequency (< 1 Hz) oscillations in the human sleep electroencephalogram"*, Achermann P. and Borbély A. A. (1997) conducted the first systematic investigation of low-frequency (< 1 Hz) components of the human sleep EEG, which had previously been identified in animal studies. The authors aimed to determine whether similar slow oscillations are present in the human EEG and how they relate to known sleep rhythms.

The study was based on full-night EEG recordings from healthy male subjects (n = 8), selected according to strict criteria (absence of sleep disorders and abstinence from caffeine and alcohol prior to the study). To analyze the signal spectrum, methods compensating for low-frequency amplifier attenuation were applied, enabling accurate assessment of activity below 1 Hz.

The authors found that during episodes of slow-wave sleep (non-REM), the EEG power spectrum exhibits a distinct peak around 0.7–0.8 Hz (varying approximately from 0.55 to 0.95 Hz). This activity differed markedly from classical delta rhythms (> 2 Hz), which decrease during the second half of sleep, whereas the < 1 Hz component maintained its power.

To identify slow components, a new time series was also constructed based on successive 0.5-second EEG segments with low-pass filtering (< 4.5 Hz) or band-pass filtering (12–15 Hz, corresponding to sleep spindle frequency). Spectral analysis of this time series revealed variable periodicity of approximately 20–30 seconds for slow waves and about 4 seconds for spindle-frequency activity, reflecting the complex dynamics of slow sleep rhythms.

Thus, the study demonstrates that EEG components below 1 Hz are a stable characteristic of human sleep, reflecting sequences of recurring phases of cortical neuron hyperpolarization and depolarization and possible cyclic influences on spindle activity. These low-frequency oscillations exhibit dynamics distinct from traditional delta waves and are consistent with observations in animals, indicating a fundamental role of slow rhythms in sleep organization and sleep-regulating processes.

In the classic monograph *"The Healthy and Diseased Human Brain"* by Natalia Petrovna Bekhtereva (1988), the structure and functions of the human brain in normal and pathological conditions are examined, along with principles of neurophysiological research and general concepts of nervous system function.

1.4. The Modern Stage of Electroencephalography Development

The modern stage of electroencephalography (EEG) development is characterized by a qualitative expansion of the method's capabilities, driven by digital technologies, advances in mathematical analysis, integration with other neuroimaging techniques, and a shift in the conceptual framework for interpreting brain activity.

1.4.1. Full Digitalization and Technical Advancement of EEG

The transition from analog to digital EEG recording has significantly increased the accuracy, reproducibility, and informational value of the method. Modern systems provide high sampling rates, multichannel recording (64–256 electrodes), improved signal-to-noise ratio, and automated data processing.

This has transformed EEG into not only a clinical tool but also a high-precision research instrument (Britton J. W., Frey L. C., Hopp J. L., et al., 2016).

1.4.2. Transition from Visual to Quantitative Analysis (qEEG)

Whereas EEG interpretation was previously based mainly on visual inspection of waveforms, the modern stage is characterized by the active implementation of quantitative EEG (qEEG), including spectral, time–frequency, correlation, and nonlinear analyses.

Quantitative methods allow the detection of latent changes in brain bioelectrical activity, the creation of normative databases, and the use of EEG as an objective diagnostic marker (Niedermeyer E., Lopes da Silva F., 2018).

1.4.3. Development of Source Localization and Spatial Analysis

Modern EEG actively employs inverse problem methods (LORETA, sLORETA, eLORETA), enabling estimation of the probable sources of electrical activity within the cerebral cortex.

This brings EEG closer to neuroimaging techniques and significantly expands its applications in neurosurgery, epileptology, and cognitive research (Pascual-Marqui R. D. *Standardized low-resolution brain electromagnetic tomography (sLORETA): technical details*. Methods Find Exp Clin Pharmacol. 2002;24(Suppl D):5–12).

1.4.4. Integration of EEG with Other Neuroimaging Methods

A defining feature of the modern stage is the multimodal approach, particularly the integration of EEG with MRI, fMRI, PET, and MEG. Combining the high temporal resolu tion of EEG with the spatial precision of MRI has enabled the study of the dynamics of functional brain networks. The EEG–fMRI method has gained particular importance (Laufs H., 2012).

1.4.5. Expansion of Clinical and Functional-Diagnostic Applications

Modern EEG is used not only for the diagnosis of epilepsy, but also for:
assessment of the level of consciousness,
monitoring in intensive care units (continuous EEG),
diagnosis of metabolic and toxic encephalopathies,
monitoring the depth of anesthesia,
functional diagnostics of cognitive impairments
(Herman S. T., Abend N. S., Bleck T. P., et al., 2015).

1.4.6. Development of EEG Research Applications

The modern stage is characterized by the active use of EEG in cognitive neuroscience. Processes such as attention, memory, perception, and decision-making are studied through the analysis of event-related potentials (ERPs) and neuronal oscillations.

EEG has become a key tool for investigating the temporal organization of mental processes (Luck S. J., 2014).

1.4.7. Implementation of Artificial Intelligence and Machine Learning

Modern EEG is increasingly integrated with machine learning and artificial intelligence methods, enabling automated pattern recognition, outcome prediction, and the development of personalized diagnostic algorithms (Roy Y., Banville H., Albuquerque I., et al., 2019).

Thus, the modern stage of EEG development is characterized by:

1. full digitalization of the method;
2. transition to quantitative and automated analysis;
3. development of source localization techniques;
4. integration with neuroimaging methods;
5. expansion of clinical and functional-diagnostic applications;
6. active use in cognitive research;
7. implementation of artificial intelligence methods.

Chapter 2. Electroencephalographic Rhythms

EEG analysis began with the identification of its frequency bands: the alpha rhythm by H. Berger (1929) and the delta rhythm by G. Walter (1937). Somewhat later, attempts were made to investigate the structure of the EEG itself (Genkin A. A., 1971).

In children during the first 2–3 months of life, waves with frequencies of 1–3 Hz, 4–7 Hz, and 8–12 Hz can already be distinguished; however, the dominant rhythm remains in the range of 0.5–3 Hz. At the same time, slow waves are occasionally superimposed with faster oscillations (13–15–19 Hz). Between 4 and 6 months of age, the number of theta waves increases. Activity at 6–7 Hz, preceding the alpha rhythm, is consistently observed on EEG by the age of 4 years. A pronounced alpha rhythm appears in the parieto-occipital region at the age of 4–5 years and becomes stable at later ages (7–8 years).

Electroencephalogram (EEG) recordings are performed under conditions of operational rest (OR)—eyes open—and psychophysiological rest (PR)—eyes closed.

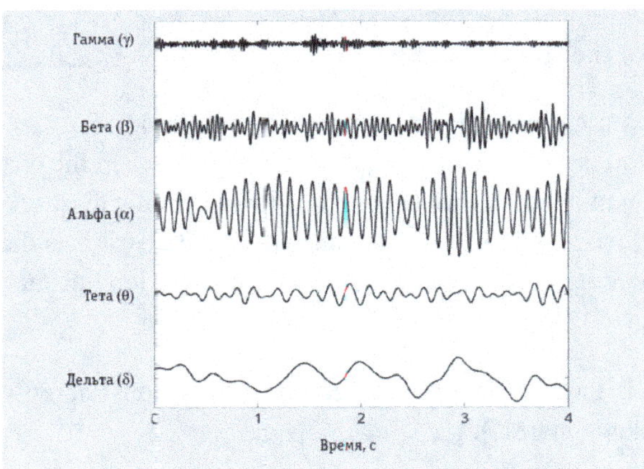

Figure 15. Electroencephalographic rhythms.

The EEG includes rhythms ranging from 0–0.5 up to 35 (70) Hz. In clinical practice, the following EEG rhythms are described: delta 0.5–4 Hz, theta 4–8 Hz, alpha 8–12 (13) Hz, beta 12 (13)–30 Hz, and gamma 30–70 Hz.

2.1. Delta Rhythm

The **delta rhythm** consists of oscillations with frequencies below 3.5 Hz (Berger, H., 1931; Walter, G., 1936). In clinical EEG, the lower boundary of the delta range is typically 0.3–0.5 Hz. Depending on the level of wakefulness and cortical localization, delta oscillations may indicate either local or diffuse cerebral dysfunction (tumor, hemorrhage, coma, etc.) or reflect a physiological reduction in the level of brain activation (sleep).

An isolated slow wave may also be a component of pathological complexes, such as epileptiform spike–wave patterns.

The delta rhythm consists of high-amplitude oscillations (20–200 μV) with frequencies of 0.5–4 Hz. It predominates in cases of cortical brain damage or in the EEG of individuals in deep sleep. The system generating the delta rhythm is considered phylogenetically the most ancient and is involved in supporting vital and biological needs (Niedermeyer, E., Lopes da Silva, F. H. L., 2005).

Delta activity is formed during deep sleep (Loomis, A. L., Harvey, E. N., Hobart, G., 1937) and in pathological conditions. It is associated with alternating depolarization and hyperpolarization of cortical neurons and reflects a high degree of synchronization and a reduced level of central nervous system activation.

Origin of the Delta Rhythm: Levels of Analysis

1. Corticothalamic mechanisms (primary generator)
The delta rhythm is generated through interactions between the cortex and thalamus. Thalamic neurons are capable of slow rhythmic discharges in a hyperpolarized mode, while the cortex amplifies and distributes the rhythm over large areas, resulting in slow waves synchronized over long distances (Steriade, M., McCormick, D. A., Sejnowski, T. J., 1993).

A key feature is the alternation between cortical neuronal activity ("up-states") and silence ("down-states").

2. Cortical generation (local delta rhythm)

Contemporary data indicate that delta activity may be generated locally within the cortex and may reflect temporary functional "shutdown" of a cortical region. This is particularly relevant for slow-wave sleep, restorative processes, and focal pathological delta activity.

3. Cellular and ionic mechanisms

At the microlevel, the following are involved: prolonged membrane hyperpolarization, T-type calcium channels, potassium currents, and synchronization of large populations of pyramidal neurons. As with other EEG rhythms, the delta rhythm reflects summed postsynaptic potentials rather than individual action potentials.

4. Ontogenesis

In newborns and infants, the delta rhythm predominates, reflecting cortical immaturity. With age, its proportion during wakefulness decreases. In the mature brain, delta activity during wakefulness is atypical.

Functional Interpretations

Sleep and recovery

The delta rhythm is a marker of deep slow-wave sleep, associated with restoration of energy resources and involved in synaptic "recalibration" (homeostatic plasticity).

Plasticity and learning

During sleep, delta waves coordinate hippocampal–cortical interactions, participate in memory consolidation, and create conditions for neural network reorganization.

Clinical Significance

Localized delta activity during wakefulness may indicate a tumor, stroke, trauma, or inflammatory process (Zhirmunskaya E. A., Losev V. S.). Therefore, the delta rhythm is an important diagnostic marker in clinical EEG.

Contemporary Concepts

Oscillatory model: EEG rhythms result from the activity of neuronal generators (Achermann, P., Borbély, A. A., 1997).

Dynamic network model: rhythms emerge as manifestations of self-organization in neuronal networks.

Cross-frequency interactions: different rhythms interact (e.g., theta–gamma coupling).

Summary

The EEG delta rhythm is generated by corticothalamic and cortical networks, reflects slow cycles of excitation and inhibition, serves as a key marker of deep sleep and recovery, and during wakefulness often indicates localized cerebral dysfunction.

2.2. Theta Rhythm

The **theta rhythm** ranges from 4–7.5 Hz (Walter & Dovey, 1944). Similar to delta oscillations, theta-range activity may reflect either local or diffuse cerebral dysfunction or a physiologically determined reduction in the level of wakefulness.

An increase in theta activity is observed during drowsiness, as well as during deep relaxation and meditative states. According to modern concepts, theta rhythm recorded during cognitive task performance reflects processes of memory encoding and retrieval. G. G. Knyazev emphasized its association with behavioral regulation and the comparison of current motivations with emotionally significant life experience.

Theta activity is an integral and important component of the human EEG and is characteristic of all mammals (Vanderwolf, C. H., 1969).

Pathological Slow-Wave Activity

The appearance of slow rhythms (theta and delta) on EEG is considered pathological. The lower the frequency and the higher the amplitude, the more pronounced the pathological process. Slow-wave activity is commonly associated with dystrophic processes, demyelinating and degenerative brain disorders, compression of brain tissue, intracranial hypertension, as well as states of reduced alertness, deactivation phenomena, and diminished activating influences from the brainstem.

As a rule, unilateral localized slow-wave activity is a sign of focal cortical damage. Bursts and paroxysms of generalized slow-wave activity in awake adults are associated with pathological changes in deep brain structures.

Dominance of a flattened EEG may also be associated with either increased cortical activation or cortical deactivation. Differentiation between these states is possible only through the use of functional activation procedures.

High-frequency, asynchronous, low-amplitude activity may result either from cortical irritation processes or from increased activating influences of the reticular activating system. Differentiation of these conditions is also achieved using functional tests.

Origin of the Theta Rhythm: Levels of Analysis

Hippocampal generator (key mechanism)

The primary source of the theta rhythm is the hippocampus and its associated structures (Green, J. D., Arduini, A. A., 1954).

Mechanisms include rhythmic activity of pyramidal neurons, inhibitory interneurons (GABAergic), and interactions within the CA1–CA3–dentate gyrus circuitry. Hippocampal theta rhythm is especially pronounced during navigation and during memory encoding and retrieval.

Septohippocampal system

The medial septum acts as a "pacemaker": cholinergic and GABAergic neurons impose rhythmic activity on the hippocampus. Damage to the medial septum leads to the disappearance of theta rhythm (Buzsáki, G., 2002).

Thalamocortical and frontal mechanisms

Cortical Theta Rhythm

In the cerebral cortex, the **theta (θ) rhythm** is not always a direct reflection of hippocampal theta activity and may be generated locally within frontal networks.

Frontal theta rhythm is associated with cognitive control, error processing, and working memory.

Neurotransmitter Regulation

Key neuromodulatory systems include:

acetylcholine, which enhances theta rhythm;

norepinephrine, which modulates theta activity;

dopamine, which is associated primarily with frontal theta rhythm.

Ontogenesis

In children, the theta rhythm predominates and reflects cortical immaturity. With age, it is gradually replaced by the alpha rhythm. In adults, theta activity emerges in specific functional states.

Functional Interpretations

Memory and learning

The theta rhythm coordinates neuronal ensembles, links distant brain regions, and provides a "temporal framework" for neural coding.

Relationship with the gamma rhythm

According to the **theta–gamma coupling model**, theta oscillations define the phase, while gamma oscillations encode content. This interaction is considered a fundamental mechanism of episodic memory.

States of consciousness

Theta rhythm is characteristic of transitions between sleep and wakefulness, meditation, and hypnagogic states (Buzsáki, G., 2006).

2.3. Alpha Rhythm

The **alpha (α) rhythm** ranges from 8 to 13 Hz and predominates in posterior brain regions. In adults, it typically has an average amplitude of up to 70–80 μV, is blocked by eye opening, and is associated with visual brain structures (Berger, 1929). The alpha rhythm develops during the first months and years of life, initially having a frequency of 3–4 Hz and gradually reaching adult values by approximately 3 years of age. It was the first EEG rhythm to be described and remains the most extensively studied. It is most prominent in the normal EEG of relaxed wakefulness, and EEG interpretation traditionally begins with its description.

This rhythm is characterized by spontaneous changes in amplitude (alpha rhythm modulation), manifested as alternating increases and decreases in wave amplitude, forming so-called **spindles**, the duration of which most commonly ranges from 2 to 8 seconds. A distinction is made between **alpha activity** (consisting of alpha waves with durations of 80–125 ms and recorded in various brain structures) and the **alpha rhythm** proper (regular oscillatory activity with a frequency of approximately 10 Hz, predominantly recorded in the occipital regions).

According to N. Wiener, G. Walter, and P. V. Simonov, the rhythmicity and clear periodicity of the alpha rhythm determine its possible role in scanning and quantizing incoming information.

According to data reported by L. A. Novikova, in individuals with congenital or long-term blindness, as well as in cases where only light perception is preserved, the alpha rhythm is absent. Disappearance of the alpha rhythm has also been observed in optic nerve atrophy. Novikova suggested that the alpha rhythm is associated with the presence of object vision.

In addition to the classical alpha rhythm most prominently expressed in the occipital regions, several other rhythms have been described. These rhythms operate at the same frequency as the alpha rhythm but are most pronounced in other brain areas and exhibit different waveform characteristics, such as the **mu rhythm**, **kappa rhythmm**, and **tau rhythm**.

In animals, alpha-like activity has been demonstrated in monkeys and rabbits. Its role is thought to involve functional stabilization of brain states and the maintenance of readiness to respond. The alpha rhythm is believed to reflect the reverberation of excitatory processes encoding intrinsic brain information and to create an optimal background for the reception and processing of afferent signals.

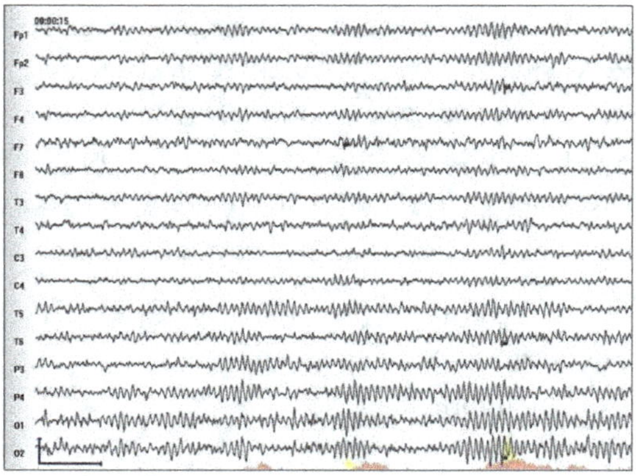

Figure 16*. Alpha rhythm.*

A detailed analysis of EEG parameters obtained from a large number of subjects demonstrated a fairly strong association between the characteristics of the alpha rhythm and other EEG components, on the one hand, and individual psychological traits, on the other (Malkin et al., 1967; see also a review of related studies in Vasilevsky et al., 1988). In particular, individuals with a well-defined, relatively monofrequency alpha rhythm during eyes-closed conditions tend to exhibit passivity and introversion, whereas individuals with highly labile alpha rhythm and reduced EEG amplitude are more likely to show frequent neurotic reactions, increased anxiety, and related features (Vasilevsky et al., 1988).

The relationship between alpha activity characteristics and psychological traits may manifest differently depending on functional load. For example, the neuroticism score was negatively correlated with mid-frequency alpha rhythm in EEG recorded during quiet wakefulness and positively correlated with alpha rhythm in EEG recorded while subjects performed a reaction-time task (Becker-Carus, 1971).

Functional or morphological disturbances primarily affect alpha rhythm parameters. The following criteria are considered indicative of pathology in alpha rhythm assessment:

1. persistent presence of alpha rhythm (index > 50%) in the frontal brain regions during bipolar recordings with electrodes placed along sagittal lines at small interelectrode distances;
2. interhemispheric amplitude asymmetry exceeding 30%;
3. frequency asymmetry greater than 1 Hz;

4. waveform abnormalities: absence of modulation, appearance of paroxysmal or arcuate alpha rhythm, and loss of sinusoidal waveform;
5. changes in quantitative parameters: lack of frequency stability; reduction of amplitude below 20 μV or increase above 90 μV; reduction of the alpha rhythm index below 50%, up to its complete absence.

Summary — Alpha rhythm (8–13 Hz):

The alpha rhythm arises predominantly in the occipital cortex and is associated with thalamocortical oscillations. It is enhanced during quiet wakefulness with eyes closed and is regarded as a rhythm of functional inhibition and selective attention.

Modern concept: the alpha rhythm reflects an active process of suppression of irrelevant sensory information.

2.4. Beta Rhythm

The **beta (β) rhythm** consists of oscillations at frequencies of 14 Hz and above. In practice, the upper boundary of beta activity is usually considered to be 30–35 Hz; frequencies above 30 Hz are sometimes classified as gamma rhythm. In healthy adults, beta activity is observed during relaxed wakefulness (Jasper, H. H., Penfield, W., 1949).

The amplitude of the beta rhythm is typically much lower than that of the alpha rhythm, most often below 20–30 μV, with a tendency toward maximal expression in anterior brain regions (Adrian, E. D., Matthews, B. H. C., 1934).

Dominance of beta activity may result from the effects of various medications. It is important to distinguish genuine beta activity of cerebral origin from electromyographic artifacts, which often occur within the same frequency range.

Certain alterations in the beta frequency band also indicate pathological processes. The criteria for pathology include:

1. dominance of low-frequency beta rhythm across the entire convexital surface of the brain;
2. paroxysmal beta rhythm discharges;
3. focal localization of beta rhythm, especially when accompanied by increased amplitude;
4. marked interhemispheric amplitude asymmetry exceeding 50%;

5. transformation of the beta rhythm into an alpha-like, rhythmic sinusoidal waveform;
6. increase in beta rhythm amplitude above 7 μV.

Beta Rhythms (β1 and β2)

Two beta rhythms are distinguished: **β1** and **β2**.

β1 EEG Rhythm: Characteristics

Frequency: approximately 13–20 Hz

Maximum expression: frontal and central cortical regions

Amplitude: moderate, usually lower than that of the alpha rhythm

Functionally associated with: wakefulness, attentional focus, cognitive activity, and sensorimotor preparation

Enhancement of β1 activity is observed during active mental work, whereas suppression occurs during relaxation or eye closure.

Origin of the β1 Rhythm

Cortical mechanisms

The β1 rhythm is formed predominantly in frontal and sensorimotor cortical areas. Its generation occurs through synchronization of pyramidal neurons and interneurons at the local network level and reflects fine balancing between excitation and inhibition.

Thalamocortical loops

Thalamic nuclei, particularly relay nuclei, participate in maintaining beta activity. Thalamocortical loops provide rhythm synchrony and stability.

Neurotransmitter regulation

Glutamate: principal excitatory neurotransmitter

GABA: inhibitory modulation maintaining synchrony

Dopamine: particularly important for frontal β1 rhythm associated with cognitive activity

Functional Interpretation

The β1 rhythm is associated with attentional activation, working memory, and motor preparation (Jasper, H. H., Penfield, W., 1949). It differs from the **β2 rhythm (20–30 Hz)**, which more often reflects sensorimotor activation and excitation. In pathological conditions, β1 abnormalities may manifest as an imbalance between excitation and inhibition, for example in stress-related states or cortical dysfunction.

Summary

β1 EEG rhythm formation involves local cortical networks (frontal and sensorimotor cortex), thalamocortical loops, and excitation–inhibition balance mediated by glutamate and GABA. Functionally, it reflects activation, attention, action preparation, and cognitive activity.

β2 EEG Rhythm: Characteristics

Frequency: approximately 20–30 Hz

Maximum expression: central (sensorimotor) and frontal cortical regions

Amplitude: low, usually lower than alpha and delta rhythms

Functionally associated with: sensorimotor system activation, motor functions, wakefulness, attention, and stress

Distinction from β1 rhythm (13–20 Hz):

β1 primarily reflects cognitive activity and attention, whereas β2 reflects sensorimotor activation and excitation (Jasper & Penfield, 1949; Pfurtscheller & Lopes da Silva, 1999).

Origin of the β2 Rhythm

Cortical mechanisms

The primary generator is the sensorimotor cortex (precentral and postcentral regions). β2 activity arises from synchronization of pyramidal neurons and interneurons, particularly during motor preparation and maintenance of posture.

Thalamocortical loops

β2 rhythm is modulated by thalamocortical loops, ensuring oscillatory stability and coherence. The thalamus supports resonant cortical interactions, especially during sensorimotor activity.

Neurotransmitter regulation

Glutamate: excitation of pyramidal neurons

GABA: inhibitory modulation of interneurons

Dopamine and norepinephrine: modulation of sensorimotor excitation, particularly during movement and attention

Functional Interpretation

β2 rhythm increases during movement, posture maintenance, and motor preparation. During relaxation or rest, its amplitude decreases (event-related desynchronization). In cognitive contexts, β2 reflects sensorimotor excitation and readiness for action, in contrast to β1, which is associated with attention and concentration (Salmelin & Hari, 1994).

Summary

β2 EEG rhythm formation involves local sensorimotor cortical networks supported by thalamocortical loops and excitation–inhibition balance (glutamate, GABA, dopamine). Functionally, it reflects motor preparation, posture control, and sensorimotor activation.

Other EEG Rhythms and Patterns

Phi (φ) rhythm: slow delta-range oscillations in posterior regions, typically emerging during eye closure (Belsh et al., 1983).

Sigma (σ) rhythm: analogous to sleep spindles (Kugler, 1981).

Rho (ρ) rhythm: analogous to positive occipital sharp transients (POSTS) (Kugler & Laub, 1973).

Under conditions of psychophysiological rest but not during sleep, the alpha rhythm is recorded, particularly clearly in the occipital region, with a frequency of 8–13 Hz and an amplitude of approximately 50 μV. Sensory stimulation (e.g., sound) or transition to activity with eyes open leads to a shift from alpha rhythm to beta rhythm with higher frequency (14–30 Hz) and lower amplitude (~25 μV). This phenomenon is known as **EEG desynchronization**.

The transition from wakefulness to sleep is accompanied by the emergence of theta rhythm (4–7 Hz). During deep sleep, delta rhythm with a frequency of 0.5–3.5 Hz is recorded. The amplitude of these slow waves ranges from 100 to 300 μV.

Mu (μ) rhythm: has the same frequency as alpha rhythm but differs in spatial organization (maximum in central regions), waveform, and reactivity; it is blocked by voluntary movements and is associated with the sensorimotor cortex (Jasper & Andrews, 1938).

Lambda waves: oscillations occurring in posterior regions during visual tracking eye movements (Gastaut, 1951; Evans, 1952).

Kappa (κ) rhythm: alpha-range oscillations with maximum expression in frontotemporal regions (Laugier & Liberson, 1937).

Pi (π) rhythm: slow oscillations (3–4 Hz) in posterior brain regions (Dutertre, 1977), distinct from the primary occipital rhythm and not its harmonic.

Special EEG Activity Patterns

EEG may also display special forms of bioelectrical activity, including:

flat EEG,

high-frequency asynchronous low-amplitude ("shaggy") activity,

low-amplitude slow polymorphic activity (LASPA),

polyrhythmic activity.

Periodically occurring EEG graphoelements are referred to as **pathological EEG patterns**. These include spikes, sharp waves, slow spikes, spike–wave complexes (spike–wave, wave–spike, spike–slow wave, helmet-shaped waves, multiple spike complexes, multiple spike–slow wave complexes), as well as bursts, paroxysms, and bursts of hypersynchronization.

Chapter 3. Genesis of the EEG

The widespread use of EEG in clinical practice presupposes an understanding of the nature and mechanisms underlying the generation of the electroencephalogram. Research on the nonspecific systems of the reticular formation and the limbic complex—structures that determine the level of functional brain activity—has been of crucial importance for understanding the mechanisms of normal EEG generation and for using EEG as a tool of functional diagnostics (Anokhin, P. K., 1964; Jasper, H., 1949; Magoun, H. W., 1958).

The EEG represents a complex oscillatory electrical process; however, the mechanisms of its generation are not yet fully understood. Contemporary concepts of EEG genesis are based on data from neurophysiology, biophysics, and computational neuroscience and differ substantially from earlier simplified models.

3.1. General Principles of EEG Formation

It is now generally accepted that the EEG reflects the summed, synchronized postsynaptic activity of neuronal populations in the cerebral cortex rather than the action potentials of individual neurons.

The principal sources of EEG signals are excitatory and inhibitory postsynaptic potentials (EPSPs and IPSPs), which arise predominantly on the dendrites of cortical pyramidal neurons.

Classical formulation:

The EEG is the result of spatially and temporally summed slow postsynaptic potentials of cortical neurons organized into functional ensembles (Niedermeyer & Lopes da Silva, 2018).

3.2. Role of Cortical Pyramidal Neurons

Modern concepts emphasize that pyramidal neurons in layers III and V of the neocortex are the primary generators of EEG activity because they:

have parallel dendritic orientation (perpendicular to the cortical surface), form open electrical dipoles, are capable of synchronous activation in large populations.

Interneuronal activity is important for rhythm modulation, but its contribution to scalp EEG is minimal due to the closed geometry of their dipoles (Buzsáki, Anastassiou, & Koch, 2012).

3.3. Postsynaptic Potentials as the Main Contribution

The contemporary view rejects the notion that action potentials play a leading role in EEG formation. Action potentials: have very short duration (≈1 ms), are not synchronized across large neuronal populations, contribute mainly to local field potentials (LFPs) rather than to EEG signals.

In contrast, slow EPSPs and IPSPs: last tens of milliseconds, readily summate in time and space, generate stable oscillations that can be recorded on the scalp (da Silva, 2013).

3.4. Synchronization of Neuronal Ensembles

A key condition for EEG emergence is the synchronization of activity across large numbers of neurons. Modern models conceptualize EEG as a manifestation of the collective dynamics of neuronal networks rather than the activity of individual cells.

EEG rhythms reflect: the degree of synchronization, the nature of interactions between neuronal ensembles, the functional state of the brain (Buzsáki, *Rhythms of the Brain*, 2006).

3.5. Thalamocortical and Corticocortical Mechanisms

Current theories emphasize the critical role of thalamocortical circuits in generating rhythmic EEG activity:

Alpha rhythm: results from interactions between the visual cortex and the thalamus,

Sleep spindles: arise from thalamoreticular networks,

Delta and theta rhythms: are associated with cortico-thalamic synchronization.

Thus, EEG reflects not only cortical but also subcortical–cortical network activity (Steriade, McCormick, & Sejnowski, 1993).

3.6. Role of Volume Conduction

Modern biophysical models of EEG genesis account for the phenomenon of volume conduction. Electrical fields generated in the cortex propagate through: brain tissue, cerebrospinal fluid, skull, scalp.

This leads to: reduced spatial resolution of EEG, spatial smoothing of local sources, the need for source modeling approaches (Nunez & Srinivasan, 2006).

3.7. Contemporary Network and Dynamic Concepts of EEG

At present, EEG is viewed as: a reflection of the dynamics of functional brain networks, the result of nonlinear interactions, a manifestation of self-organizing processes within neuronal ensembles.

EEG rhythms are interpreted as functional modes of brain operation rather than purely local phenomena (Breakspear, 2017).

Summary

Modern concepts of EEG genesis can be summarized as follows:

1. EEG is generated primarily by slow postsynaptic potentials.
2. The main generators are cortical pyramidal neurons.
3. Synchronization of neuronal ensembles is a key prerequisite.
4. Thalamocortical networks play a substantial role.
5. EEG reflects the dynamics of distributed functional brain networks.
6. The spatial structure of EEG signals is distorted by volume conduction.
7. EEG represents a macroscopic manifestation of collective neuronal dynamics.

Alpha EEG Activity and Its Origin

Alpha EEG activity (≈8–13 Hz in adults) is one of the most extensively studied brain rhythms, yet it remains an incompletely resolved topic. Today, researchers generally speak not of a single origin, but of several complementary theories.

3.7.1. Thalamocortical Theory (Classical)

This is the most widespread and foundational theory.

Core idea: The alpha rhythm arises from interactions between the thalamus and the cerebral cortex.

Mechanism: Thalamic neurons—especially relay and reticular nuclei—are capable of endogenous oscillations. Through thalamocortical and corticothalamic loops, this rhythmic activity is imposed on the cortex. Synchronization of large neuronal populations gives rise to the alpha rhythm observable in the EEG.

Supporting evidence:

Alpha activity increases with eye closure (reduced sensory input to the thalamus),

Thalamic lesions severely disrupt alpha activity,

Intracranial recordings demonstrate alpha oscillations in the thalamus.

Currently, the thalamus is regarded as a key—but not the sole—source of alpha rhythm generation.

3.7.2. Cortical Theory (Local Generators)

Alpha as a Product of the Cortex Itself

Core idea: The alpha rhythm can be generated locally within the cerebral cortex without the obligatory involvement of a thalamic "conductor."

Mechanism: Alpha oscillations arise from interactions between excitatory pyramidal neurons and inhibitory interneurons. Local cortical networks are capable of producing alpha-band oscillations, which are subsequently spatially synchronized across cortical areas.

Supporting evidence:

Alpha activity is observed in isolated cortical slices.

Multiple types of alpha rhythms exist (occipital, sensorimotor, parietal).

MEG and intracranial EEG studies demonstrate local cortical alpha sources.

Currently, this view is most often framed as **multifocal cortical generation coordinated by the thalamus**, rather than purely autonomous cortical activity.

3.7.3. Active Inhibition Theory (Inhibition Hypothesis)

One of the most influential contemporary interpretations.

Core idea: The alpha rhythm does not reflect "rest," but rather **active functional inhibition**.

Functional meaning:

High alpha power corresponds to suppression of information processing in a given cortical area.

Alpha desynchronization indicates readiness for stimulus processing.

Examples: With eyes closed, alpha power increases in the visual cortex, indicating functional disengagement of the visual system.

During attention to a stimulus, alpha power decreases specifically in task-relevant regions.

Alpha activity can be lateralized, selectively inhibiting processing

in one hemisphere.

This is not strictly a theory of origin but a **functional model** closely linked to mechanisms of alpha generation.

3.7.4. Pacemaker Theory

Closely related to the thalamic theory but more mechanistic.

Core idea:

Specialized neurons act as "pacemakers" that determine the alpha frequency.

Proposed candidates:

Neurons of the thalamic reticular nucleus.

Neurons expressing T-type Ca^{2+} channels, which are prone to rhythmic bursting.

Today, this theory is generally regarded as a **specific mechanism within the broader thalamocortical framework**.

3.7.5. Neuronal Ensemble and Synchronization Theory

A systemic, network-based approach.

Core idea:

The alpha rhythm emerges from the self-organization of large-scale neuronal networks.

Key principles: Alpha does not arise in a single structure but emerges from network synchronization.

Conduction delays, feedback loops, and excitation–inhibition balance are critical.

Alpha represents a **network operating mode**, not an isolated generator.

This framework aligns well with combined EEG–fMRI findings and modern theories of brain network dynamics.

3.7.6. Evolutionary–Adaptive Theory

A more conceptual perspective.

Core idea:

The alpha rhythm represents an optimal brain mode for:

energy conservation,

maintaining readiness for action,

protection against sensory overload.

This theory is usually treated as a conceptual overlay on neurophysiological models rather than a standalone mechanistic explanation.

3.7.7. Contemporary Consensus (Brief)

Today, alpha rhythm is most commonly described as:

The result of interactions between thalamocortical circuits and local cortical generators, reflecting active functional inhibition and large-scale network synchronization of the brain.

3.8. Lobasyuk B. A. Hypothesis on the Genesis of the EEG

Neuronal systems of the cerebral cortex exhibit filtering properties with respect to the electrical activity of their constituent elements, while simultaneously possessing properties of self-generating systems.

The distributed nature of alpha rhythm sources in ECoG–EEG recordings has led to the hypothesis of the existence of multiple discrete oscillatory sources in the alpha frequency range, termed **"alphons."**

According to the proposed hypothesis (Lobasyuk, B. A., 2005), it may be assumed that similar hypothetical generators exist in the cerebral cortex for beta-2, beta-1, theta, and delta rhythms (and possibly other EEG rhythms).

The positive and negative relationships between the amplitudes of different ECoG rhythms identified using multiple linear regression and correlation analyses suggest that, although multiple hypothetical generators of various ECoG rhythms may exist, they are simultaneously integrated by certain control mechanisms that ensure the overall organization of the ECoG.

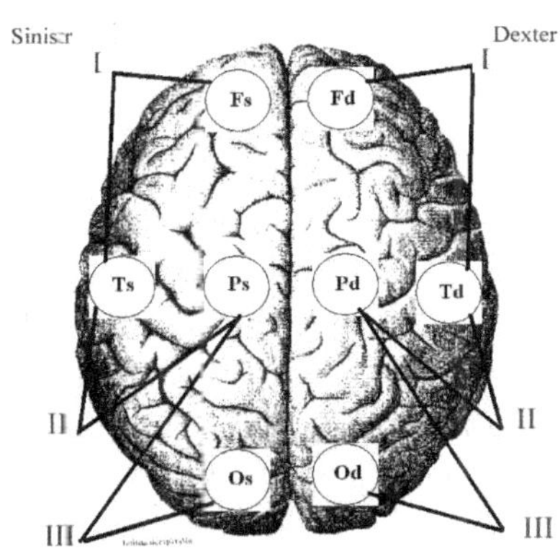

Figure 17. *EEG Electrode Placements*

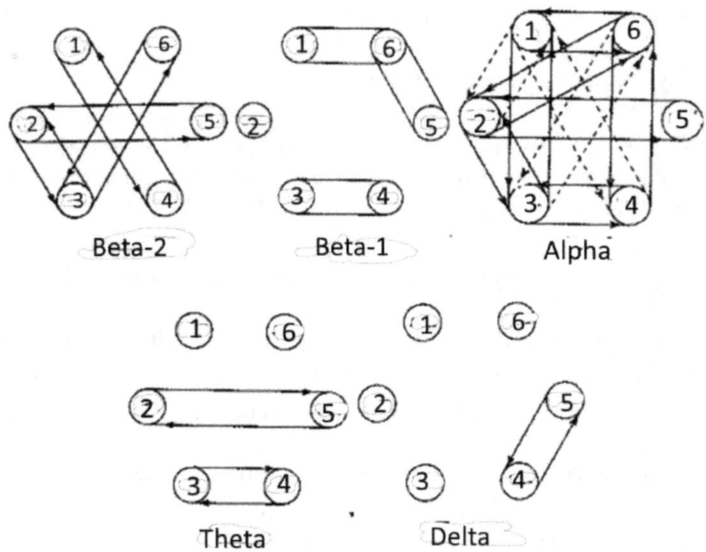

Figure 18. *Polycyclic graphs describing the relationships between the amplitude indicators of EEG rhythms based on calculations of multiple regression and correlation analysis. Notations: leads: 1 – right frontal-temporal, 2 – right temporal-parietal, 3 – right parietal-occipital, 6 – left frontal-temporal, 5 – left temporal-parietal, 4– left parietal-occipital.*

Analyzing the polycyclic graph describing the relationships between alpha-activity indicators in different EEG leads (Fig. 18), both positive and negative connections can be noted. This may indicate the presence of multiple stationary generators (at least two) of the alpha rhythm, operating at similar frequencies but with different phases. It can also be suggested that the generation of alpha activity in different leads is carried out by different alpha activity generators, and the positive and negative relationships observed between alpha activity indicators in different leads reflect the presence of control mechanisms within this system of generators.

It should be emphasized that the magnitudes of the regression relationships originating from the graph vertex corresponding to the right temporal-parietal lead were larger in absolute value than the incoming relationships to this vertex. This may indicate that the alpha rhythm generator, whose electrical activity is projected to this lead, is system-forming relative to the other alpha activity generators, whose electrical activity is projected to the remaining studied leads. All amplitude indicators of the alpha rhythm from all leads used in constructing the polycyclic graph were interconnected, suggesting that these amplitude indicators belong to a single set and supporting the hypothesis that all possible alpha activity generators are unified into a single system by control mechanisms.

When calculating two-dimensional correlation coefficients between alpha amplitude indicators from different leads, it was found that all analyzed indicators are in correlated relationships. In the right parietal-occipital lead, bilateral positive mutual influences of theta and delta rhythms were observed, showing the facilitating effect of delta rhythm on theta rhythm generation in the cortex.

The electrical activity of beta-2, beta-1, and theta rhythms appears to be provided by two generators. For the beta-2 rhythm, electrical activity in the left frontal-temporal, right parietal-occipital, right temporal-parietal, and left temporal-parietal leads forms the first beta-2 activity construct, which is presumably controlled by its own generator. The second construct includes the right frontal-temporal and left parietal-occipital leads, whose beta-2 activity is also presumably generated by a separate generator.

For the beta-1 rhythm, electrical activity in the right frontal-temporal, left frontal-temporal, and left temporal-parietal leads forms the first beta-1 activity construct, presumably generated by its o

wn generator. The second construct consists of the left and right parietal-occipital leads, also presumably controlled by a separate beta-1 rhythm generator.

Electrical activity in the left-right temporal-parietal leads and left-right parietal-occipital leads in the theta range was associated with mutual positive influences (Fig. 18). This suggests that theta-range EEG activity is likely generated by two generators.

During regression analysis of beta-2, beta-1, theta, and delta rhythms, polycyclic multigraphs were not constructed, which may indicate that the generators of these EEG rhythms are multiple.

3.9. Structures Forming EEG

In Zhirmunskaya's work, six main structures of the limbic-reticular complex that shape the EEG pattern were considered:

1. Brainstem reticular formation (RF);
2. Nonspecific thalamic nuclei (NT);+
3. Associative thalamic nuclei (AT);

4. Posterior hypothalamus (PH);
5. Anterior hypothalamus (AH);
6. Caudate nucleus (CN).

Each of these structures can exist in two states (activated and inhibited) or three states (activated, resting, and inhibited).

Numerous animal experiments and human studies have shown that excitation of the activating reticulocortical systems leads to EEG desynchronization, manifested as high-frequency, low-amplitude, irregular electrical activity. The strong association between increased functional activity and EEG desynchronization has led to the literature often referring to brain arousal systems as "desynchronizing," which is partly accurate. Theoretical and experimental data indicate that the link between increased functional activity and EEG desynchronization is not accidental.

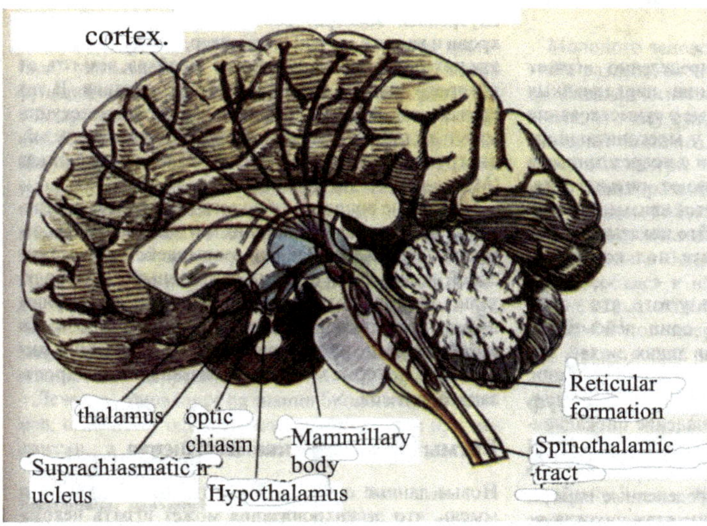

Figure 19. *Reticular formation of the brain.*

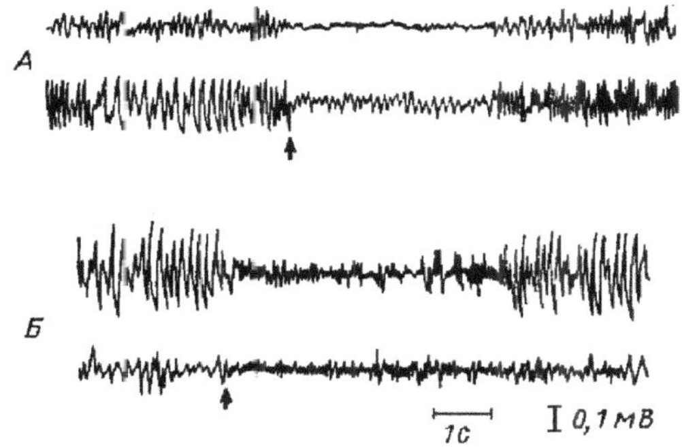

Figure 20. *Desynchronization response induced by peripheral afferent stimulation (A) or direct stimulation of the reticular formation (B). The moment of stimulation is indicated by the arrow (after Bremer).*

A high level of functional brain activity, corresponding to emotional arousal, focused attention, or performing a new task that requires intellectual mobilization, is characterized by an increase in the volume of information perceived and processed by the brain, as well as higher demands on the flexibility and mobility of brain systems.

All of this requires greater autonomy of neurons in carrying out their functions, which corresponds to a higher informational content of the processes occurring within them. This increase in freedom and autonomy of individual neurons over time is manifested as desynchronization in the overall electrical activity.

A decrease in functional activity is accompanied by a reduction in afferent input and greater dependence of the organization of neuronal activity on endogenous mechanisms. Under these conditions, individual neurons, forming large synchronized groups, become more dependent on the activity of the large populations of neurons with which they are connected. Brain systems, in this state, operate somewhat in resonant modes, which limits the ability of neurons to engage in new activity and respond to incoming external stimuli.

Such synchronized activity, reflected in the EEG as regular, high-amplitude but slow oscillations, corresponds to a lower informational content of brain processes, characteristic of dreamless sleep, anesthesia, or deep coma.

Continuous fluctuations in the level of functional brain activity, depending on the organism's internal needs and changes in the environment, determine both the complex spectral composition of the EEG and its substantial variations under specific conditions.

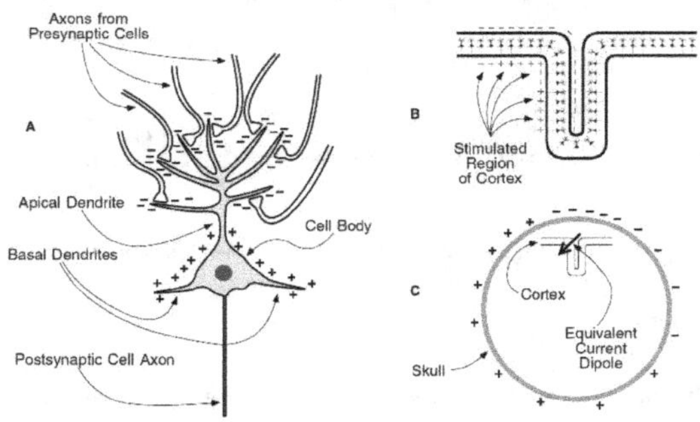

Figure 21. *Principle of EEG and ERP generation.*

(A) *A cortical pyramidal cell at the moment of an excitatory postsynaptic potential on its dendrites; the cell becomes a tiny dipole.*

(B) *With synchronous activation of a large number of pyramidal cells in a cortical area, the dipoles of individual cells sum up.*

(C) *The sum of dipoles from individual cells can be approximated by a single equivalent dipole (indicated by the arrow).*

3.10. Biophysics and Signal Propagation

How a measurable signal arises. The EEG signal is the cumulative electric field of thousands of neurons, passing through neural tissue, cerebrospinal fluid, skull bone, and scalp. These media attenuate and filter the signal, which is why EEG has relatively low spatial resolution but high temporal resolution.

Oscillations as a result of network synchronization. EEG rhythms (α, β, θ, δ) emerge through dynamic interactions between the cortex and subcortical structures (e.g., the thalamus) and due to the synchronization of neuronal ensembles.

Table 1. Key Insights into the Generation of EEG

Aspect	Mechanism
Sources	EEG primarily arises from postsynaptic potentials in cortical pyramidal neurons.
Surface detectability	Synchronous activation of thousands of neurons produces a summated dipole detectable at the scalp.
Role of action potentials	Individual action potentials are too brief and do not sum effectively to contribute to the scalp-recorded EEG.
Biophysical propagation	Electrical currents spread through brain tissue, cerebrospinal fluid, skull, and scalp, forming measurable potentials.
Rhythmic activity	Interactions between cortical and subcortical networks generate oscillations across distinct frequency bands.

Chapter 4. EEG Research Methods

4.1. Conditions for EEG Recording

EEG recording must be conducted under strictly controlled conditions, as EEG is a highly sensitive method easily affected by external and internal factors. Below are the current standards and conditions for EEG recording used in clinical and functional diagnostics.

4.1.1. Environmental Conditions

Recording Room

EEG should be performed in a quiet, isolated room, with dim, diffuse lighting, a comfortable and stable temperature (~20–23 °C), and minimal external stimuli (noise, bright light).

Purpose: To minimize nonspecific cortical activation.

4.1.2. Subject Preparation

General Condition

The patient should be physically and mentally relaxed, free from pain, significant anxiety, or stress, and adequately informed about the procedure to reduce emotional tension.

Pre-recording Regimen

It is recommended that the patient:

Have normal sleep (unless sleep deprivation is part of the protocol)

Avoid alcohol for 24 hours

Avoid caffeine, energy drinks, and nicotine for 3–6 hours

Eat 1.5–2 hours before the recording to prevent hypoglycemia

Patient Positioning

EEG can be recorded in a lying or seated position, with relaxed muscles, head support, and no active movements. Muscle tension, particularly in facial and neck muscles, should be minimized.

Wakefulness State

Standard EEG is performed during relaxed wakefulness with eyes closed (main recording) and periodic eye opening to assess rhythm reactivity. Sleep, drowsiness, and awakening can also be recorded if necessary.

4.1.3. Technical Recording Conditions

Electrodes

Placed according to the international 10–20 (or 10–10, 10–5) system. Electrode-skin impedance is usually ≤5 kΩ (up to 10 kΩ is acceptable with modern amplifiers), using gel or paste to improve contact.

Equipment

Reliable grounding

Minimization of mains interference (50/60 Hz)

Calibration before recording

Artifact Control

During recording:

Avoid chewing or talking

Limit blinking

Prevent head and body movements

Monitor respiration (except during hyperventilation)

Minimize EMG and EOG artifacts

4.1.4. Functional Tests (during standard EEG)

EEG is often performed with activation procedures, which must be conducted in controlled conditions and documented. Common functional tests include:

1. Hyperventilation
2. Visual stimulation
3. Photostimulation
4. Auditory stimulation
5. Electrical stimulation
6. Sleep deprivation

Significant events and activation tests are marked during recording. Eye-opening and closing elicit characteristic electrooculographic artifacts, allowing assessment of the patient's alertness, level of consciousness, and approximate EEG reactivity.

External stimuli, such as brief light flashes or sound signals, are used to evaluate brain responses. In comatose patients, noxious stimuli (e.g., nail-bed pressure on the index finger) may be applied.

Since resting EEG may not always reveal pathology, functional tests are applied, including:

Assessing orienting responses

Testing resistance to external rhythms (rhythmic photostimulation)

Triggered photostimulation to detect latent or compensated pathology by presenting light flashes synchronized with intrinsic EEG rhythms (delta, theta, etc.)

Photostimulation uses short light flashes (≈150 μs) with a spectrum close to white light and intensity of 0.1–0.6 J. Series of flashes test the brain's ability to "entrain" EEG rhythms to external stimuli. In healthy individuals, entrainment is most pronounced at frequencies close to intrinsic EEG rhythms, with maximal amplitude in the occipital regions. In photosensitive epilepsy, rhythmic photostimulation can trigger a photoparoxysmal response—generalized epileptiform discharges.

Hyperventilation mainly provokes epileptiform activity. Patients are instructed to breathe deeply and rhythmically for 3 minutes at a rate of 16–20 breaths per minute. EEG recording begins at least 1 minute before hyperventilation, continues during the procedure, and extends for at least 3 minutes afterward.

4.1.5. Special Recording Conditions

Children

Parental presence, use of play-based methods, often recording during sleep.

ICU and Neurosurgical Patients

Continuous monitoring, consideration of medication effects, recording with life-support measures.

Summary

EEG should be recorded:

In a calm, controlled environment

With the patient at rest

Minimizing external and internal interference

Following standard electrode placement and technical parameters

Documenting all conditions and activation tests

Only under these conditions is EEG a reliable and interpretable tool for functional diagnostics.

4.2. Practical EEG Research Methods

EEG research methods encompass the stages of recording, analysis, and interpretation of brain bioelectrical activity and now represent a well-developed system of clinical and research approaches. Below is a structured overview of contemporary EEG methods used in neurophysiology and functional diagnostics.

4.2.1. EEG Recording Methods

Routine (Standard) EEG

Recorded at rest (eyes closed / open)

Duration: usually 20–30 minutes

Used for initial diagnosis (epilepsy, diffuse brain lesions)

Long-term and Monitoring EEG

Multi-hour and 24-hour recordings

Video-EEG monitoring

Used for epilepsy, paroxysmal events, and sleep disorders

Ambulatory EEG

Recorded in naturalistic conditions

Used for rare seizure or syncope episodes

Invasive Recording Methods

Electrocorticography (ECoG)

Intracranial EEG (iEEG)

Stereo-EEG (SEEG)

Primarily used in neurosurgery (epilepsy, tumors)

4.3. Functional Tests (Activation Methods)

Functional loads increase the diagnostic value of EEG.

Hyperventilation

Rhythmic photic stimulation

Sleep deprivation

Cognitive and sensory stimuli

Pharmacological tests

4.4. Methods of Mathematical EEG Analysis

4.4.1. Time-Domain Analysis

This is the classical method in which the researcher studies the raw EEG signal over time.

What is analyzed: signal waveform, amplitude, and frequency of oscillations.

Parameters:

Amplitude — the magnitude of voltage fluctuations

Frequency — the number of oscillations per second (Hz)

Patterns:

Alpha (8–13 Hz)

Beta (13–30 Hz)

Theta (4–7 Hz)

Delta (0.5–4 Hz)

Applications:

Detection of epileptic discharges

Identification of abnormal activity

Analysis of sleep stages

4.4.2. Frequency-Domain Analysis

In this approach, EEG is analyzed in terms of its frequency spectrum.

Methods:

Fast Fourier Transform (FFT) — shows which frequencies are present in the signal and their power

Power Spectral Density — a quantitative measure of the energy at each frequency

Applications:

Analysis of dominant brain rhythms

Assessment of brain activity during cognitive tasks or pathological conditions

4.4.2.1. Fourier Transform

The mathematical basis of frequency analysis is the Fourier transform. This transform was formulated in 1822 by the French mathematician Jean-Baptiste Joseph Fourier. It exists in various forms depending on the type of signal being analyzed. The general assumption is that the studied processes (signals) consist of a certain number (possibly infinite) of sinusoidal and/or cosinusoidal components (harmonics) with successively increasing frequencies.

The Fourier transform decomposes a signal into a series of harmonic components without any loss of information (if all harmonics are summed arithmetically, the original signal is reconstructed). Each harmonic is characterized by three parameters: amplitude, initial phase, and frequency. The dependence of harmonic amplitude and phase on frequency is called the spectrum.

For a continuous signal of infinite duration, the spectrum is also continuous and infinite in the frequency domain. In practice, however, signals are time-limited and their amplitudes are measured at equal time intervals (digitized by an analog-to-digital converter). As a result, the obtained spectrum is discrete and limited in the frequency domain, consisting of separate spectral lines. This type of decomposition is achieved using a modified method known as the Discrete Fourier Transform (DFT).

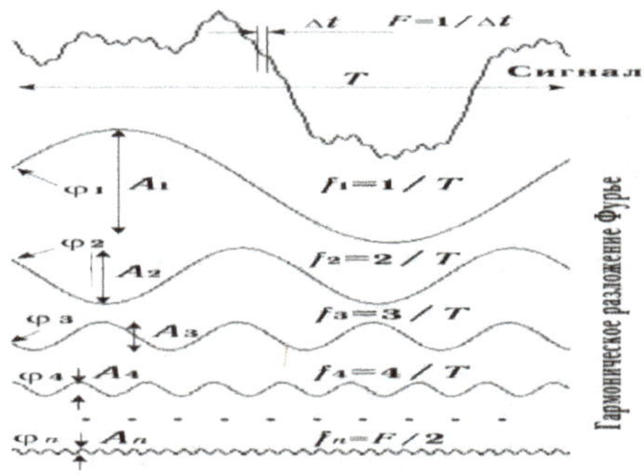

Figure 22. *Fourier analysis.*

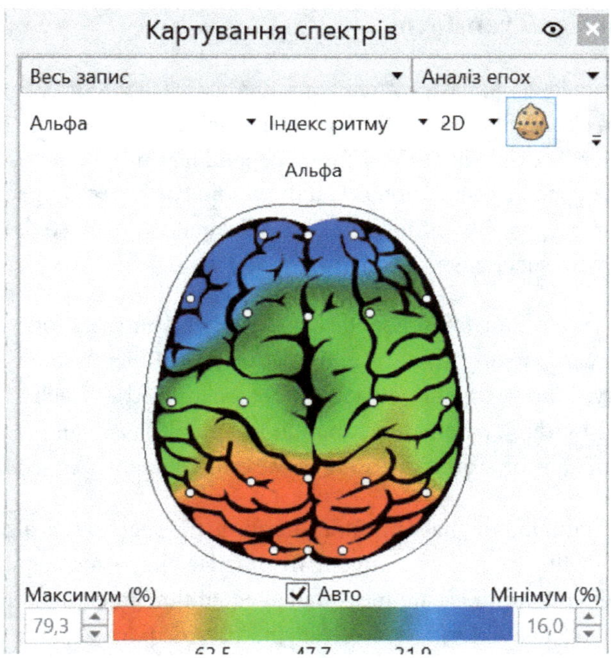

Figure 23. *Spectral mapping.*

4.4.2.2. Periodometric Analysis

Periodometric analysis originated and became widely used in the pre-computer era, when manual measurements of paper EEG recordings were predominant.

The aim of periodometric analysis is to study the distribution of amplitudes and frequencies of a given rhythm. A rhythm is understood as harmonic oscillations within any specified frequency range, in particular within the standard frequency bands. The analysis is preceded by signal filtering, which isolates the harmonic components within the selected frequency range.

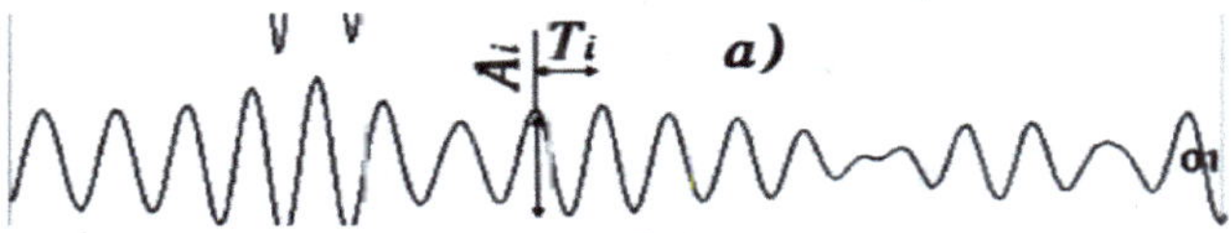

Figure 24. *In periodometric analysis, wave amplitude is measured peak-to-peak.*

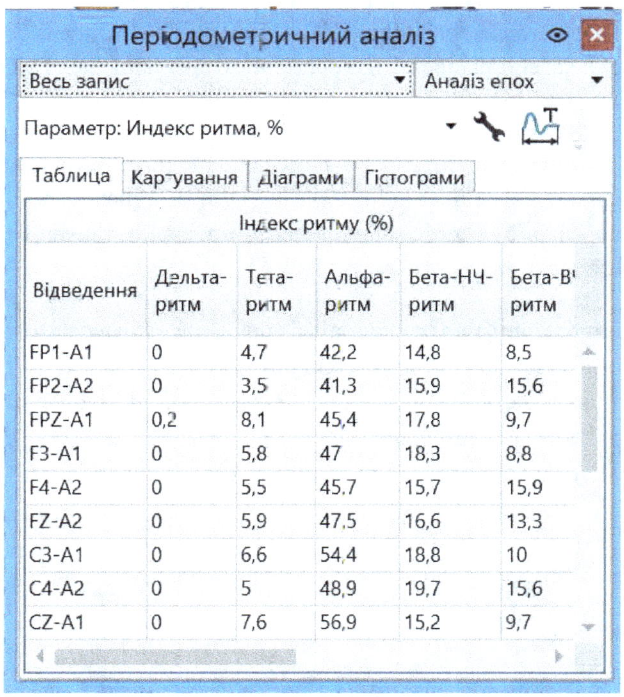

Індекс ритму (%)					
Відведення	Дельта-ритм	Тета-ритм	Альфа-ритм	Бета-НЧ-ритм	Бета-В' ритм
FP1-A1	0	4,7	42,2	14,8	8,5
FP2-A2	0	3,5	41,3	15,9	15,6
FPZ-A1	0,2	8,1	45,4	17,8	9,7
F3-A1	0	5,8	47	18,3	8,8
F4-A2	0	5,5	45,7	15,7	15,9
FZ-A2	0	5,9	47,5	16,6	13,3
C3-A1	0	6,6	54,4	18,8	10
C4-A2	0	5	48,9	19,7	15,6
CZ-A1	0	7,6	56,9	15,2	9,7

Figure 25. *Periodometric analysis.*

Although this method originated and was widely used before the introduction of spectral analysis techniques, it allows a more detailed investigation of the distribution of rhythm amplitudes and frequencies within a specified frequency range. This includes the construction of histograms, calculation of descriptive statistical parameters, percentage content and modulation of the rhythm, and its frequency instability.

As a result of periodometric analysis, the amplitude and frequency of EEG rhythms, as well as the time index (the percentage of time during which a given rhythm occupies a certain recording interval), are calculated. After obtaining the primary data, further processing is performed using digital methods. Subsequently, various EEG parameters across the entire set of recorded leads may serve as source data for topographic mapping — a visual representation of the distribution of selected parameter values over the scalp using a multicolor scale.

The following can be mapped: EEG amplitudes at a given time point, spectral parameters at a given frequency, and generalized spectral parameters (GSP) within a specified frequency range. Mapping of GSP can be performed either by frequency bands within the current analysis epoch or within a selected frequency range across epochs into which the EEG recording is divided. Such mapping may be accompanied by bar charts showing changes in EEG parameters across all leads.

Visualization of maps can be performed in three forms: a single map controlled by a movable cursor (adjustable over time, frequency, range, or epoch); a series of maps (for a specific time interval, frequencies, ranges, or epochs); or an animated series of maps.

Furthermore, any maps can be saved and averaged in a database. Averaging may be performed separately for different physiological states, tests, diseases, and other conditions. The contents of the database are of interest for statistical evaluation of pairwise differences between maps: between two native maps, between a native and an averaged map, or between averaged maps.

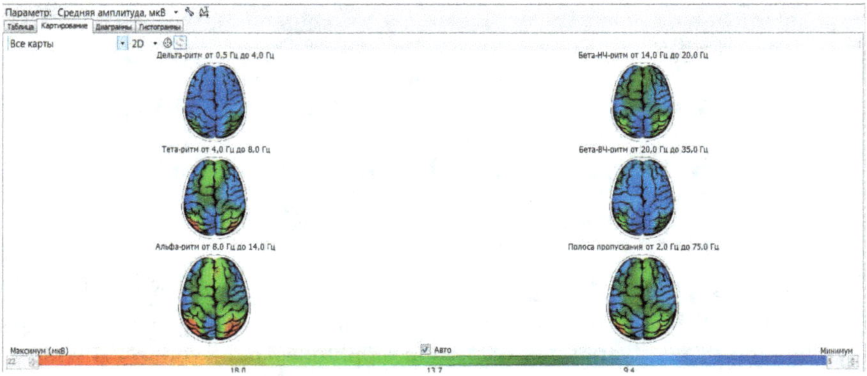

Figure 26. *Generalized spectral parameters.*

4.4.3. Time–Frequency Analysis

This approach combines time-domain and frequency-domain methods.

Methods:

Wavelet transform — suitable for the analysis of short-lasting and non-stationary signals.

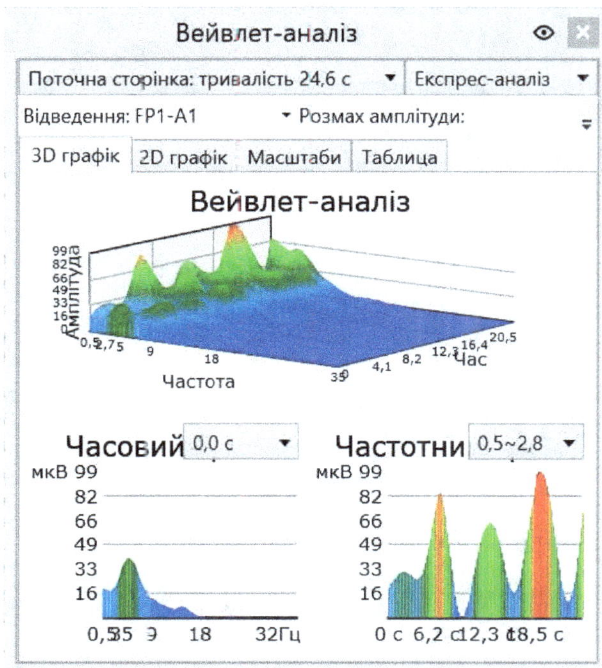

Figure 27. Wavelet analysis.

STFT (Short-Time Fourier Transform) — divides the signal into short time windows to observe changes in the spectrum over time.

Applications:

Detection of epileptic seizures

Analysis of responses to stimuli (e.g., visual or auditory)

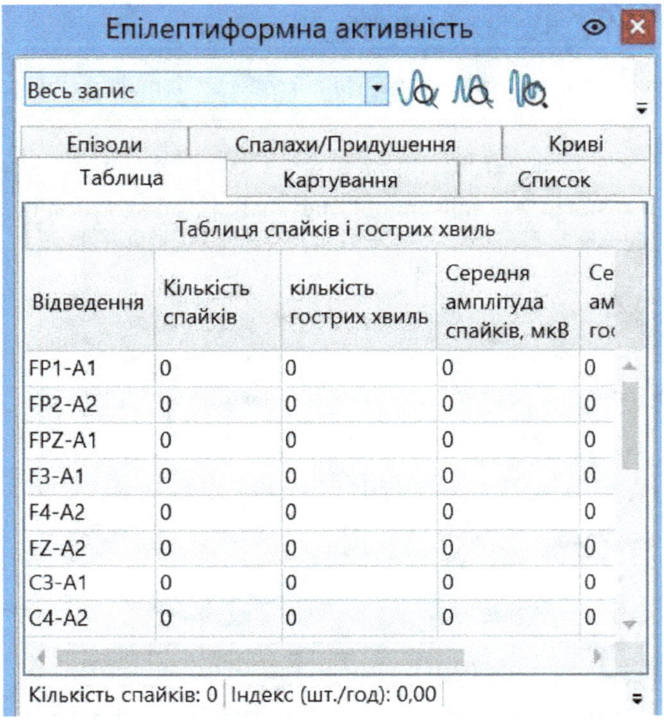

Figure 28. *Analysis of epileptic activity.*

4.4.4. Correlation and Coherence Analysis

These methods study the relationships between signals from different brain regions.

Methods:

Cross-correlation — evaluates how similar two signals are over time.

Correlation analysis includes the calculation of correlation coefficients, as well as auto- and cross-correlation functions. In the pre-computer era, correlation analysis was widely used as a substitute for spectral analysis due to the availability of analog computing devices. In modern applications, modified versions of this method are used as correlators for pattern recognition.

The **Pearson correlation coefficient (r)** (parametric) is an indicator of a linear relationship between paired variables or paired samples X and Y and is applied when the original data are normally distributed. It is calculated as the ratio of the covariance of two variables to their standard deviations. A value close to +1 or −1 indicates a strong positive or negative correlation, respectively. A value close to 0 indicates the absence of a linear relationship but does not exclude the possibility of a nonlinear relationship.

A high correlation does not necessarily imply a causal relationship between variables, as both may depend on a third variable.

In this context, paired samples correspond to two segments of equal duration belonging either to the same EEG channel (autocorrelation) or to two different channels (cross-correlation). A high positive correlation indicates in-phase or synchronous changes of two signals, where an increase in one signal corresponds to an increase in the other, and likewise for decreases. A high negative correlation indicates synchronous anti-phase behavior, where an increase in one signal corresponds to a decrease in the other. Asynchronous signal changes result in correlation values close to zero.

The statistical significance of the correlation coefficient is evaluated using **Student's t-test**, with calculation of a critical value.

Coherence refers to the degree of synchronization between two brain regions at different frequencies.

EEG coherence analysis reveals functional relationships between different brain areas. Since the electrical activity of the brain reflects its functional state, coherence makes it possible to identify the involvement of different cortical regions in specific brain functions and to provide a quantitative assessment of the level of integrative activity of brain structures.

The main measure of EEG coherence analysis is the **coherence coefficient**, which ranges from 0 to 1: the higher the coherence value, the more coordinated the activity between two regions. The degree of interaction between different brain areas must be adequate for optimal functional performance.

Applications:

Investigation of functional connectivity between brain regions

Diagnosis of disorders characterized by impaired synchronization (e.g., schizophrenia, dementia)

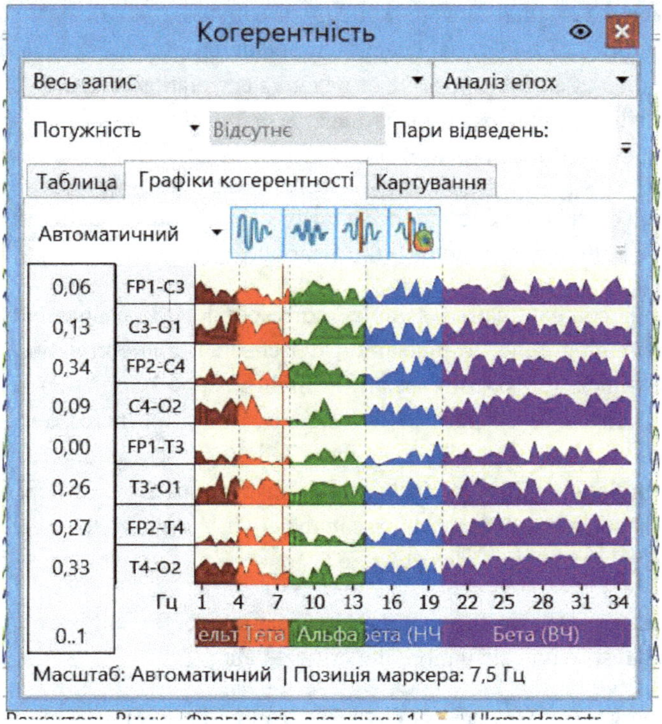

Figure 29. Coherence.

4.4.5. Nonlinear and Chaotic Analysis

EEG is considered as a complex nonlinear signal rather than simply a sum of sinusoids.

Methods:

- **Entropy** — measures the complexity of the signal
- **Fractal analysis** — evaluates the self-similarity of EEG structure

Applications:

- Assessment of brain arousal and functional state
- Detection of epileptic predisposition

4.4.6. Channel and Topographic Visualization

Methods:

Topographic mapping — shows the distribution of activity across the scalp

EEG Source Localization — attempts to determine the exact brain region generating the signal

Applications:

Localization of epileptic foci

Planning of neurosurgical interventions

Conclusion: Modern EEG analysis methods are often combined, integrating time-domain, frequency-domain, and spatial analyses, sometimes supplemented with nonlinear measures for a deeper understanding of brain function.

Table 2. EEG analysis methods with their main characteristics and applications

Analysis method	What it measures / how it works	Main metrics	Applications
Time-domain analysis	Analysis of the raw EEG signal in the time domain	Amplitude, frequency, waveform morphology (alpha, beta, theta, delta), epileptiform discharges	Epilepsy diagnosis, sleep stage identification, basic assessment of brain activity
Frequency-domain analysis	Decomposition of the signal into frequency components	Power spectral density, dominant rhythms	Assessment of brain rhythm activity, cognitive studies, pathology detection
Time–frequency analysis	Examines how the frequency spectrum changes over time	Wavelet coefficients, STFT, frequency dynamics	Detection of epileptic seizures, stimulus-related brain responses
Correlation and coherence analysis	Relationships between signals from different brain regions	Cross-correlation, coherence	Study of functional connectivity, diagnosis of synchronization disorders
Nonlinear / chaotic analysis	Signal complexity and instability	Entropy, fractal dimension, Lyapunov exponent	Assessment of arousal level, epilepsy predisposition, analysis of brain activity dynamics
Channel-based / topographic visualization	Spatial distribution of brain activity across the scalp	Topographic maps, source localization	Localization of epileptic foci, neurosurgical planning, brain network studies

Historically, early computer-based encephalographs were developed on computers with very limited memory capacities—initially 8 KB, then 16 KB, 20 KB, 40 KB, and so on. The implementation of Fourier analysis required significantly less memory than that of half-period analysis. As a result, Fourier analysis became more widely used in computer encephalographs than half-period analysis.

However, in the analysis of EEG recordings from children and rats, particularly in cases of so-called immature cortex, practical experience showed that the application of Fourier analysis was not sufficiently accurate. It was found that the results of manual analysis and automated analysis performed using Fourier analyzers differed by 20–40%.

Norbert Wiener proposed considering EEG as a stochastic signal, by analogy with the signal characteristics of any complex system (Wiener, 1961). Based on this assumption, it was suggested that the fundamental laws governing EEG dynamics could be studied using probabilistic and statistical analysis, regardless of the biophysical origin of cortical electrical processes (Lopes da Silva, 1981). This concept stimulated the emergence of a large number of studies devoted to the stochastic properties of the EEG signal.

In early studies focused on the statistical properties of EEG as a stochastic process, it was demonstrated that the distribution of EEG amplitude values corresponded to Gaussian parameters (Kozhevnikov V.A., 1958; Lion K.S., Winter D.F., 1953; Sounders M.G., 1963). This was a highly important conclusion for understanding the nature of the summed EEG signal.

According to the central limit theorem, the Gaussian properties of EEG could be explained by the mutual independence of individual sources (generators) of the cortical electric field (Elul R., 1969). This assumption would fully justify the application of parametric methods of mathematical statistics to EEG signal analysis and would significantly simplify its interpretation. However, a number of authors did not confirm the Gaussian structure of EEG (Sugimoto H., Ishii N., Iwata A. et al., 1978; Weiss M.S., 1973; Campbell J. et al., 1967). The main reason for these apparent contradictions was related to the use of EEG segments of different durations for testing. Short EEG segments, up to 10 seconds, were generally well approximated by a Gaussian distribution, whereas longer segments—up to 1 minute—usually did not follow a normal distribution. An important conclusion of these studies was the assumption that EEG can, in fact, be described by probability distributions only for relatively short realizations, not exceeding 10–20 seconds.

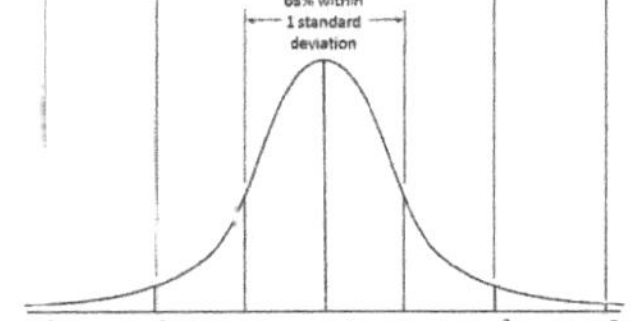

Figure 30. *Normal distribution, also known as the Gaussian distribution or the Gauss–Laplace distribution, is a probability distribution that, in the continuous case, is defined by a probability density function identical to the Gaussian function.*

The application of nonlinear dynamics methods (deterministic chaos theory) to the problem of describing the electroencephalogram has been relatively successful (Jansen, 1991; Roeschke et al., 1997; Pritchard & Herzog, 1992). This theory operates with ensembles of trajectories of dynamical systems and uses a probabilistic approach to describe observed systems. However, nonlinear dynamics methods are based on the hypothesis that the electrical activity of the brain can be described by stationary dynamical models. Such a hypothesis is unrealistic in many cases (A. Ya. Kaplan, S. L. Shishkin, 2000).

Taken together, the above facts indicate that the dynamic pattern of the EEG process can be correctly described only when sufficiently short signal segments are considered. This conclusion motivated researchers to develop specialized EEG segmentation methods.

4.4.7. Methodological aspects

Electrode placement systems (10–20, 10–10, 10–5)

Filtering and artifact suppression

Calibration and standardization

Normative databases

Summary

Modern EEG research methods include various recording techniques (routine, long-term, invasive), functional tests, visual and quantitative analysis, source and network interpretation, integration with other modalities, and the use of artificial intelligence.

EEG remains a unique method due to its high temporal resolution, noninvasiveness, and wide range of clinical and research applications.

4.4.8. Main components of a modern electroencephalograph

1. Electrodes

Modern systems use from 16 to 256 electrodes arranged according to standard layouts (e.g., 10–20 or 10–10 systems).

Types of electrodes include:

Dry electrodes — do not require gel, are quick to apply, but may produce noisier signals.

Wet electrodes (gel/paste) — provide better skin contact and cleaner signals.

Caps or helmets — allow rapid placement of multiple electrodes simultaneously.

2. Amplifier

Brain signals are very weak (approximately 10–100 microvolts), requiring amplification.

Modern EEG amplifiers are digital, featuring noise filtering and suppression of power-line interference and muscle artifacts.

3. Recording and processing system

Signals are digitized and displayed on a computer.

Modern software enables:

Real-time signal visualization

Frequency band analysis (delta, theta, alpha, beta, gamma)

Automatic detection of epileptiform discharges, artifacts, or sleep-related events

Generation of 3D brain activity maps

4. Power supply and interfaces

Modern portable EEG systems can operate on batteries and transmit data via Wi-Fi or Bluetooth.

Desktop clinical systems connect via USB or specialized interfaces and can be integrated with other systems (MRI, brain stimulation devices).

3. Functions and capabilities of modern EEG systems

Diagnostic:

Epilepsy and seizure disorders

Sleep disorders

Brain injuries and stroke

Research:

Neuropsychology

Cognitive research and attention studies

Brain–Computer Interfaces (BCI)

Prognostic and monitoring:

Anesthesia monitoring

Post-stroke rehabilitation

Monitoring of comatose patients

4. Differences between modern EEG systems and older models

Parameter	Older EEG systems	Modern EEG systems
Number of electrodes	6–20	16–256
Recording type	Paper-based, analog	Digital, with advanced analysis capabilities
Computer connectivity	Not available	USB, Wi-Fi, Bluetooth
Signal processing	Manual, visual inspection	Automated processing, noise filtering
Portability	No	Yes, compact caps and portable systems

For topographic diagnosis, a large number of leads are required, recorded in various combinations. In order to save time, modern electroencephalographs use predefined lead configurations (montage schemes, routine programs, etc.).

4.4.9. EEG lead placement and recording

Recording electrodes are positioned so that all major brain regions are represented in the multichannel recording. These regions are designated by the initial letters of their Latin anatomical names. In clinical practice, two main EEG lead systems are used: the international **10–20 system** and a modified scheme with a reduced number of electrodes. When a more detailed EEG representation is required, the **10–20 system** is preferred.

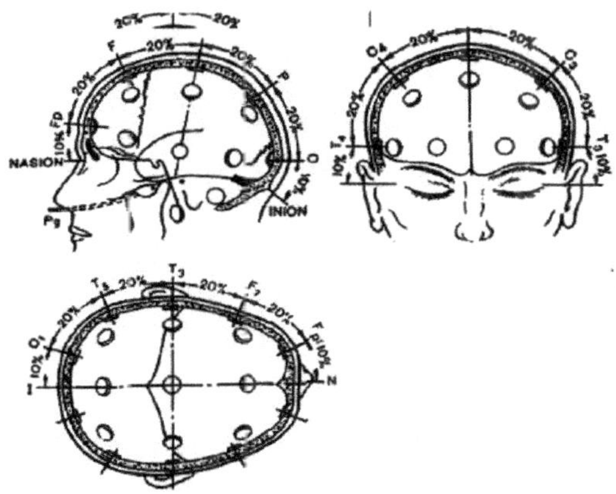

Figure 31. International "10–20" electrode placement system. *Letter indices denote the following regions:* ***O (occipitalis)*** *— occipital derivation;* ***P (parietalis)*** *— parietal derivation;* ***C (centralis)*** *— central derivation;* ***F (frontalis)*** *— frontal derivation;* ***T (temporalis)*** *— temporal derivation.*

Numeric indices specify the exact position of the electrode within the corresponding region.

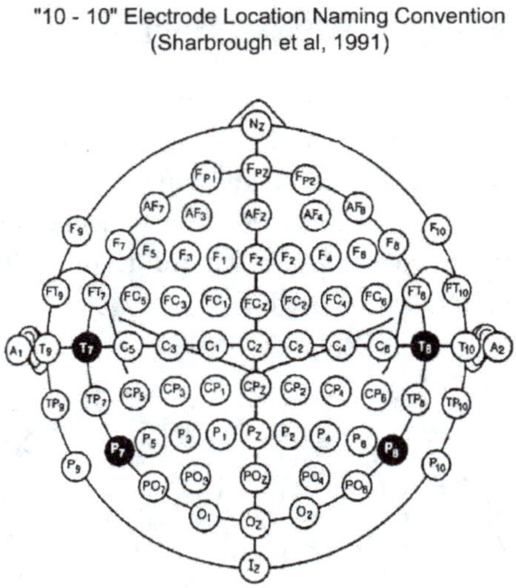

Figure 32. *Localization of electrodes during EEG recording.*

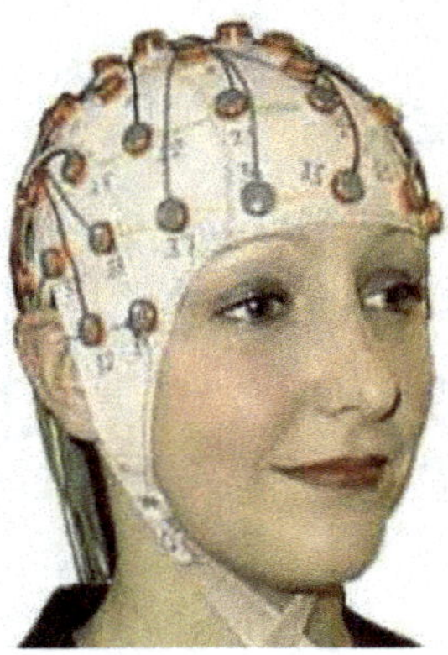

Figure 33. *EEG electrode cap for recording.*

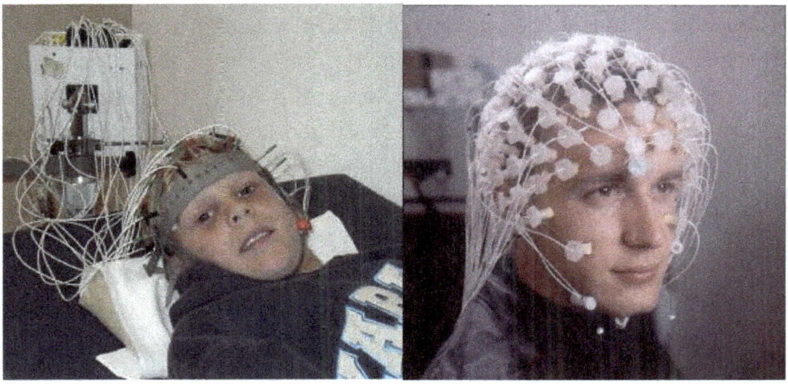

Figure 34. *EEG electrodes placed on the subject's head.*

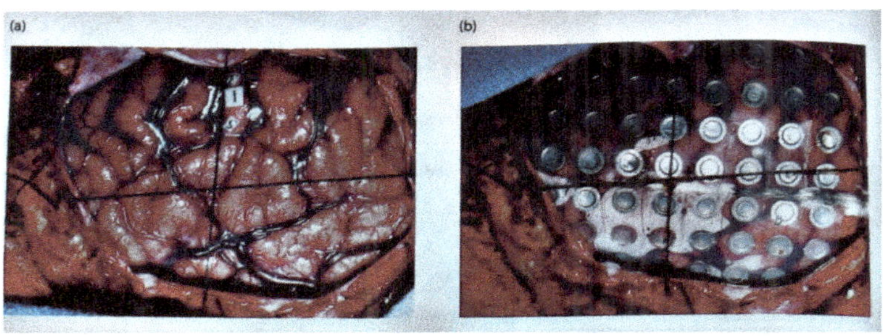

Figure 35. *Subdural electrode grid can be used to measure epileptic activity during chronic recordings over large areas of the cortical surface. Neurosurgeons use this technique during surgical procedures. The electrodes may also be used for stimulation to assess neural function.*

For topographic EEG analysis, the following principles for constructing montage schemes are considered most rational:

1. **First montage** — bipolar derivations with large interelectrode distances (the "10–20" system), with electrodes paired along sagittal and frontal lines.
2. **Second montage** — bipolar derivations with small interelectrode distances, with electrodes paired along sagittal lines.
3. **Third montage** — bipolar derivations with small interelectrode distances, with electrodes paired along frontal lines.
4. **Fourth montage** — monopolar derivations with indifferent (reference) electrodes.
5. **Fifth montage** — bipolar derivations with small interelectrode distances, with electrodes paired along sagittal lines, combined with the recording of eye movements, ECG, or skin galvanic responses during functional loads.

Since pathological features are not always evident in resting EEG, clinical electroencephalography—similar to other functional diagnostic methods—employs physical or functional loads, some of which are mandatory. These include tasks to assess the orienting response and tests to evaluate resistance to external rhythms, such as rhythmic photic stimulation. Another mandatory procedure, effective for detecting latent (compensated) pathology, is **triggered photic stimulation**, in which stimulation is delivered at frequencies corresponding to the brain's own bioelectrical activity using a trigger-based converter of EEG waveform components into light flashes.

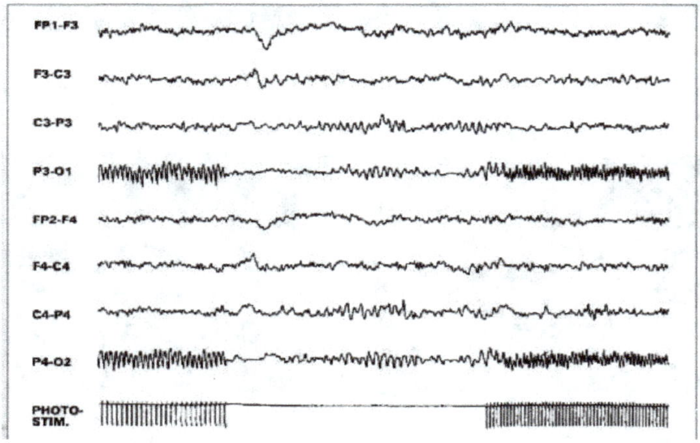

Figure 36. *Normal EEG of an awake subject during photic stimulation.*

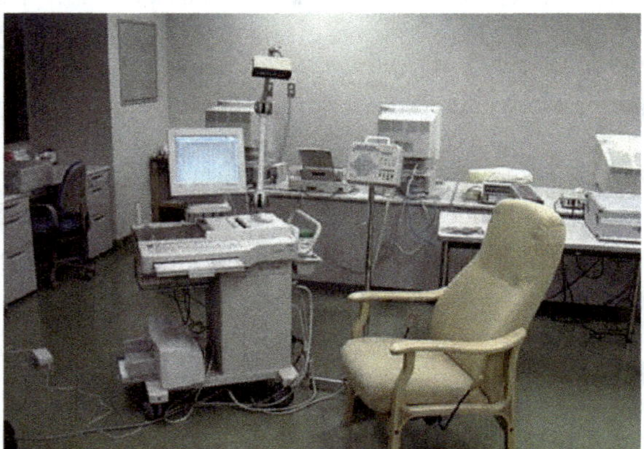

Figure 37. *A modern EEG system.*

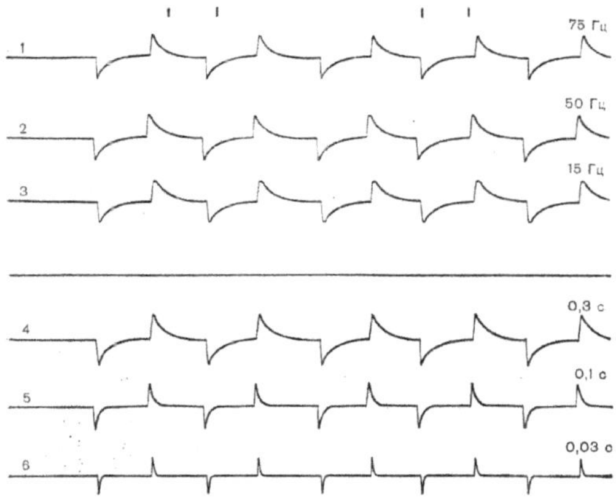

Figure 38. *Signal filtering.*

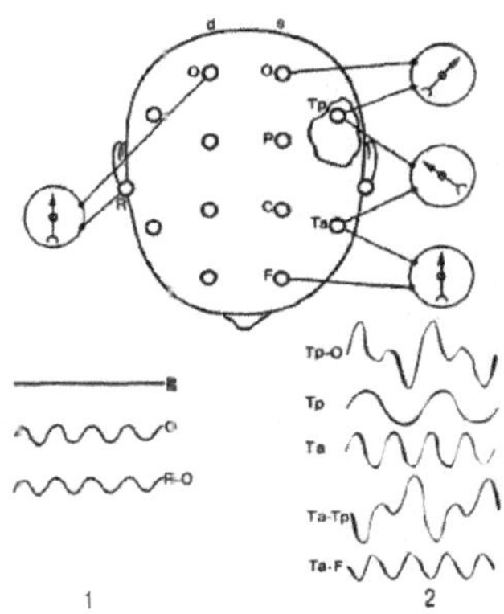

Figure 39. *EEG recording scheme for monopolar (1) and bipolar (2) derivations.*

In monopolar derivation, the reference electrode (R) is placed on the earlobe, while bipolar derivations use pairs of electrodes on the scalp. In a reduced-lead system, letter indices indicate brain regions: ***O*** *— occipital derivation;* ***P*** *— parietal derivation;* ***C*** *— central derivation;* ***F*** *— frontal derivation;* ***Ta*** *— anterior temporal derivation;* ***Tr*** *— posterior temporal derivation.*

- ***1-R*** *— potential under the active electrode relative to the reference electrode.*
- ***R-O*** *— recording obtained from monopolar derivation from the right occipital region.*
- ***Tr*** *— potential under an electrode over a pathological focus;* ***Ta*** *— potential under an electrode over normal brain tissue.*
- ***Ta-Tr, Tr-O, Ta-F*** *— recordings obtained from bipolar derivations of the corresponding electrode pairs.*

A **reference derivation** is defined as a recording where the potential from an electrode over the brain is applied to "input 1" of the amplifier, and the potential from an electrode distant from the brain is applied to "input 2." The electrode over the brain is called the **active electrode**, while the distant electrode is termed **indifferent**. Often, the reference consists of a combined electrode from the left and right earlobes. The active electrode connects to input 1 of the amplifier, while the reference electrode connects to input 2. In some cases, a reference electrode consists of two shorted electrodes (AA) on the earlobes.

Since EEG records the potential difference between two electrodes, changes under each electrode influence the waveform in equal but opposite directions.

A **bipolar derivation** connects electrodes over the brain to both inputs of the amplifier. The recorded waveform reflects the potential difference between the electrodes. Therefore, the activity of each individual electrode cannot be determined from a single bipolar derivation. However, analyzing EEG from multiple electrode pairs in various combinations allows localization of potential sources contributing to the composite waveform.

For example, if there is a local slow-wave source in the posterior temporal region, connecting the anterior and posterior temporal electrodes (Ta, Tr) to the amplifier will produce a recording containing the slow component corresponding to Tr, overlaid by faster oscillations from normal tissue at Ta. To determine which electrode contributes to the slow component, additional channels are connected with one electrode from the original pair (Ta or Tr) and another electrode from a non-temporal region (e.g., F or O). The pair including Tr over the pathological focus (Tr-O) will still display the slow component, whereas the pair over intact brain tissue (Ta-F) will show normal EEG. This allows precise localization of pathological sources.

In reference derivations, the active electrode generates the brain's variable potential. The reference electrode, being distant from the brain, has a constant potential that does not pass through the AC amplifier and does not affect the recording. The potential difference reflects the true brain oscillations under the active electrode. However, any intense source asymmetrically located between the active and reference electrodes will affect the recording, making source localization less reliable in reference derivations.

4.4.10. EEG segmentation

Electroencephalography is a primary method for epilepsy diagnosis; thus, increasing the informativeness of EEG studies in epileptic patients is crucial (Gnezditsky, 2000). A major limitation of conventional spectral analysis is averaging highly heterogeneous data, making it impossible to distinguish a single high-amplitude wave from many smaller waves (Jansen, 1978).

Consequently, digital analysis of EEG containing both background activity and seizure phenomena averages the signals, obscuring paroxysmal events. Recognizing EEG and electrocorticogram (ECoG) as non-stationary processes that can be interpreted as piecewise-stationary, **segmental description methods** are employed for accurate analysis of electrical phenomena (Kaplan, 1999).

For instance, in rats after cerebellar hemisphere removal, ECoG registers both background and paroxysmal seizure activity (Hiroko Ohishi et al., 2003). This experimental model was used to develop an EEG segmentation algorithm to separate seizure from background activity.

Model formalism: Previous studies (Lobasyuk, 2005) using multiple regression, correlation analysis, and graph theory demonstrated relationships between ECoG rhythm amplitudes within a single derivation. It was hypothesized that mass EEG reflects the interaction of hypothetical beta-2, beta-1, theta, and delta rhythm generators. Positive and negative amplitude relationships suggested regulatory mechanisms organizing the ECoG. Pathological seizure activity is generated by hyperexcitable neuronal generators (Kryzhanovsky, 1980, 1997, 2002), forming a pathological network. Therefore, control mechanisms in normal and pathological functional systems differ, and in ECoG segments with paroxysmal activity, rhythm amplitude relationships do not match those of background activity. This pragmatic concept underpins the current work.

Experimental methodology: White rats (210–220 g) were anesthetized with nembutal (40 mg/kg, i.p.), and recording electrodes were bilaterally implanted in the frontal and occipital cortices. Vacuum aspiration of cerebellar hemispheres was performed in five animals under nembutal anesthesia (AP group). A control group included four rats (IM group). ECoG was recorded to a computer hard disk using an analog-to-digital converter at 256 Hz. Recordings were obtained from the following derivations: Frontal cortex — left occipital cortex, Frontal cortex — right occipital cortex, Left frontal cortex — right frontal cortex, Left occipital cortex — right occipital cortex. The amplifier time constant was 0.3 or 1.0 s.

Analysis of the ECoG files was performed after the experiments using the **"Analist 2"** software, applying a **periodometric approach** (half-period analysis algorithm). Five physiological ECoG rhythms were distinguished: **beta-1, beta-2, alpha, theta, and delta**.

For each frequency band, the following parameters were measured and calculated: **mean amplitude** (μV), **modal frequency** (Hz), and **duration index** (the normalized duration of oscillations in the analyzed ECoG segment for each frequency band relative to the analysis epoch). ECoG recordings were continuously obtained for 30 minutes. During statistical analysis, **mean values, standard deviations, and standard errors** were calculated.

ECoG segmentation was performed using the **fixed-interval method** (Kaplan, 1999) based on the following sequence of procedures:

1. **Half-period analysis** of fixed short ECoG epochs (segments) of 2 s duration.
2. **Classification of these epochs** using **cluster analysis** with the **k-means algorithm**, resulting in two or more clusters.
3. **Statistical analysis** of ECoG parameters corresponding to each cluster.

For segments included in the same cluster, **mean values, standard deviations, and standard errors** of the parameters were calculated.

Relationships between the amplitudes of ECoG rhythms were analyzed using **multiple linear regression and correlation analysis** (Mannheim & Rich, 1997). **Statistical significance** was accepted at $\mathbf{p < 0.05}$ and $\mathbf{p < 0.1}$.

To construct mathematical models, each amplitude parameter selected for analysis was considered as a **dependent variable (Y)**, and the remaining parameters as **independent variables (X)**. Using **multiple linear regression**, directional influences were determined, resulting in regression equations of the form:

$Y' = a0 + b1X1 + b2X2 + \cdots + bnXn + e$,

where:

a0 — intercept,

b1,b2,…,bnb_1, b_2, \dots, b_nb1,b2,…,bn — regression coefficients reflecting the influence of the independent variables (X1, X2, …, Xn) on the analyzed parameter,

eee — error term representing any variation in Y' not caused by the independent variables.

Regression coefficients were evaluated using their **standard deviations**, and the overall regression effectiveness was assessed via the **multiple correlation coefficient**. Geometrically, multiple linear regression equations were interpreted using **polycyclic multigraphs** (Zykov, 1987).

In this approach, **graph nodes** represent ECoG parameters; **solid lines** indicate positive regression coefficients, while **dashed lines** indicate negative coefficients.

Own research:

After segmentation, ECoG parameters of intact rats were divided into **two clusters** (Figure 40). The amplitude of the **beta-2 rhythm** in synchronized fragments was **statistically significantly higher** than in desynchronized fragments: by **1.08 times** in the left hemisphere and **1.12 times** in the right hemisphere (Figure 1, I, II). The **beta-1 rhythm amplitude** was higher by **1.18 and 1.34 times**, respectively.

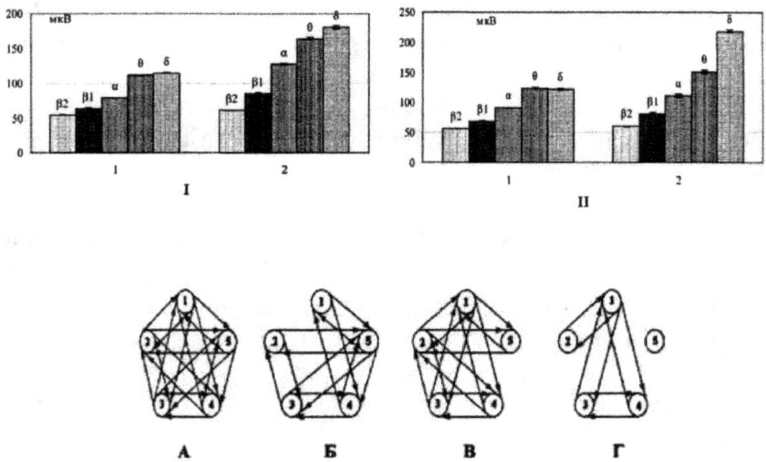

Figure 40. *Diagrams of the mean amplitudes of* ***β2, β1, α, θ, and δ ECoG rhythms*** *recorded from the* ***left (I)*** *and* ***right (II) hemispheres*** *of the intact brain, within* ***desynchronization (1)*** *and* ***synchronization (2)*** *segments, and mathematical models reflecting the relationships between ECoG rhythm amplitudes in the* ***left (A, B)*** *and* ***right hemispheres (C, D)*** *of intact rats during* ***desynchronization (A, C)*** *and* ***synchronization (B, D)*** *periods.*

Notation:

1 — beta-2 rhythm amplitude, 2 — beta-1 rhythm amplitude, 3 — alpha rhythm amplitude, 4 — theta rhythm amplitude, 5 — delta rhythm amplitude.

Accordingly, the **alpha rhythm amplitude** was **1.32 and 1.62 times higher**, the **theta rhythm amplitude** was **1.22 and 1.47 times higher**, and the **delta rhythm amplitude** was **1.79 and 1.58 times higher**, respectively.

Analysis of the relationships between ECoG rhythm amplitudes in the intact rat during desynchronization segments (Figure 40, A, C) revealed **more connections** than in synchronization segments (Figure 40, B, D). It should be noted that **all identified connections were positive**.

In the ECoG of rats after **cerebellar hemisphere aspiration**, there was a predominance of **high-amplitude, generalized slow-wave delta rhythm**, episodes of **hypersynchronous alpha rhythm against a background of desynchronization**, low-amplitude **theta- and delta-range slow rhythms**, and **rapid, island-like high-amplitude seizure activity**.

After segmentation, the ECoG parameters of rats with cerebellar hemisphere aspiration were divided into **seven clusters** (Figure 41).

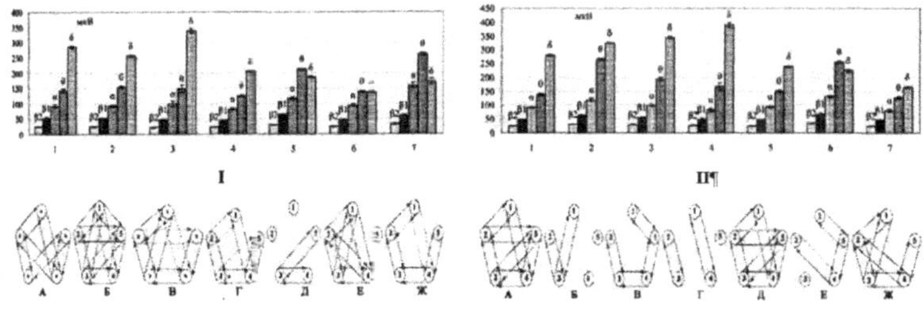

Figure 41. *Diagrams of the mean amplitudes of **β2, β1, α, θ, and δ rhythms** of **segmented ECoG**, recorded from the **left (I)** and **right (II) hemispheres** of rats after cerebellar hemisphere aspiration, and mathematical models reflecting the relationships between ECoG rhythm amplitudes in **seven clusters**.*

Notation:

A — first cluster, B — second cluster, C — third cluster, D — fourth cluster, E — fifth cluster, F — sixth cluster, G — seventh cluster.

I — ECoG of the left hemisphere, II — ECoG of the right hemisphere.

1 — beta-2 rhythm amplitude, 2 — beta-1 rhythm amplitude, 3 — alpha rhythm amplitude, 4 — theta rhythm amplitude, 5 — delta rhythm amplitude.

***Solid lines** indicate positive influences, **dashed lines** indicate negative influences.*

The cluster representing the **desynchronization phenomenon in the left hemisphere** was identified as **cluster two**. The structure of the polycyclic multigraph relationships in cluster two (Figure 41, B) was identical to that observed in the analysis of relationships in desynchronization segments of the intact rat (Figure 40, A). Notably, this cluster contained the **largest number of relationships — 18** — between ECoG rhythm amplitudes, with the alpha rhythm amplitude measuring **93.38 ± 3.06 μV**.

The cluster representing the **synchronization phenomenon in the left hemisphere** was identified as **cluster seven**. The alpha rhythm amplitude in this cluster was the **highest** compared to other clusters, measuring **158.93 ± 9.31 μV**, while the number of relationships between ECoG rhythm amplitudes was **10**, fewer than in the desynchronization cluster.

In the **right hemisphere**, the cluster representing the **desynchronization phenomenon** was identified as **cluster five**, which exhibited the **largest number of relationships between ECoG rhythm amplitudes — 14** (Figure 41, D), with the alpha rhythm amplitude **93.45 ± 3.13 µV**. The structure of the polycyclic multigraph relationships in cluster two (Figure 41, B) was identical to that observed in the synchronization segments of the right hemisphere in the intact rat (Figure 40, C).

The cluster representing **synchronization in the right hemisphere** was identified as **cluster six** (Figure 41, E), with **6 relationships** and an alpha rhythm amplitude of **130.70 ± 4.12 µV**.

It should be noted that in clusters **3–5 of the left hemisphere**, where the delta rhythm amplitude exceeded **300 µV** (which may indicate paroxysmal activity), **polycyclicity was absent**, meaning that the relationships between ECoG rhythm amplitudes were not fully formed.

Based on these findings, it can be suggested that the **generator organization of background and seizure (paroxysmal) activity is not identical**, which in turn supports their **discrete description as simultaneously occurring EEG phenomena**.

Chapter 5. EEG in the Normal State

5.1. EEG Development by Age Periods

Newborn Period. The electroencephalogram of a full-term newborn in the waking state is **polymorphic**, lacking organized rhythmic activity, and is represented by **generalized, irregular, low-amplitude slow waves** (up to 20 μV), predominantly in the **delta range (1–3 cycles/s)**, with **no regional differences or clear symmetry** (Farber D.A., 1969; Zenkov L.R., 1996).

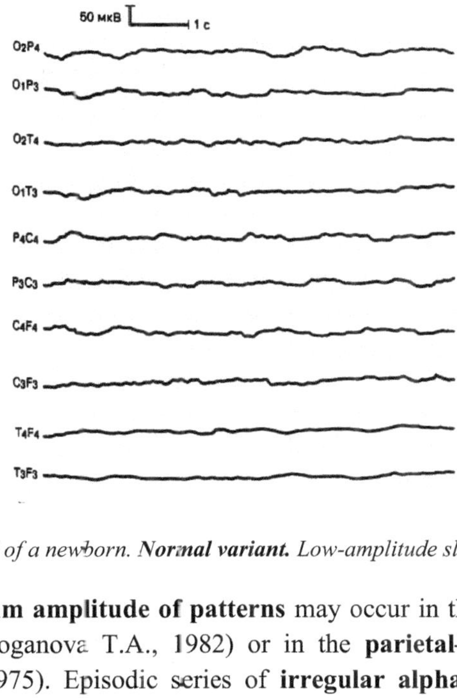

Figure 43. *EEG of a newborn.* ***Normal variant.*** *Low-amplitude slow oscillations.*

The **maximum amplitude of patterns** may occur in the **central regions** (Posikera I.N., Stroganova T.A., 1982) or in the **parietal–occipital regions** (Dreyfus-Brisac, 1975). Episodic series of **irregular alpha oscillations** with amplitudes of up to **50–70 μV** may also be observed (Kalab Z., 1969) (Figure 44).

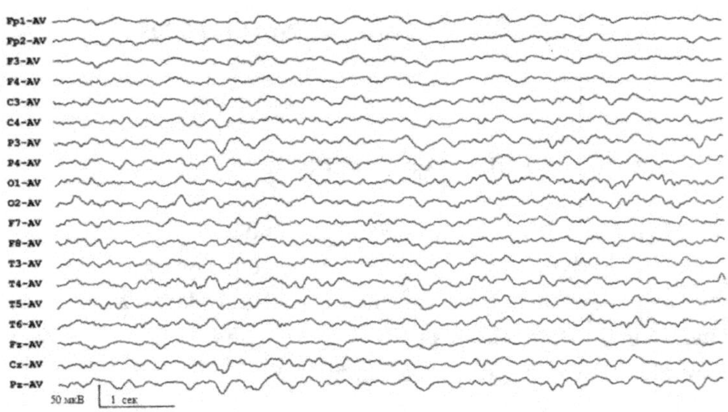

Figure 44. *Girl, 1 week old. Healthy. The EEG during wakefulness is* ***low-amplitude and polymorphic****, with* ***predominant delta activity*** *(64% index) at a frequency of* ***1.5–3 cycles/sec*** *and an amplitude of* ***up to 25–30 μV*** *in the occipital–parietal regions. Theta activity is also present* ***diffusely in groups of waves****.*

Source: Atlas of Childhood Epilepsies, N.V. Korolyova, S.I. Kolesnikov, S.V. Vorobyov, 2011.

By **1–2.5 months**, the **amplitude of bioelectrical potentials increases up to 50 μV**. Rhythmic activity with a frequency of **4–6 cycles/sec** may be observed in the **occipital and central regions**. Predominant delta waves acquire a **bilateral-synchronous organization** (Figure 45).

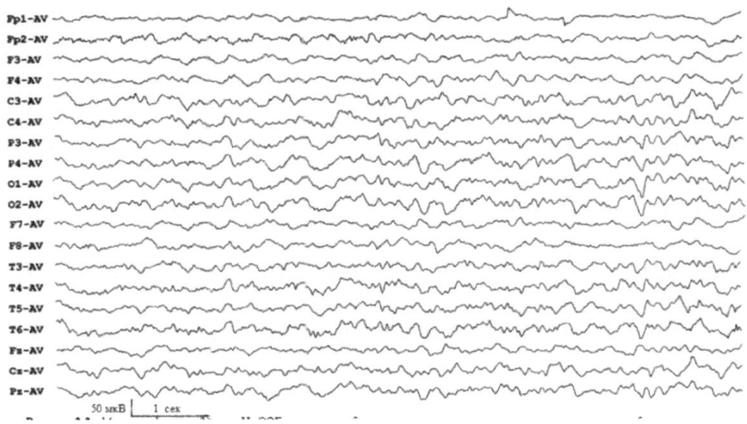

Figure 45*. *Boy, 1 month old. Healthy. In the EEG during wakefulness with eyes closed, a bilaterally synchronous, poly-rhythmic pattern is recorded, with the highest amplitude of biopotentials (up to 50 μV) in the parietal–occipital regions. Delta activity predominates at a frequency of 1.5–3 cycles/sec, interspersed with diffuse theta waves at 4–5 cycles/sec and groups of low-amplitude (up to 15–20 μV) fast activity at 10–20 cycles/sec. In the central–parietal regions, bilaterally synchronous groups of theta waves with a frequency of 5.5–6.5 cycles/sec and an amplitude of up to 40 μV are observed.*
Korolyova N.V., Kolesnikov S.I., Vorobyov S.V., 2011

From 3 months of age, a mu rhythm can appear in the central regions, with a frequency ranging from 6–10 cycles/sec (mu rhythm frequency mode 6.5 cycles/sec) and amplitude of 20–50 μV, sometimes showing moderate interhemispheric asymmetry. *Pampiglione G., 1972; Dreyfus-Brisac, 1975; Stroganova T.A., Posikera I.N., 1993*

From 3–4 months, a rhythm of about 4 cycles/sec is recorded in the occipital regions, which reacts to eye opening. Overall, the EEG remains unstable, with the presence of oscillations of various frequencies. *Blume W.T., 1982; Blagoslonova N.K., Novikova L.A., 1994* (Figure 46).

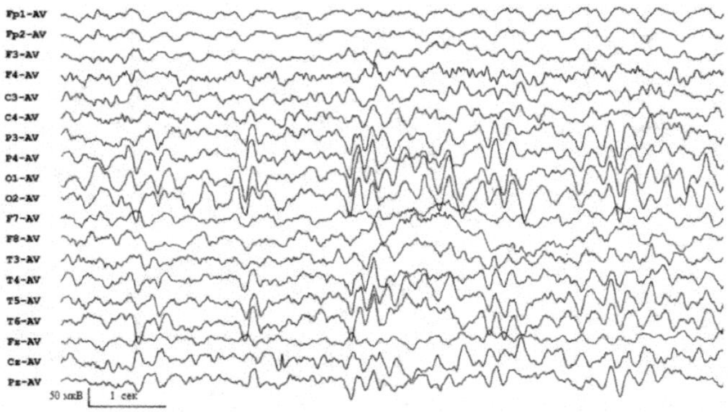

Figure 46. *Boy, 3 months old. Healthy. In the* ***EEG during wakefulness with eyes closed****, a* ***high-amplitude pattern*** *is recorded, predominantly in the* ***parietal–temporo–occipital regions****, consisting of* ***bilaterally synchronous oscillations*** *at* ***3.5–4.5 cycles/sec*** *with amplitudes up to* ***100 µV****, alternating with* ***delta waves*** *at* ***2–3 cycles/sec*** *and amplitudes up to* ***70 µV****.* ***Theta oscillations*** *at* ***4–6 cycles/sec*** *with amplitudes up to* ***60 µV*** *are diffusely present in groups of waves. Superimposed on the slow activity are* ***isolated bursts of faster oscillations*** *at* ***10–18 cycles/sec*** *with amplitudes up to* ***10–15 µV****. Korolyova N.V., Kolesnikov S.I., Vorobyov S.V., 2011*

By **4 months of age**, children show **diffuse delta and theta activity**, and rhythmic activity at **6–8 cycles/sec** may appear in the occipital and central regions. From **6 months**, the EEG is **dominated by a rhythm of 5–6 cycles/sec**. *Blagoslonova N.K., Novikova L.A., 1994* (Figure 47)

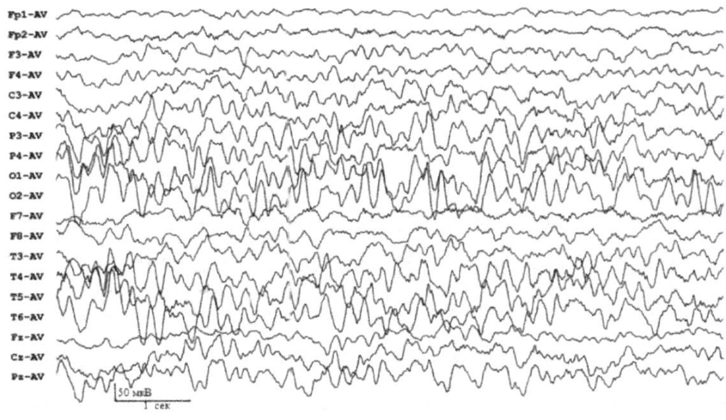

Figure 47. *Girl, 6 months old. Normal variant. In the* ***EEG during wakefulness with eyes closed****, a* ***high-amplitude pattern*** *is observed (up to* ***100 µV in the posterior regions****) and is predominantly represented by* ***theta activity****, along with* ***delta waves*** *exhibiting a zonal gradient. In the* ***parietal–temporo–occipital regions****,* ***theta activity*** *at* ***4.5–6 cycles/sec*** *predominates, alternating with* ***delta waves*** *at* ***1.5–3 cycles/sec****. Diffusely present are* ***isolated oscillations*** *at* ***7–8 cycles/sec*** *with amplitudes up to* ***60 µV****, and* ***groups of beta waves*** *at* ***25–35 cycles/sec*** *with amplitudes up to* ***10 µV****.*

Korolyova N.V., Kolesnikov S.I., Vorobyov S.V., 2011

According to T.A. Stroganova et al. (2005), the **average peak frequency of alpha activity** is **6.24 cycles/sec at 8 months** and **6.78 cycles/sec at 11 months**. The **frequency mode of the mu rhythm** from **5–6 months to 10–12 months** is **7 cycles/sec**, and after **10–12 months** it reaches **8 cycles/sec**.

The **EE*G of a 1-year-old child** is characterized by **pronounced sinusoidal oscillations** of **alpha-like activity** (ontogenetic variant of the alpha rhythm) across all recorded regions, with frequencies from **5–7 cycles/sec**, occasionally **8–8.5 cycles/sec**, alternating with **isolated higher-frequency waves** and **diffuse delta waves** (Farber D.A., Alferova V.V., 1972; Zenkov L.R., 1996). Alpha activity is **unstable**, and despite its broad regional presence, it generally does **not exceed 17–20% of the total recording time**. The **majority of activity** is represented by **theta rhythm* (22–38%)** and **delta rhythm (45–61%)**, over which alpha and theta oscillations may be superimposed.

The **amplitudes of the main rhythms in children up to 7 years old** vary within the following ranges: **Alpha activity**: 50–125 µV, **Theta rhythm**: 50–110 µV, **Delta rhythm**: 60–100 µV *Korolyova N.V., Kolesnikov S.I., 2005* (Figure 48)*

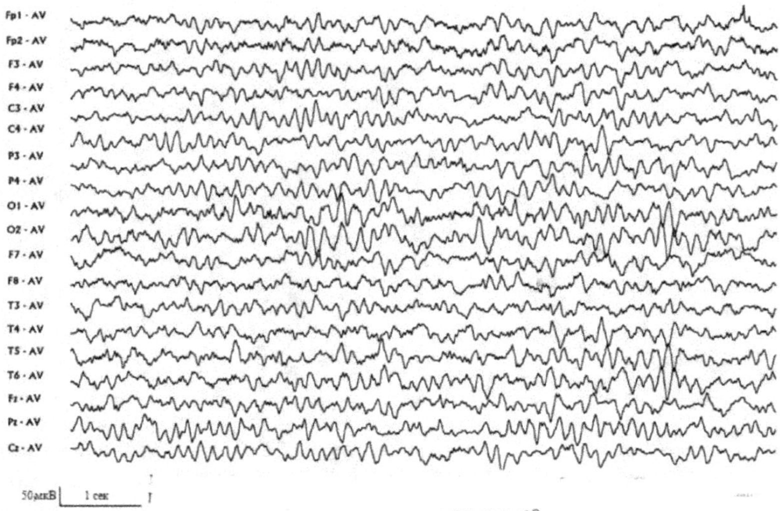

Figure 48. *Girl, 1 year old. Normal variant. In the* ***EEG during quiet wakefulness****, all leads show* ***unstable sinusoidal alpha activity*** *without clear regional predominance, with an* ***index of 18%, frequency 5.5–7.5 cycles/sec****, and* ***amplitude up to 70 μV****, alternating with* ***diffuse theta and delta waves*** *with amplitudes up to* ***80 μV****, and* ***beta oscillations*** *with amplitudes up to* ***15 μV****.*

Korolyova N.V., Kolesnikov S.I., Vorobyov S.V., 2011

By the age of **2 years, alpha activity** is also present in all regions, although its exp*ression **decreases toward the frontal areas** of the cerebral cortex. Alpha oscillations have a **frequency of 6–8 cycles/sec** and alternate with **groups of high-amplitude waves** at **2.5–4 cycles/sec. Beta waves** with frequencies of **18–25 cycles/sec** may also be present in all recorded regions (Farber D.A., Alferova V.V., 1972; Blagosklonova N.K., Novikova L.A., 1994; Korolyova N.V., Kolesnikov S.I., 2005).

The **indices of the main rhythms at this age** are **similar to those of 1-year-old children** (Figure 49).

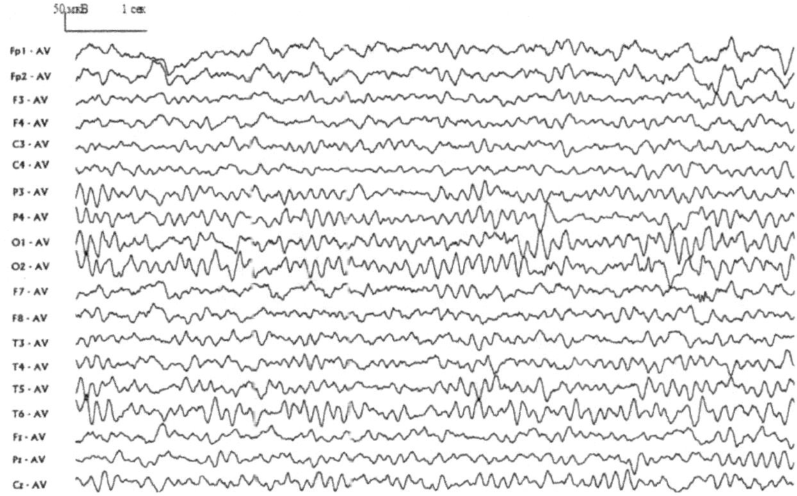

Figure 49. *Boy, 2 years old. Normal variant. In the* ***EEG during quiet wakefulness, unstable alpha activity*** *is recorded with an* ***index up to 20%, frequency 6–8 cycles/sec****, predominating in the* ***parieto-occipital regions****. Alpha activity coexists with* ***theta and delta oscillations****, which have the highest amplitudes in the* ***parieto-occipital and posterior-temporal regions****, and* ***diffuse beta activity*** *in groups of waves with a* ***frequency of 18–25 cycles/sec*** *and* ***amplitude up to 10 μV****.*
Korolyova N.V., Kolesnikov S.I, Vorobyov S.V., 2011

Starting at **2 years of age**, in the EEG, **polyphasic potentials** may be observed within the alpha activity, more often in the **parieto-occipital region**. These represent a combination of an alpha wave with a preceding or following slow wave. Polyphasic potentials can be **bilaterally synchronous, slightly asymmetric**, or **predominant alternately in one hemisphere** (Blagosklonova N.K., Novikova L.A., 1994).

In **3–4-year-old children, theta-range oscillations dominate**. At the same time, alpha activity, predominating in the **occipital leads**, continues to coexist with a significant number of **high-amplitude slow waves** with frequencies of **2–3 cycles/sec and 4–6 cycles/sec** (Zislina N.N., Tyukov V.L., 1968). The **alpha activity index** at this age ranges from **22–33%**, the **theta rhythm index** is **23–34%**, and the **representation of delta rhythm** decreases to **30–45%**. The **frequency of alpha activity** averages **7.5–8.4 cycles/sec**, ranging from **7 to 9 cycles/sec**, indicating the emergence of an **alpha focus at 8 cycles/sec**. Simultaneously, the **frequency of theta oscillations increases** (Farber D.A., Alferova V.V., 1972; Korolyova N.V., Kolesnikov S.I., 2005, Normal..., 2006).

Alpha activity has its **highest amplitudes in the parieto-occipital regions** and may acquire a **sharpened form** (Figure 50).

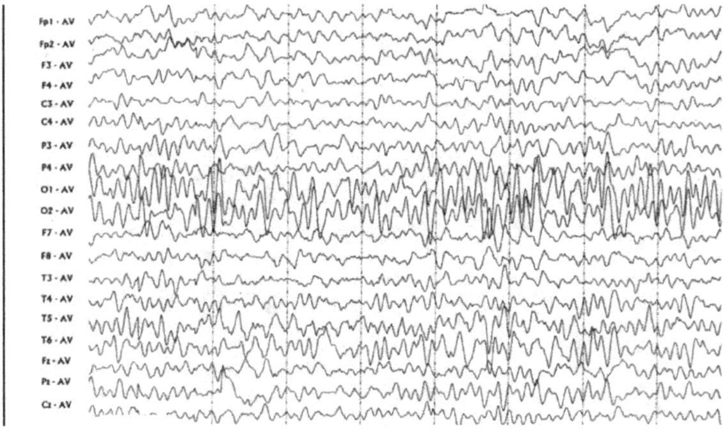

Figure 50. *Boy, 3.5 years old. Normal variant. In the* ***EEG during quiet wakefulness****, the majority of the recording time belongs to* ***theta-range activity****.* ***Alpha activity*** *predominates in the* ***occipital regions****, showing a* ***sharp amplitude gradient****. The* ***alpha activity index*** *is 2%, with a* ***frequency of 7–9 cycles/sec*** *and an* ***amplitude up to 120 µV****.* ***Theta*** *and* ***delta oscillations*** *are diffusely distributed, but have their* ***highest amplitude in the posterior-temporal regions****. Korolyova N.V., Kolesnikov S.I., Vorobyov S.V., 2011*

In **children up to 10–12 years old**, the **EEG** typically shows **high-amplitude bilateral synchronous bursts** of oscillations with frequencies **2–3 cycles/sec** and **4–7 cycles/sec** superimposed on the main activity. These bursts are predominantly expressed in the **frontal-central**, **central-temporal**, or **parieto-occipital regions** of the cortex (Blume W.T., 1982; Blagosklonova N.K., Novikova L.A., 1994) or may have a **generalized character** without a pronounced focus. In practice, these **paroxysms** are considered signs of **hyperactivity in the brainstem structures**. These paroxysms are most commonly observed during **hyperventilation**.

At the age of **5–6 years**, there is a noticeable improvement in the **organization of the primary rhythm**, and **alpha rhythm** typical for adults becomes established. The **alpha activity index** is **greater than 27%**, the **theta index** is **20–35%**, and the **delta index** is **24–37%. Slow rhythms** have a **diffuse distribution** and do not exceed the amplitude of **alpha activity**, which predominates in the **parieto-occipital regions** both in terms of amplitude and index. The **alpha frequency** within a single recording may range from **7.5 to 10.2 cycles/sec**, with an average frequency of **8 cycles/sec or more** (Bernhard C.G., Skoglund C.R., 1939; Henry

C.E., 1944; Gorbacheva T.G., 1969; Korolyova N.V., Kolesnikov S.I., 2005) (Figure 51).

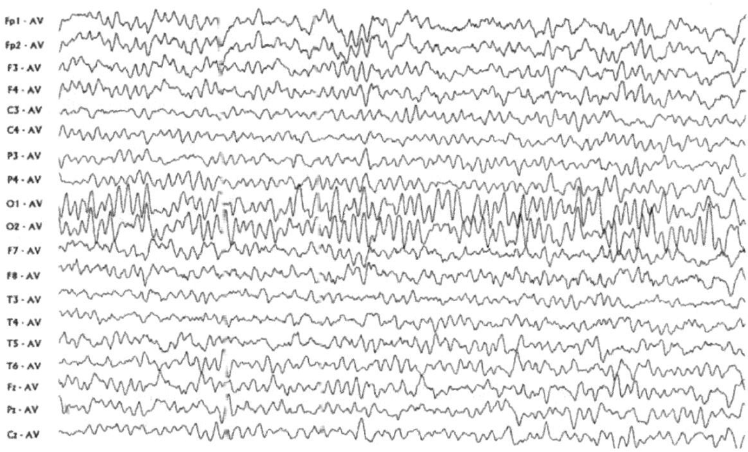

Figure 51. *Boy, 5.5 years old. Normal variant. The* ***EEG during quiet wakefulness*** *shows an* ***organized pattern****. In all leads, a* ***well-defined sinusoidal alpha activity*** *is present, with an* ***index of 41%, frequency 7.5–9 cycles/sec****, and* ***amplitude up to 90 μV****, predominating in the* ***occipital regions****.* ***Theta*** *and* ***delta oscillations*** *are represented diffusely and have* ***lower amplitudes than alpha activity*** *(up to 60 μV).* ***Beta rhythm*** *is also diffusely distributed, with emphasis in the* ***frontal and temporal regions****. Korolyova N.V., Kolesnikov S.I., Vorobyov S.V., 2011*

In the **EEGs of children aged 7–9 years**, **alpha rhythm** is present in all regions, with the **highest prominence in the parieto-occipital areas**. The recordings are dominated by **alpha and theta rhythms**, while the index of slower activity does not exceed **35%**. **Alpha index values** range from **35–55%**, and **theta index values** range from **15–45%**. **Beta rhythm** appears in the form of **wave groups**, recorded either diffusely or with emphasis in the **fronto-temporal regions**, at a **frequency of 15–35 cycles/sec** and **amplitude up to 15–20 μV**.

Among **slow rhythms**, oscillations with frequencies **2–3 cycles/sec** and **5–7 cycles/sec** predominate. The **dominant alpha rhythm frequency** at this age is **9–10 cycles/sec**, with its **highest amplitudes in the occipital regions**. **Alpha amplitude** varies between **70–110 μV** among individuals. **Slow waves** may reach their highest amplitude in the **parieto-posterior-temporal-occipital regions**, but always remain **lower than alpha amplitudes**. By around **9 years of age**, **modulations of alpha rhythm** may begin to appear in the occipital regions, although not clearly expressed (Figure 52).

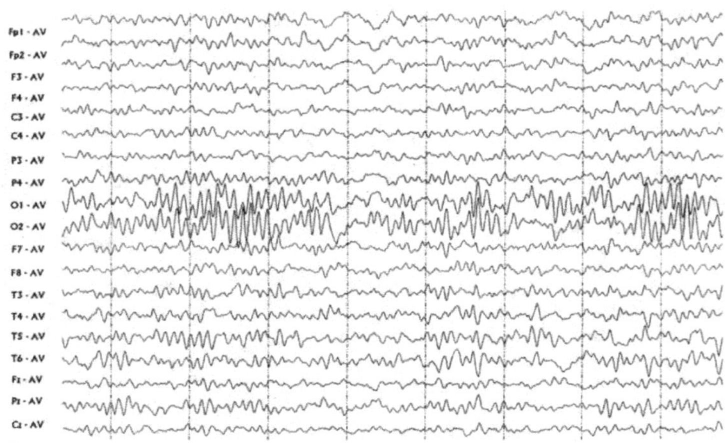

Figure 52. *Boy, 7 years old. Normal variant. In the EEG during quiet wakefulness, alpha rhythm predominates, in combination with theta rhythm. The alpha rhythm has an index of 47%, frequency 8.5–10 cycles/sec, and amplitude up to 100 μV. It is well-defined, rhythmic, and shows a tendency to form modulations in the occipital regions. Korolyova N.V., Kolesnikov S.I., Vorobyov S.V., 2011*

In the EEGs of children aged 10–12 years, alpha rhythm maturation is largely complete. The recordings show a well-organized, clearly expressed alpha rhythm, which dominates over other main rhythms both in recording time and index, ranging from 45–60%. In terms of amplitude, alpha rhythm predominates in the parieto-occipital or posterior-temporo-parieto-occipital regions, where alpha oscillations may cluster into still not clearly expressed modulations.

Alpha rhythm frequency varies from 9–11 cycles/sec, most commonly around 10 cycles/sec. In the frontal regions, alpha rhythm is less organized, more uniform, and noticeably lower in amplitude. Against the background of dominant alpha rhythm, isolated theta waves are observed with frequencies of 5–7 cycles/sec, and their amplitude does not exceed other EEG components.

From around 10 years of age, beta activity increases in the frontal leads. Bilateral generalized paroxysmal bursts, which may occur in earlier developmental stages, are no longer normally recorded in adolescents (*Blagosklonova N.K., Novikova L.A., 1994; Sokolovskaya I.E., 200)* (Figure 53)

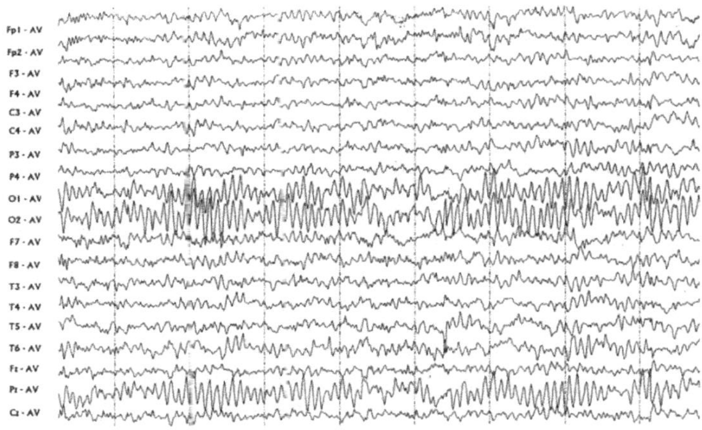

Figure 53. *Boy, 10 years old. Healthy. In the* ***EEG during quiet wakefulness****, a* ***well-expressed, slightly sharpened alpha rhythm*** *dominates, with an* ***index of 52%, frequency 9-10.5 cycles/sec****, and* ***amplitude up to 115 µV****. The* ***alpha rhythm is modulated*** *and predominates in the* ***occipital regions****. In the* ***frontal and temporal regions, beta rhythm*** *is recorded with an* ***index of up to 12%, frequency 18-25 cycles/sec****, and* ***amplitude up to 20 µV. Theta and isolated delta oscillations****, closer to the anterior regions, are associated with a* ***less organized alpha rhythm****. Korolyova N.V., Kolesnikov S.I., Vorobyov S.V., 2011*

EEG of adolescents aged 13-16 years continues to show the processes of **bioelectric activity formation** in the brain. **Alpha rhythm becomes the dominant form of activity** and predominates in all regions of the cortex. The **average frequency of the alpha rhythm** is **10-10.5 cycles/sec** (*Sokolovskaya I.E., 2001*).

In some cases, along with the **pronounced alpha rhythm in the occipital regions, less stability** of the rhythm is observed in the **parietal, central, and frontal areas**, often **combined with low-amplitude slow waves**. During this age period, the **degree of similarity between the alpha rhythm** in the **occipital-temporal and central-frontal regions** of the cortex increases, reflecting an **increase in the coordination of different cortical regions** during ontogenesis. The **amplitudes of the main rhythms decrease**, approaching those of adults, and there is a **reduction in the sharpness of regional differences** in the primary rhythm when compared to younger children (Figure 54).

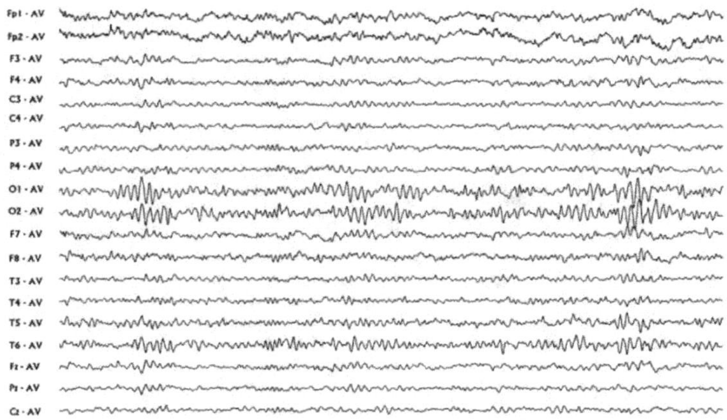

Figure 54. *Girl, 15 years old. In the* ***EEG during quiet wakefulness****, the* ***alpha rhythm dominates****, with an* ***index of 55%, frequency 10–12 cycles/sec****, and* ***amplitude up to 55 µV****. The* ***alpha rhythm is combined with beta rhythm****, with an* ***index up to 20%, frequency 14–25 cycles/sec****, and* ***amplitude up to 20 µV****, and is interspersed with* ***polymorphic theta and delta oscillations****, represented as* ***single waves or groups of medium-amplitude waves*** *(up to 30 µV). Korolyova N.V., Kolesnikov S.I., Vorobyov S.V., 2011*

After age 15, in adolescents:

Polyphasic potentials gradually disappear from the EEG, appearing only as occasional single oscillations.

Sinusoidal rhythmic slow waves with frequencies of **2.5–4.5 cycles/sec** cease to be recorded.

The **degree of expression of low-amplitude slow oscillations** in the **central cortical regions decreases**.

By **18–22 years**, the EEG reaches **full maturity**, characteristic of adults (*Blagosklonova N.K., Novikova L.A., 1994*).

5.2. Adult EEG

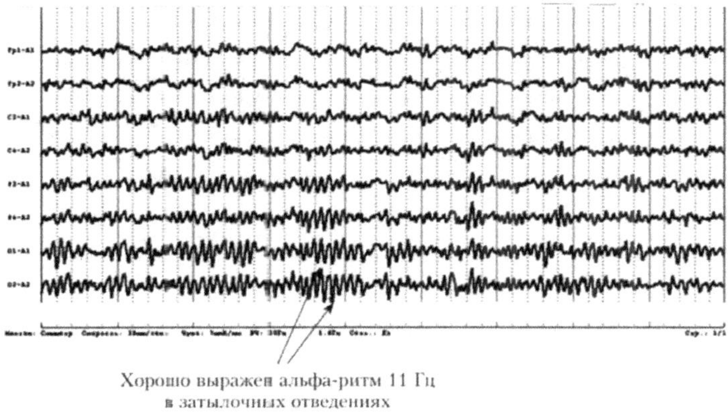

Figure 55. Normal EEG of a healthy adult at rest with eyes closed. *Alpha rhythm, modulated in amplitude, predominates in the parieto-occipital leads.*

High-frequency beta-band activity predominates in the frontal regions.

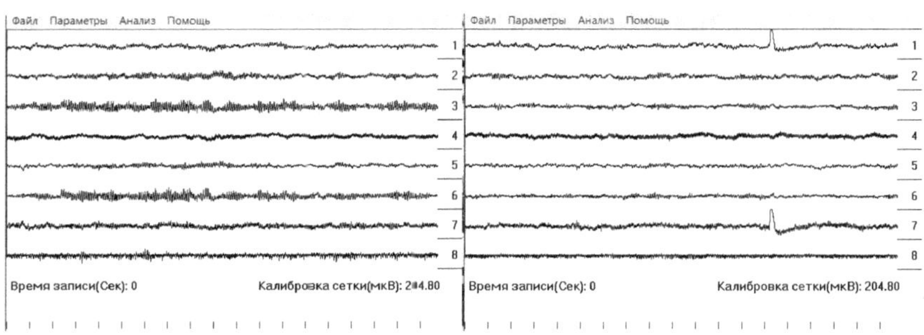

A **B**

Figure 56. Activation response on EEG. Age 19.
A – psychosensory rest, eyes closed; B – alert wakefulness, eyes open.
Legend:
1 – frontal–temporal; 2 – temporal–parietal; 3 – right parietal–occipital;
4, 5, 6 – corresponding regions on the left.

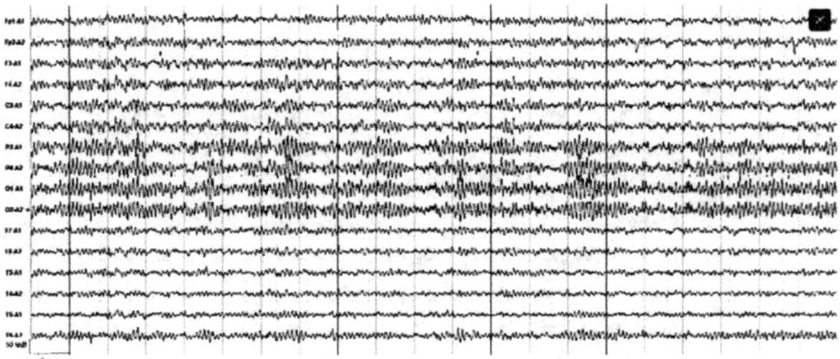

Figure 57. Normal electroencephalogram during passive wakefulness.

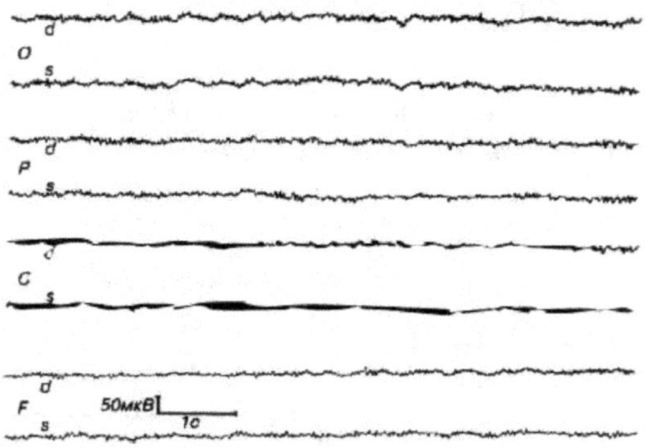

Figure 58. *Variant of the EEG of an awake adult.*

Beta (β) activity is recorded in all leads, with some predominance in the parietal (P) and central (C) regions.

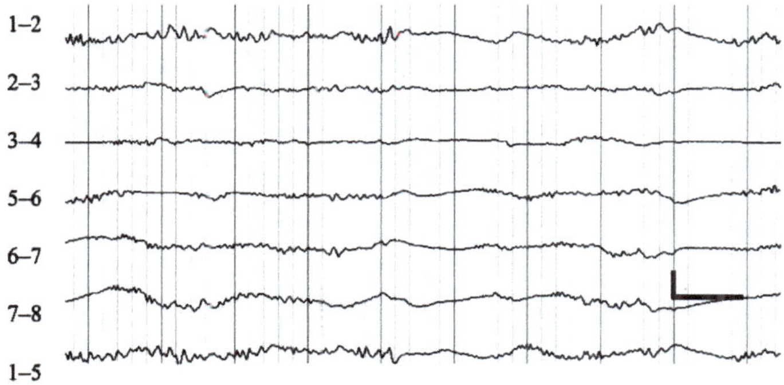

Figure 59. *Variant of a normal electrocorticogram recorded over the frontal cortex. Calibration signal: amplitude 500 μV, duration 1 s.*

5.3. Quantitative Analysis (qEEG) Under Normal Conditions

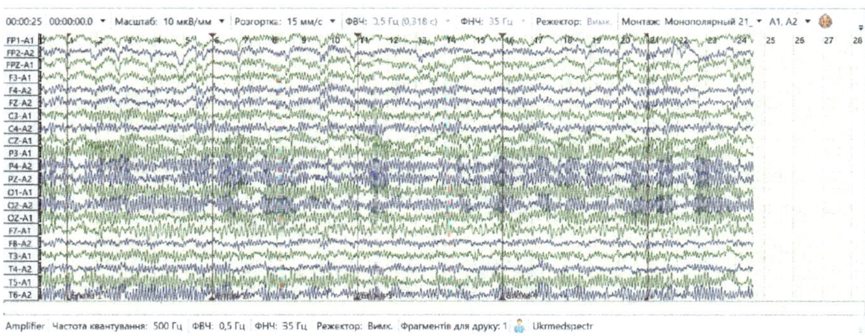

Figure 60. *Normal EEG of a healthy adult at rest with eyes closed. The alpha rhythm, modulated in amplitude, predominates.*

Table 5. *Periodometric Analysis (Entire Recording)*
Rhythm Index (%)

Lead	Delta Rhythm	Theta Rhythm	Alpha Rhythm	Beta LF Rhythm	Beta HF Rhythm	Total Rhythm Band (%)	Alpha/Theta	Theta/Beta	Mu Rhythm	Theta + Alpha
FP1–A1	0	4.7	42.2	14.8	8.5	100	8.98	0.20	31.4	54.4
FP2–A2	0	3.5	41.3	15.9	15.6	100	11.8	0.11	29.8	51.8
FPZ–A1	0.2	8.1	45.4	17.8	9.7	100	5.6	0.29	31.6	59.7
F3–A1	0	5.8	47.0	18.3	8.8	100	8.1	0.21	33.4	58.6
F4–A2	0	5.5	45.7	15.7	15.9	100	8.31	0.17	31.6	56.7
FZ–A2	0	5.9	47.5	16.6	13.3	100	8.05	0.20	34.0	57.1
C3–A1	0	6.6	54.4	18.8	10.0	100	8.24	0.23	39.0	64.2
C4–A2	0	5.0	48.9	19.7	15.6	100	9.78	0.14	31.8	56.0
CZ–A1	0	7.6	56.9	15.2	9.7	100	7.49	0.31	37.2	67.7
P3–A1	0	7.9	70.4	13.5	5.6	100	8.91	0.41	48.7	79.2
P4–A2	0	6.6	65.8	15.1	8.9	100	9.97	0.27	42.5	73.5
PZ–A2	0	5.1	68.7	14.1	8.6	100	13.47	0.22	46.5	75.6

Lead	Delta Rhythm	Theta Rhythm	Alpha Rhythm	Beta LF Rhythm	Beta HF Rhythm	Total Rhythm Band (%)	Alpha/Theta	Theta/Beta	Mu Rhythm	Theta + Alpha
O1–A1	0	8.0	77.1	7.3	3.4	100	9.64	0.75	51.2	86.8
O2–A2	0	8.3	69.7	12.6	6.6	100	8.40	0.43	47.7	78.2
OZ–A1	0	7.4	68.8	12.3	5.7	100	9.30	0.41	45.3	77.1
F7–A1	0.3	25.4	38.1	10.5	11.7	100	1.50	1.14	25.6	68.9
F8–A2	0	2.0	36.1	19.2	18.8	100	18.05	0.05	26.0	44.6
T3–A1	0	4.3	45.8	22.8	12.7	100	10.65	0.12	35.3	54.6
T4–A2	0	3.1	38.1	19.1	19.7	100	12.29	0.08	31.2	44.8
T5–A1	0	10.2	67.4	11.5	5.9	100	6.61	0.59	44.1	78.7
T6–A2	0	8.0	58.2	14.5	12.1	100	7.28	0.30	37.3	68.4

Periodometric Analysis

Periodometric analysis aims to investigate the distribution of amplitudes and frequencies of a given rhythm. A rhythm is understood as harmonic oscillations within any specified frequency range, particularly within the standard frequency bands.

The analysis itself is preceded by filtering, which isolates the harmonic components of the signal within the selected frequency range.

The EEG signal is the electrical activity of the brain recorded from the scalp surface. It consists of a combination of oscillations of different frequencies and amplitudes.

The purpose of periodometric analysis is to determine the amplitude of oscillations and the frequency characteristics of each EEG rhythm.

Procedure

The EEG signal is divided into short segments.

The frequency spectrum is calculated for each segment.

The results are displayed graphically as amplitudes and frequencies — this representation is called a periodogram.

Clinical Significance

Periodometric analysis allows the physician to:

Identify dominant brain rhythms (for example, alpha rhythm during relaxed wakefulness with eyes closed).

Detect pathological oscillations, such as epileptic spikes or changes associated with encephalopathies.

Perform quantitative assessment of brain dynamics during treatment or patient monitoring.

Applications

Diagnosis of epilepsy and seizure disorders

Assessment of brain function in trauma, stroke, and disorders of consciousness

Sleep studies

Research in cognitive activity and neurobiology

Example of Interpretation

If alpha rhythm (8–13 Hz) predominates in an adult at rest with eyes closed, this is considered normal.

An increase in delta rhythm (0.5–4 Hz) during wakefulness may indicate pathology.

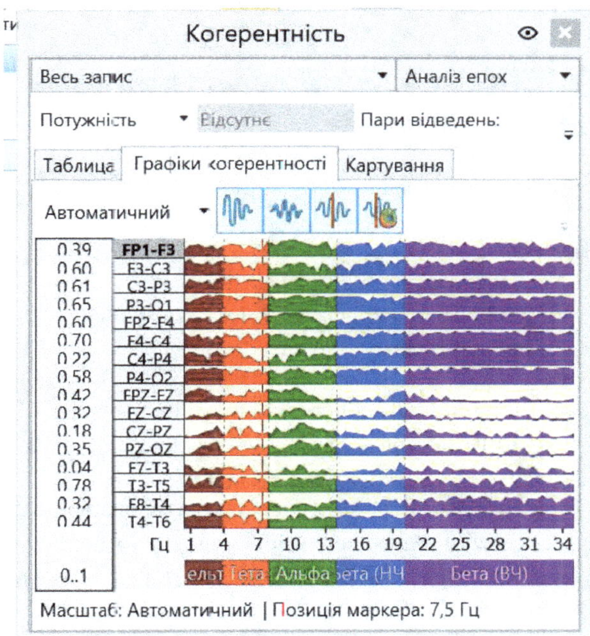

__Figure 51.__ Coherence, longitudinal montage 21.

EEG Coherence

EEG coherence is a measure of functional connectivity between different brain regions, that is, how consistently (in terms of phase and frequency synchronization) neuronal ensembles recorded by different electrodes operate together.

Simply put, coherence shows how well different brain regions "communicate" with each other.

Longitudinal Coherence Montage

The longitudinal montage in EEG refers to the analysis of coherence between electrodes positioned along the anterior–posterior axis of the brain: frontal – central – parietal – occipital regions (for example: Fp–F, F–C, C–P, P–O).

Interpretation

Longitudinal coherence reflects the integration of cortical activity along the "frontal–occipital" axis. It is associated with:

regulation of attention

cognitive control

sensory information processing

executive functions

High longitudinal coherence indicates coordinated functioning of cortical regions and functional integrity.

Reduced longitudinal coherence may indicate impaired interregional interaction (e.g., asthenic states, organic lesions, functional disorders, etc.).

Thus, the longitudinal EEG coherence montage characterizes the degree of functional connectivity between cortical regions located along the anterior–posterior axis of the brain and reflects the integration of cognitive and sensory processes.

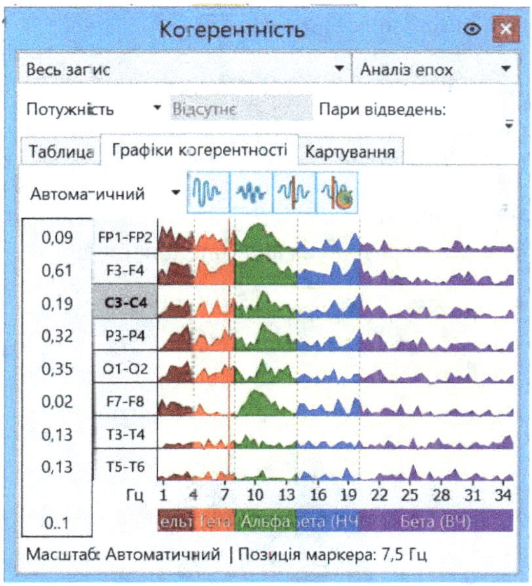

Figure 62. *Transverse Montage 16*

"Coherence, Transverse Montage" in EEG refers to the analysis of functional connectivity between symmetrically or laterally positioned brain regions, primarily between the left and right hemispheres.

Transverse Coherence Montage

The transverse (or lateral) montage evaluates coherence along the left–right axis of the brain:

Frontal: left–right (F3–F4)

Central: (C3–C4)

Parietal: (P3–P4)

Temporal: (T3–T4)

Occipital: (O1–O2)

What Transverse Coherence Reflects

Interhemispheric interaction

Degree of symmetry in functional activity

Role of the corpus callosum in information transfer

Functional lateralization (speech, attention, emotions)

Interpretation Normal or increased transverse coherence indicates good synchronization between hemispheres and functional integrity.

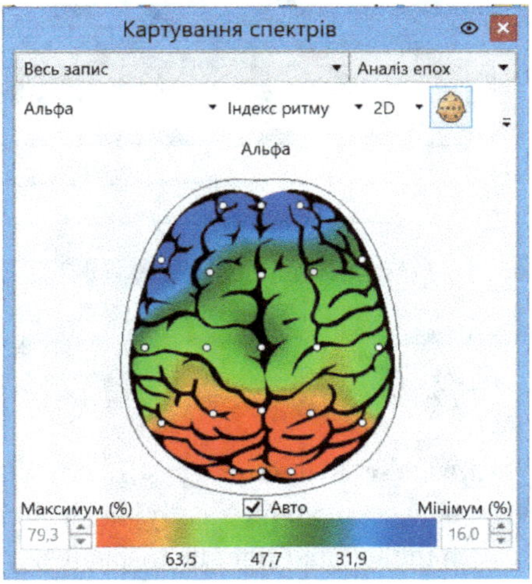

Figure 63. *Frequency Analysis, Spectral Mapping, Alpha Rhythm*

Reduced or asymmetric coherence may indicate possible local disturbances, focal changes, consequences of traumatic brain injury, epileptiform activity, or functional asymmetry.

Thus, the transverse EEG coherence montage reflects the degree of functional connectivity between symmetrical regions of the left and right hemispheres and characterizes interhemispheric interaction.

Frequency Analysis and Spectral Mapping in EEG

Frequency analysis and spectral mapping provide information about the brain's functional state, showing the distribution and strength of rhythms across different cortical areas.

EEG frequency analysis shows:

Dominant rhythms (delta, theta, alpha, beta, gamma)

Their power (amplitude)

Frequency shifts (slowing or acceleration of activity)

Ratios between rhythms

Spectral Mapping (Topographic Mapping)

Displays the spatial distribution of EEG frequency components across the scalp

Allows identification of:

Alpha rhythm localization (usually occipital)

Foci of pathological slow activity

Interhemispheric asymmetries

Areas of functional tension or depletion

Clinical Significance

Frequency analysis and spectral mapping indicate:

Level of cortical activation

Maturity and integrity of cortical rhythms

Presence of diffuse or focal changes

Functional disturbances (asthenia, neuroinfections, TBI)

Possible epileptiform predisposition (indirectly)

In summary, EEG frequency analysis and spectral mapping reflect the distribution and amplitude of major brain rhythms and provide insight into cortical functional state as well as local or diffuse abnormalities.

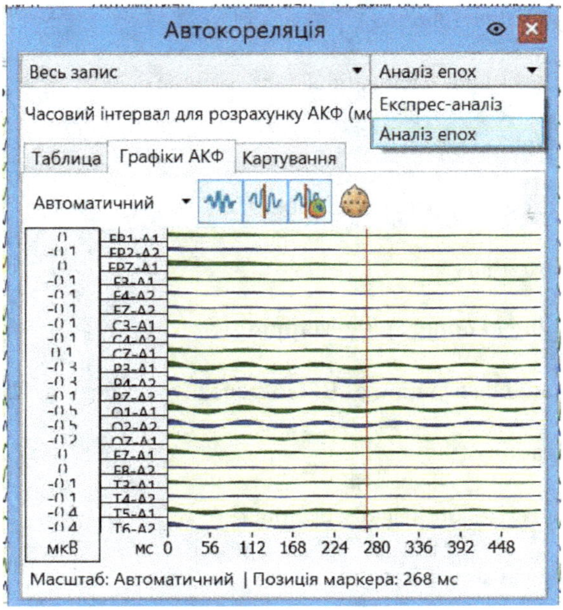

Figure 64. *Autocorrelation*

Autocorrelation in EEG reflects the degree of regularity, periodicity, and stability of the brain's electrical activity over time.

What EEG Autocorrelation Shows:

Rhythm and stability of waves

Presence of periodic oscillations

Degree of orderliness or, conversely, chaotic activity

Preservation of the dominant rhythm (most often alpha rhythm)

Stability of rhythmic activity generators

Interpretation:

Strong autocorrelation indicates regular, well-organized rhythmic activity, functional maturity, and cortical integrity.

Reduced autocorrelation suggests rhythm disorganization, functional instability, asthenia, or diffuse changes.

Short-period peaks may indicate possible paroxysmal or epileptiform predisposition (indirect sign).

Clinical Significance:

Autocorrelation helps assess:

The functional state of the central nervous system

Balance between excitatory and inhibitory processes

Presence of pathological rhythm generators

Dynamics of changes during treatment or stress testing

In summary, EEG autocorrelation reflects the temporal orderliness and rhythmicity of brain bioelectrical activity and allows evaluation of the stability of dominant rhythms and cortical functional state.

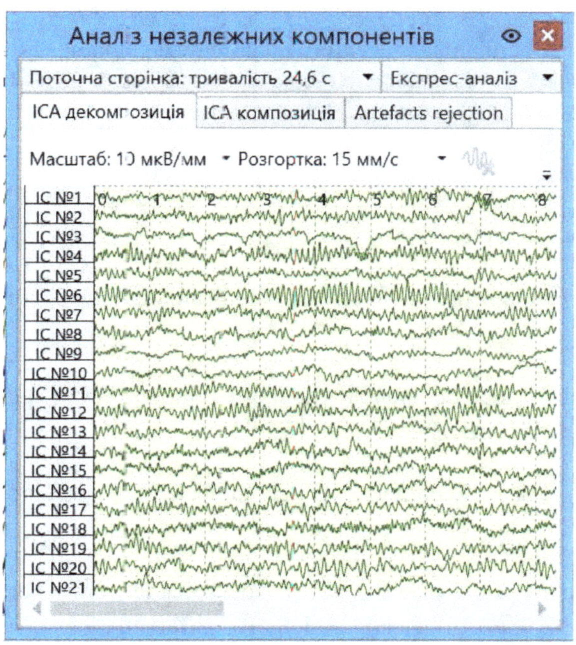

Figure 65. *Independent Component Analysis (ICA)*

Independent Component Analysis (ICA) in EEG provides information about the structure of the brain's bioelectrical activity sources and their independent contributions to the recorded signal.

What ICA Shows in EEG:

Separation of the mixed EEG signal into independent sources

Identification of neuronal components versus non-cerebral artifacts

Localization of functional activity generators

Contribution of individual components to the overall EEG pattern

Practical Significance:

ICA allows:

Detection and removal of artifacts (blinking, eye movements, EMG, ECG)

Separation of background activity from pathological components

Clarification of the origin of paroxysmal or epileptiform activity

Assessment of the functional organization of brain networks

Clinical Interpretation:

Well-defined, stable neuronal components indicate organized, preserved cortical activity

Dominance of artifact components suggests low recording quality or strong muscular/vegetative influences

Pathological independent components may indicate local generators of abnormal activity

In summary, ICA of EEG allows identification and characterization of independent sources of bioelectrical activity, differentiation of neuronal versus artifact components, and clarification of functional brain organization.

5.4. Interhemispheric EEG Asymmetry

Since the 1950s, evidence has accumulated demonstrating functional asymmetry or specialization of the cerebral hemispheres (Baben'kova, 1970; Mosidze, 1973, 1983, 1990; Simmernitskaya, 1978; Balonov, 1979; Bragina & Dobrokhotova, 1981).

It is assumed that the phenomenon of human functional asymmetry cannot be understood outside the general laws of evolution of inanimate and living nature (Y.A. Urmantsev, 1978) and has become an interdisciplinary problem (Bragina & Dobrokhotova, 1981).

In the preface to the recently published book *Functional Interhemispheric Asymmetry: Reader* (2004, ed. Bogolepov N.N., Fokin V.F.), functional interhemispheric asymmetry is described as one of the most enigmatic phenomena of the brain.

The control of dynamic properties of interhemispheric asymmetry remains insufficiently studied, despite its relevance.

Population Statistics:

The proportion of right-handed individuals is estimated at 80–95%, with the remainder being left-handed or ambidextrous.

Over the past 50 years, the proportion of left-handers in Europe has increased 3–4 times, attributed to reduced forced retraining and adaptation of tools and equipment.

Left-handedness has become a focus of research in neurophysiology, psychology, and sociology.

Practical implications include child development, education, and career choice. Left-handers often show artistic, musical, and cognitive abilities, sometimes excelling in mathematics, architecture, and other sciences.

Functional Interhemispheric Asymmetry (FIA):

FIA is now considered a fundamental principle of human and animal brain function.

Calculation of Interhemispheric Asymmetry Coefficients (FIA):

Uas=(L−R)/(L+R)×100U_

Where:

L – value for the left hemisphere

R – value for the right hemisphere

Positive values indicate left-hemisphere predominance

Negative values indicate right-hemisphere predominance

Error Estimation of FIA Coefficients:

$mUas=Uas\times((mL/ML)^2+(mR/MR)^2)^{1/2}$

Where:

mUasm – error of the asymmetry coefficient

Uas – interhemispheric asymmetry coefficient

mL– error of the left hemisphere measurement

MR – right hemisphere value

Interpretation:

Depends on frequency band, particularly important for alpha rhythm.

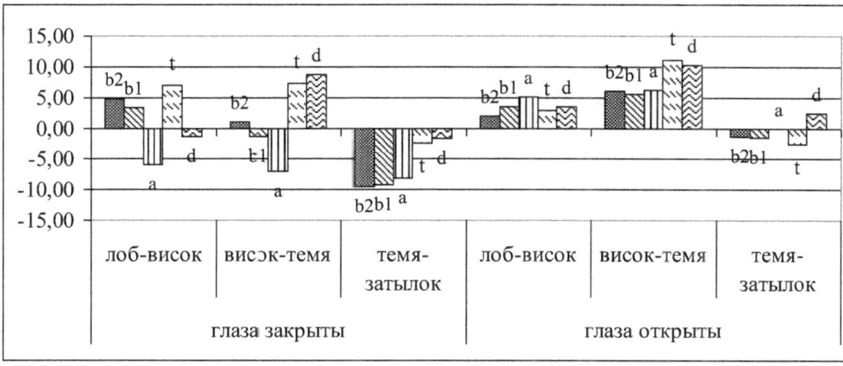

Figure 66. *Functional Interhemispheric Asymmetry in Operative and Psychosensory Rest in Right-Handed Individuals*

Legend: b2 *– FIA of beta-2 rhythm amplitude,* ***b1*** *– FIA of beta-1 rhythm amplitude,* ***t*** *– FIA of theta rhythm amplitude,* ***d*** *– FIA of delta rhythm amplitude*

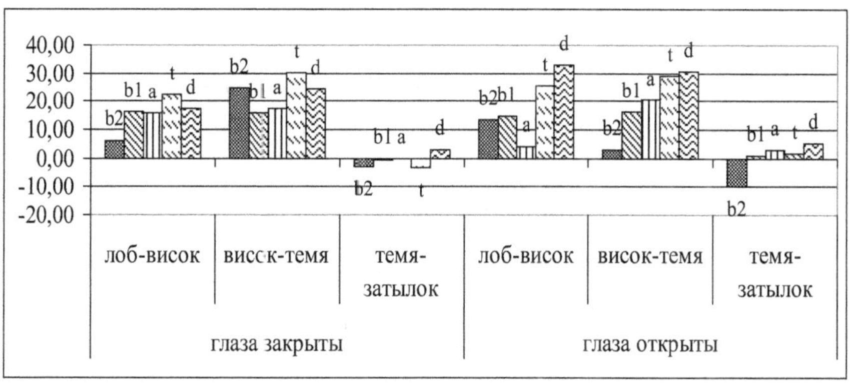

Figure 67. *Functional Interhemispheric Asymmetry in Operative and Psychosensory Rest in Left-Handed Individuals.*

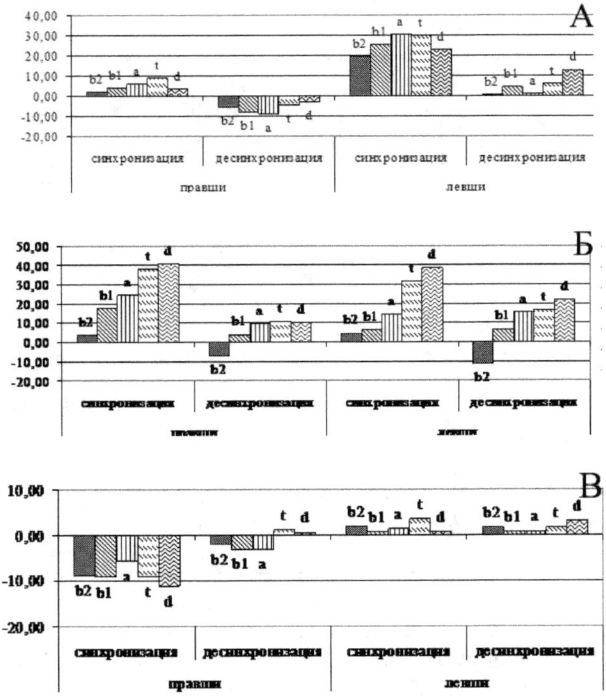

Figure 68. *Functional Interhemispheric Asymmetry of EEG Amplitudes in Right-Handed and Left-Handed Individuals during Synchronization and Desynchronization Fragments*

***Legend: b2** – Beta-2 rhythm amplitude, **b1** – Beta-1 rhythm amplitude, **a** – Alpha rhythm amplitude, **t** – Theta rhythm amplitude, **d** – Delta rhythm amplitude, **A** – Frontal–temporal derivation, **B** – Temporal–parietal derivation, мC – Parietal–occipital derivation*

Summary of Findings:

Studies indicate that left-handers, compared to right-handers, show enhanced synchronization processes, manifested by increased EEG rhythm amplitudes both without segmentation and in desynchronization segments.

During synchronization segments, left-hemisphere amplitudes are larger in left-handers, while in the right hemisphere, increased synchronization is observed in the temporal–parietal derivation.

Under conditions of enhanced synchronization, left-handers show positive functional interhemispheric asymmetry (FIA) values in both synchronization and desynchronization fragments.

Interhemispheric EEG Asymmetry: Overview

Definition:

Interhemispheric EEG asymmetry reflects differences in electrical activity between the left and right hemispheres, as recorded by EEG. It is a key concept in neurophysiology and cognitive neuroscience.

What Is Compared:

Homologous electrode pairs: F3–F4 (frontal), C3–C4 (central), P3–P4 (parietal), O1–O2 (occipital)

Parameters: amplitude, spectral power, frequency

Asymmetry index often uses logarithmic ratios of power

Frequency Bands and Asymmetry:

Alpha (8–13 Hz): Most studied in asymmetry research

Frontal alpha asymmetry lower alpha power corresponds to higher cortical activation

Interpretation examples:

Greater left frontal activation → positive affect, approach motivation

Greater right frontal activation → anxiety, avoidance

Note: probabilistic correlations, not direct diagnoses

Beta (13–30 Hz): Linked to cognitive load and attention

Asymmetry may reflect task-solving strategies or lateralization of motor control

Theta and Delta: No strong asymmetry expected in awake adults; asymmetry may indicate local functional impairment (trauma, stroke, tumors)

Physiological vs. Pathological Asymmetry:

Physiological:

Related to handedness, language lateralization, task, or state

Can change over time and conditions

Pathological:

Suspected if persistent, pronounced (>30–40% difference), or accompanied by slowed rhythms

Seen in focal brain lesions, epilepsy, or post-traumatic conditions

Limitations and Common Errors:

Misinterpreting alpha as "activity" rather than inhibition

Ignoring artifacts (EMG, EOG)

Drawing conclusions without considering state (eyes open/closed)

Extrapolating group-level correlations to individuals

Applications:

Cognitive neuroscience, affective research, neurofeedback

Clinical EEG as supplementary information

Interhemispheric Asymmetry and Consciousness

Key Points:

The brain is functionally asymmetric:

Left hemisphere: speech, logic, sequential information processing, abstract symbols

Right hemisphere: holistic perception, spatial imagery, emotions, intonation, intuitive understanding

Consciousness arises from integration of specialized but interconnected hemispheres

Corpus callosum, subcortical structures, and neuronal synchronization mediate this integration

Neuropsychological Evidence (Split-Brain Studies):

Each hemisphere can process information and exhibit awareness

Unified subjective "self" requires interhemispheric interaction

Left hemisphere often acts as an "interpreter" creating coherent narrative

Asymmetry and Levels of Consciousness:

Reflective consciousness (self-awareness, inner dialogue) → left hemisphere

Perceptual/body-centered consciousness → right hemisphere

Emotional consciousness → dependent on limbic asymmetry

Cognitive and Philosophical Implication:

Interhemispheric asymmetry does not divide consciousness but creates a multi-level structure of subjective experience

Ensures balance between analysis vs. holistic perception, symbols vs. emotions, control vs. spontaneity

Conscious unity arises from integration of asymmetric functions; disconnection leads to fragmented subjective experience

Handedness and Cortical Dominance Distribution:

Studies show lateralization patterns differ between right- and left-handers (Grüsser O.J., Selke T., Zinda B., 1995)

Left Hemisphere	Right Hemisphere
1. Spoken language	Metaphorical meaning of speech
2. Reading	Sense of humor
3. Writing	Emotional tone of speech
4. Verbal thinking	Intonation of spoken language (prosody)
5. Prose and poetry meter	Pitch relations, timbre, and harmony in music
6. Musical rhythm	Spatial concepts and representations, stereoscopic vision, spatial rotation
7. Color naming	Spatial coordinates, general spatial orientation
8. Color classification	Geometry, chess playing
9. Counting	Perception of "gestalts"
10. Right side of external space	Left and right sides of external space
11. Interpretation of facial expressions and gestures	Recognition of facial expressions and gestures, face recognition, emotional reactions

Numerous studies have now accumulated showing that, in every individual, regardless of the profile of asymmetry, one hemisphere of the brain differs from the other in a number of morphological, functional, and biochemical parameters, which are reflected in specific features of mental activity. A common characteristic for all Homo sapiens is that brain asymmetry progressively increases during childhood, supporting normal mental development, reaches its peak in adulthood when brain function is most efficient, and diminishes in old age as its productivity declines. It should be noted that, thanks to the rapid development of modern research methods—such as positron emission tomography—we now have a better understanding of the mechanisms underlying these complex processes.

Over the past decades, many findings have emerged regarding another aspect of brain asymmetry—neurochemical. In right-handed individuals, various biochemical substances, including neurotransmitters, are distributed asymmetrically between the right and left hemispheres. For example, dopamine—a neurotransmitter and neurohormone that is a biochemical precursor to norepinephrine and epinephrine—is found in greater concentrations in the basal ganglia (an anatomically distinct group of paired subcortical structures that facilitate cortex-initiated movements and inhibit unnecessary associated movements) of the left hemisphere compared to the right. The asymmetry of dopamine levels across different brain structures increases with maturation.

Analyses of cortical enzymatic activity in right-handers have shown higher acetylcholine (a neurotransmitter that, when released into the bloodstream, lowers blood pressure, slows heart rate, etc.) content in the left hemisphere, particularly in the precentral and frontal cortical areas, compared to the right. Conversely, neurochemical studies of serotonin metabolites (serotonin—a neurotransmitter involved in the transmission of nerve impulses across synapses; neurons using it participate in the regulation of many behaviors, sleep processes, and thermoregulation) revealed a predominance in the right hemisphere, especially in the mediofrontal regions

The substantive hypothesis regarding selective involvement of the right or left hemisphere in specific activities during activation of certain subcortical structures was first proposed globally by T.A. Dobrokhotova and N.N. Bragina (1981). The study of the role of individual regulatory cerebral structures in forming different functional states of the brain in humans and animals, both in health and pathology, remains a fundamental problem in neurophysiology (Boldyreva G.N., Sharova E.V., Dobronravova I.S., 2000).

For many years, the existence of functional interhemispheric asymmetry in animals was questioned because it was believed that such asymmetry is primarily a feature of hominid evolution, particularly humans, and arose from the development of socially oriented behavior (Adrianov O.S., 1979, 1983). Indeed, if functional interhemispheric asymmetry is calculated using the standard formula, it appears that asymmetry in rats is not apparent (Figure 69):

$$Uas=(L-R)/(L+R)\times 100U\_$$

where L is the measure for the left hemisphere and R is the measure for the right hemisphere. Positive values indicate left-hemisphere dominance, while negative values indicate right-hemisphere dominance.

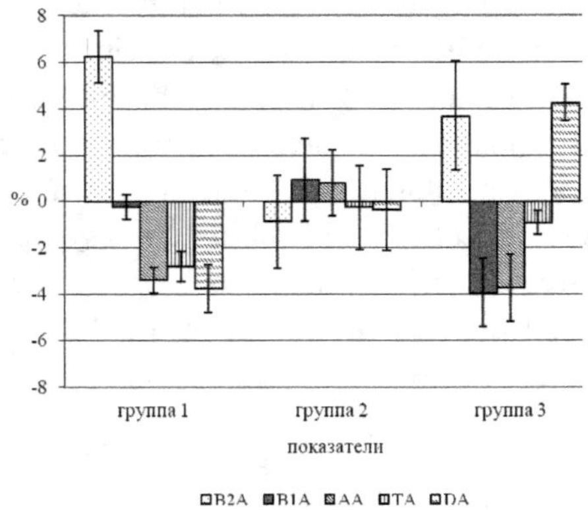

Figure 69. *Functional interhemispheric asymmetry in rats from three groups, determined using the classical formula.*

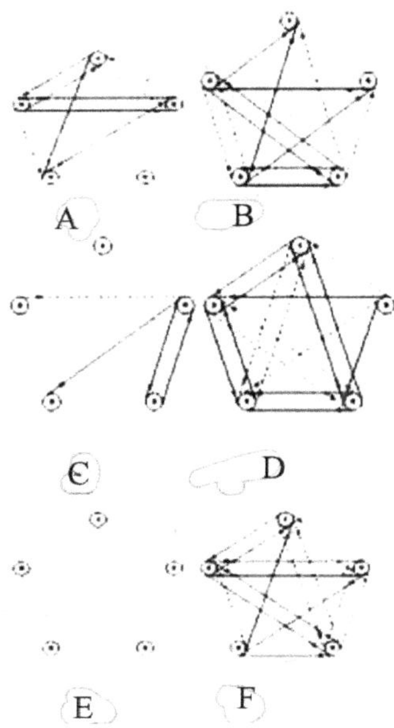

Figure 70. *Functional interhemispheric asymmetry in three groups of rats, determined using multiple regression analysis.*

EEG recordings were obtained in the classical fronto-occipital derivations on the left and right sides. Polycyclic multigraphs reflect mutually oriented influences between the amplitudes of ECoG rhythms.

Legend: *A and B – left and right hemispheres of rats in Group 1? C and D – left and right hemispheres of rats in Group 2? E and F – left and right hemispheres of rats in Group 3. Graph nodes: 1 – beta-2 rhythm, 2 – beta-1 rhythm, 3 – alpha rhythm, 4 – theta rhythm, 5 – delta rhythm/*

Solid lines indicate positive influences; dashed lines indicate negative influences

Using the developed EEG analysis method with multiple regression, it was found that the left hemispheres exhibit fewer regression connections between EEG rhythm amplitudes. This demonstrates the presence of interhemispheric asymmetry in rats. Many studies consider interhemispheric asymmetry as a marker of consciousness.

To investigate the role of the brainstem reticular formation in shaping interhemispheric asymmetry, experiments were conducted using an "isolated forebrain" preparation, in which the brainstem was transected, effectively disconnecting the influence of the reticular formation on the cortex.

Under these conditions, functional interhemispheric asymmetry showed significantly higher positive values than in the intact brain, indicating that the amplitude of biopotentials in the left hemisphere increased substantially. This suggests an enhancement of inhibitory processes in the left hemisphere, surpassing those in the right hemisphere, and demonstrates that the brainstem reticular formation exerts an activating influence on the left hemisphere.

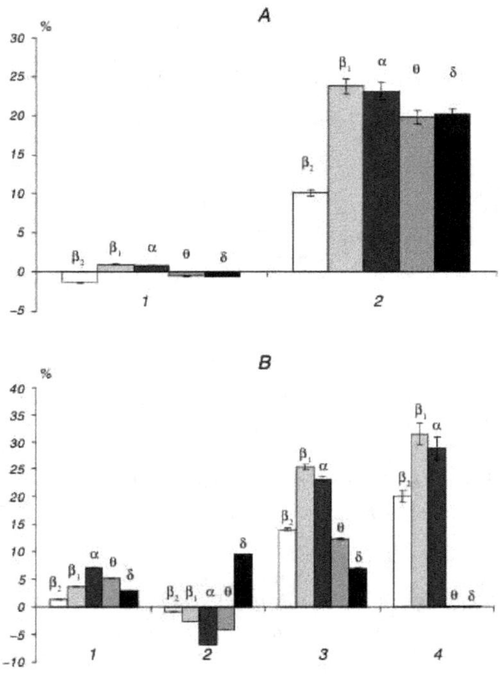

Figure 71. *Diagrams of functional interhemispheric asymmetry coefficients for the amplitudes of beta-2, beta-1, alpha, theta, and delta rhythms in ECoG recorded from the intact brain (A1, B1, B2) and from the isolated forebrain preparation (A2, B3, B4), without (A) and with (B) segmentation of the ECoG; B1 and B3 correspond to desynchronization segments, whereas B2 and B4 correspond to synchronization segments.*

In our experiments, the transition from desynchronization to synchronization in ECoG recordings from the intact rat brain was accompanied by a shift from pronounced left-sided lateralization of beta-2, beta-1, alpha, and theta rhythm amplitudes to right-sided lateralization, while the delta rhythm amplitude showed increased left-sided lateralization. Studies by L. Goldstein et al. (1972) demonstrated that in right-handed subjects, the transition from REM sleep to slower sleep phases is accompanied by changes in the relative spectral power between the two hemispheres.

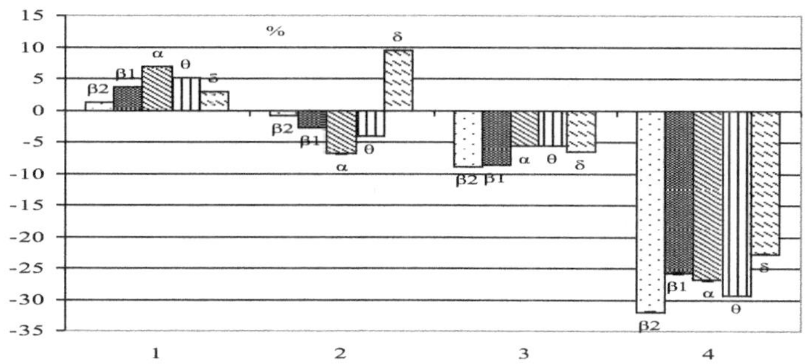

Figure 72. *Diagram of functional interhemispheric asymmetry coefficients for the amplitudes of β2, β1, α, θ, and δ rhythms in ECoG, recorded from the intact brain (1,2) and from a preparation with removed cerebellar hemispheres on the third day of observation (3,4), within desynchronization segments (1,3) and synchronization segments (2,4).*

Following cerebellar damage, functional interhemispheric EEG asymmetry is characterized by negative values, meaning that EEG wave amplitudes are higher in the right hemisphere than in the left. These results indicate that the functional state of the brainstem and cerebellum influences functional interhemispheric EEG asymmetry.

6. Influence of EEG rhythms on extraversion–introversion and SMIL test scores in left- and right-hemisphere-dominant individuals

The relationship between mental acts and states, individual psychological traits, and the functional state of the central nervous system (CNS) is a fundamental problem in brain and psychological sciences. Psychology studies the neuropsychological process (Bekhterev, 1991; Bekhtereva, 1974) and the holistic psychophysiological reality (Vygotsky, 1984), which underlies all mental processes, including higher cognitive functions (Rubinstein, 1976).

Many researchers have attempted to correlate personality test scales with EEG characteristics, often finding only weak associations. For example, K. Becker-Carus, using the Minnesota Multiphasic Personality Inventory (MMPI), found a positive correlation between the neuroticism scale and alpha rhythm indices and frequency. However, A. Gasto did not confirm this relationship in larger datasets (Novikova, 1978).

EEG parameters are considered stable for individual subjects (Eysenck, 1967) and may reflect the degree of expression of psychological traits and cognitive styles (Dunn, 1991). Following Eysenck's biological theory of personality (Eysenck, 1967; 1976; 1985), research focused on correlations between EEG activity parameters and the extraversion–introversion construct, primarily using the Eysenck Personality Inventory (EPI) (Eysenck, 1964). Correlations between EEG data and MMPI scores were also studied (Kullaev et al., 2013).

Earlier studies often relied on two-dimensional correlation coefficients, which are now considered insufficient for testing hypotheses about relationships among variables (Mannheim & Rich). Multivariate analysis, considering three or more interrelated variables simultaneously, is required to properly evaluate such influences.

Study goal: To identify probable regulatory influences of CNS functional states, as reflected in EEG, on individual psychological traits assessed using EPI and SMIL tests, employing multivariate regression and correlation analysis.

Methods: EEG was recorded in 48 healthy participants (mean age 20 ± 0.5 years) during psychosensory rest (eyes closed) for 2 minutes. Bipolar EEG recordings were made in the following derivations: frontal–temporal (F–T), temporal–parietal (T–P), parietal–occipital (P–O), left and right hemispheres, with a time constant of 0.1 s. EEG signals were digitized at 256 Hz and analyzed using "Analist2" software via amplitude–interval (semi-period) analysis. Five physiological rhythms were extracted: β2 (21–32 Hz), β1 (14.22–18.3 Hz), α (8–12.8 Hz), θ (4–7.53 Hz), δ (0.5–3.87 Hz). For each frequency band, amplitude (μV), frequency (Hz), and time index (%) were calculated.

EEG segmentation used the fixed-interval method (Kaplan, 1999), followed by clustering with k-means to classify epochs into two clusters. Mean values, standard deviations, and standard errors were computed for each cluster. Psychological tests (EPI and SMIL) were conducted electronically in standardized form.

Regression analysis: EEG rhythm amplitudes (X variables) were used to predict psychological test scores (Y variables) via multiple linear regression:

Y1=a0+b1X1+b2X2+...+bnXn

where a0 is the intercept, b1,...,bnb_1, ..., b_nb1,...,bn are regression coefficients reflecting the influence of each EEG parameter on the target variable. Statistical significance of coefficients was assessed via standard deviations, and the overall model was evaluated using the multiple correlation coefficient.

This approach allows the construction of a mathematical model to analyze EEG data in terms of CNS regulatory influences on individual psychological traits.

Results of the Study:

Right-Handed Individuals:

During EEG desynchronization periods, right-handed subjects showed a significantly higher number of statistically meaningful regression coefficients between EEG rhythm amplitudes and psychological test scores, with 96 coefficients compared to 48 during synchronization periods. In desynchronization conditions, the greatest number of regression relationships from EEG rhythm amplitudes were found with the "paranoia" scale (15 relationships) and the "extraversion–introversion" scale (14 relationships) (Table 6).

Out of the 15 regression relationships associated with the "paranoia" score, 6 were related to the theta rhythm amplitude: 4 were negative and 2 were positive. For the delta rhythm amplitude, 5 regression coefficients were found (3 negative, 2 positive).

Regarding "extraversion–introversion," 14 regression relationships were observed: 5 negative from the beta rhythm, 4 from the alpha rhythm (1 negative, 3 positive), and 4 from the theta rhythm (2 negative, 2 positive).

Table 6. *Statistically Significant Regression Coefficients from EEG Rhythm Amplitudes to Psychological Test Scores in Right-Handed Subjects under Desynchronization Conditions*

Таблица 6. *Statistically Significant Regression Coefficients from EEG Rhythm Amplitudes to Psychological Test Scores in Right-Handed Subjects under Desynchronization Conditions*

Psychological Test	Beta-2 (–)	Beta-2 (+)	Beta-1 (–)	Beta-1 (+)	Alpha (–)	Alpha (+)	Theta (–)	Theta (+)	Delta (–)	Delta (+)	Row Sum
Extraversion–Introversion	5	1	1	3	2	2	0	0	0	0	14
Hypochondria	2	1	2	1	1	1	0	0	0	0	8
Depression	1	1	3	1	1	2	1	1	1	0	12
Hysteria	2	2	1	2	2	1	0	0	0	0	10
Psychopathy	1	1	3	3	2	0	0	0	0	0	10
Paranoia	2	1	1	4	2	3	2	0	0	0	15
Psychasthenia	2	1	1	2	2	1	0	0	0	0	9
Schizoidism	1	2	1	4	1	1	0	0	0	0	10
Hypomania	4	2	1	2	1	0	0	0	0	0	10
Column Sum	20	13	14	19	14	10	3	1	1	0	**88**

The largest number of statistically significant regression coefficients for the **extraversion–introversion** and **SMIL test** scores under EEG desynchronization conditions was associated with the **theta rhythm amplitude** – 33 coefficients. Among these, the majority were **negative influences** (21), while 12 were positive.

In desynchronization conditions, **positive EEG rhythm influences predominated in the left hemisphere** compared to the right (30 vs. 18), whereas **negative influences predominated in the right hemisphere** compared to the left (31 vs. 19).

Under synchronization conditions, the largest number of regression relationships from EEG rhythm amplitudes was observed for the **extraversion–introversion**, **schizoid**, and **psychasthenia** scores – 9, 8, and 7 respectively (Table 7).

Table 7. *Statistically Significant Regression Coefficients from EEG Rhythm Amplitudes to Psychological Test Scores in Right-Handed Subjects under Synchronization and Desynchronization Conditions*

Psychological Test	**Beta-2 (–)**	**Beta-2 (+)**	**Beta-1 (–)**	**Beta-1 (+)**	**Alpha (–)**	**Alpha (+)**	**Theta (–)**	**Theta (+)**	**Delta (–)**	**Delta (+)**	**Row Sum**
Extraversion–Introversion	3	1	1	1	3	0	0	0	0	0	9
Hypochondria	1	0	1	0	0	1	0	0	1	0	3
Depression	2	0	0	0	0	3	0	0	0	0	5
Hysteria	3	0	0	1	0	0	0	0	0	0	4
Psychopathy	1	0	2	0	1	0	0	0	0	0	4
Paranoia	1	0	0	0	1	0	0	0	0	0	2
Psychasthenia	2	2	1	1	1	0	0	0	0	0	7
Schizoidism	4	0	2	0	1	1	0	0	0	0	8
Hypomania	1	1	1	0	1	1	0	0	0	0	5
Column Sum	15	4	8	3	8	6	0	0	1	0	**48**

In **desynchronization** periods of EEG, left-handed subjects exhibited **82 statistically significant regression coefficients** to the psychological test scores, while in **synchronization** periods, only **22 significant regression coefficients** were observed (Tables 8 and 9). Thus, similarly to right-handed subjects, left-handed individuals also showed more statistically significant regression coefficients during **desynchronization** periods than during synchronization periods.

During **desynchronization**, the highest number of regression relationships from EEG rhythm amplitudes was found for the **"paranoia"** scale, with **12 significant relationships**. These relationships included **3 positive coefficients** each from the **beta-2** and **beta-1** rhythm amplitudes.

For the **"extraversion–introversion"**, **"psychasthenia"**, and **"schizoidism"** scales, **11 regression relationships** were identified from the EEG rhythm amplitudes.

Table 8. *Statistically Significant Regression Coefficients from EEG Rhythm Amplitudes to Psychological Test Scores in Left-Handed Subjects under Desynchronization Conditions*

Psychological Test	**Beta-2 (–)**	**Beta-2 (+)**	**Beta-1 (–)**	**Beta-1 (+)**	**Alpha (–)**	**Alpha (+)**	**Theta (–)**	**Theta (+)**	**Delta (–)**	**Delta (+)**	**Row Sum**
Extraversion–Introversion	3	2	3	1	1	1	0	0	0	0	11
Hypochondria	1	3	1	1	1	1	0	0	0	0	8
Depression	1	1	1	1	0	0	0	0	0	0	4
Hysteria	2	1	1	1	1	2	1	0	0	0	9
Psychopathy	1	2	1	0	4	1	0	0	0	0	9
Paranoia	1	3	1	3	1	2	1	0	0	0	12
Psychasthenia	1	2	1	3	1	2	1	0	0	0	11
Schizoidism	1	1	3	1	3	2	0	0	0	0	11
Hypomania	1	1	2	2	1	0	0	0	0	0	7
Column Sum	11	16	14	12	12	11	3	0	0	0	**82**

For **left-handed subjects**:

During **desynchronization**, **positive influences** of EEG rhythms predominated in **both the left and right hemispheres**.

During **synchronization**, the **highest number of regression relationships** from EEG rhythm amplitudes was observed for the **"extraversion–introversion"** scale (Table 9).

Table 9. *Statistically Significant Regression Coefficients Oriented from EEG Rhythm Amplitudes to Psychological Test Scores in Left-Handed Subjects under Synchronization Conditions*

Test Indicators	Beta-2		Beta-1		Alpha		Theta		Delta		Sum
	"–"	"+"	"–"	"+"	"–"	"+"	"–"	"+"	"–"	"+"	
Extraversion–Introversion	1	2	2	2	2	2	2	2	2	2	9
Hypochondria	1	0	1	0	1	0	0	0	0	0	3
Depression	1	0	1	0	0	0	0	0	0	0	2
Hysteria	1	0	0	0	0	0	0	0	0	0	1
Psychopathy	1	0	1	0	1	0	0	0	0	0	3
Paranoia	1	0	0	0	0	0	0	0	0	0	1
Psychasthenia	1	0	0	0	0	0	0	0	0	0	1
Schizoidism	2	0	0	0	0	0	0	0	0	0	2
Hypomania	0	0	0	0	0	0	0	0	0	0	0
Sum	1	2	0	3	1	1	5	3	3	3	22
Total	3	3	2	8	6						

The **highest number of statistically significant regression coefficients** to psychological test scores under **synchronization** in right-handed subjects was observed for the **theta rhythm amplitude** – 8 coefficients (5 negative and 3 positive).

In **left-handed subjects** under synchronization, **negative influences** of EEG rhythms predominated in **both the left and right hemispheres**.

Under **desynchronization**, in the **right hemisphere**, the number of **positive regression coefficients** in right- and left-handers differed **insignificantly** (Fig. 74), while the number of **negative coefficients** differed **substantially** – by 12 units. In the **left hemisphere**, by contrast, the number of **negative coefficients** differed **insignificantly**, whereas the number of **positive coefficients** differed **significantly** – by 5 units.

Under **synchronization**, in both the **right and left hemispheres**, right-handers had a **substantially higher number of positive regression coefficients** than left-handers, while left-handers had a **larger number of negative coefficients** than right-handers.

Discussion. In both right- and left-handers, during **desynchronization**, the number of statistically significant regression coefficients from EEG rhythm amplitudes to Eysenck and SMIL test scores was **higher** than during synchronization.

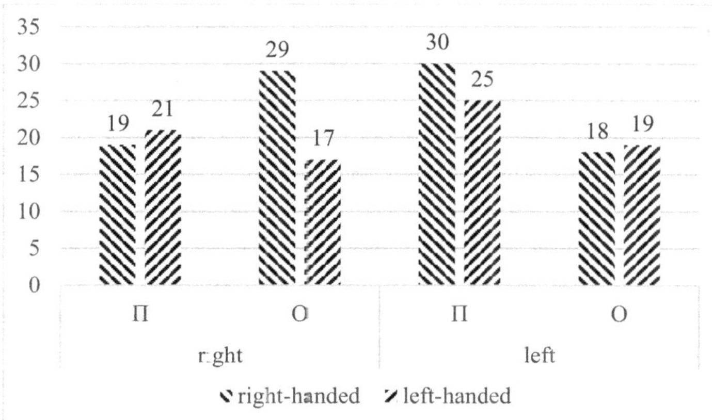

Fig. 73. *Statistically significant positive (P) and negative (N) regression coefficients directed from EEG rhythm amplitudes to extraversion–introversion indices and SMIL test scores in right-handed and left-handed individuals under desynchronization conditions.*

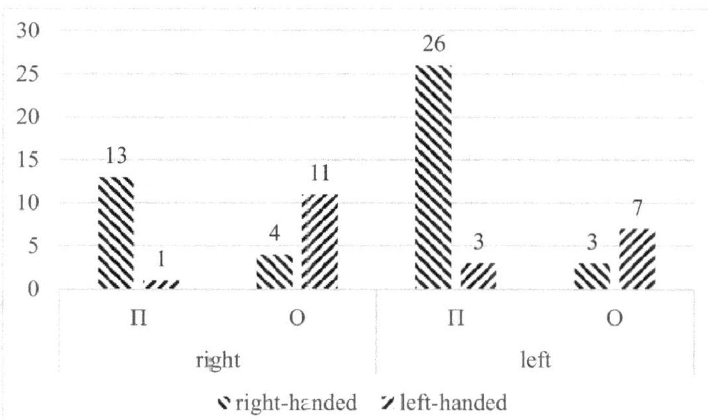

Fig. 74. *Statistically significant positive (P) and negative (N) regression coefficients directed from EEG rhythm amplitudes to extraversion–introversion indices and SMIL test scores in right-handed individuals.*

This may indicate that the implementation of mental acts and states, verifiable through the scores of the applied tests, occurs predominantly during periods of desynchronization. One might hypothesize that desynchronization periods in some way reflect episodes of consciousness, whereas synchronization periods reflect episodes of the unconscious. The greatest number of statistically significant regression coefficients from EEG rhythm amplitudes to psychological test scores during **desynchronization** in right-handed subjects was observed for **theta** and **beta-2** rhythm amplitudes, while during **synchronization**, it was seen for **beta-2** amplitude.

It has been shown that **theta rhythms** prevail when there is difficulty in EEG performance, whereas **high-frequency beta rhythms** dominate during effective work, which is associated with emotional tension (Novikova L.A., 1978). This rhythm plays a major role in human orientation during many activities. Cognitive activity and intellectual strain lead to an increase in power and spatial synchronization of **theta waves**. The expression of the **theta rhythm** depends on the nature of the activity and significantly increases during mental and emotional stress. One could assume that during the desynchronization and synchronization episodes of EEG, different components of cognitive processes and intellectual activity are realized.

In **right-handed subjects**, during both desynchronization and synchronization, **positive regression coefficients** from the amplitudes of **beta-2**, **beta-1**, and **alpha rhythms** to test scores were predominant.

In **left-handed subjects**, during **desynchronization**, **positive influences** predominated from **beta-2** and **beta-1**, while **negative influences** were more prominent from **alpha**, **theta**, and **delta rhythms**. During **synchronization**, no predominant influence was observed. The greatest number of statistically significant regression coefficients from EEG rhythm amplitudes to psychological test scores, for both right- and left-handed subjects, was found during **desynchronization** for the **"paranoia"** and **"extraversion-introversion"** indices, while during **synchronization**, it was found mainly for the **"extraversion-introversion"** index.

Out of **15 regression relations** oriented to the **"paranoia"** index in right-handed subjects during desynchronization, **8 were negative** – from **alpha**, **theta**, and **delta rhythms**.

Out of **14 regression relations** oriented to the **"extraversion-introversion"** index in right-handed subjects during desynchronization, **9 were negative** – from all EEG rhythm amplitudes. The greatest number of **negative influences** was observed from **beta-2**, **theta**, and **delta rhythms**.

During **synchronization**, for the **"extraversion-introversion"** index in right-handed subjects, **4 negative** regression relations were observed – from **beta-2** and **theta rhythms**, and **5 positive** – from **beta-1**, **alpha**, and **theta rhythms**.

Out of **12 regression relations** oriented to the **"paranoia"** index in left-handed subjects during desynchronization, the number of **positive and negative regression relations** was **equal** – **6 each**. Negative relations were identified from **all EEG rhythm amplitudes**, while positive relations were identified from **beta-2** and **beta-1** rhythms.

7. EEG in Various Pathological Forms in Adults

Modified classification by L.R. Zenkov.

1. **Normal and borderline EEG** (EEG conclusion: "EEG within normal limits").
2. **Diffuse changes in brain bioelectric activity** (irritative nature: mild, moderate, severe).
3. **Local changes in brain bioelectric activity** (mild, moderate, severe).
4. **Signs of dysfunction in nonspecific midline structures** (mild, moderate, severe dysfunction).
5. **Epileptiform activity** (local, local with secondary generalization, generalized).

If no local or diffuse changes, dysfunction in nonspecific midline structures, or epileptiform activity are registered on the EEG, the physician concludes: "EEG within normal limits". Low-amplitude EEG can also be considered a normal variant.

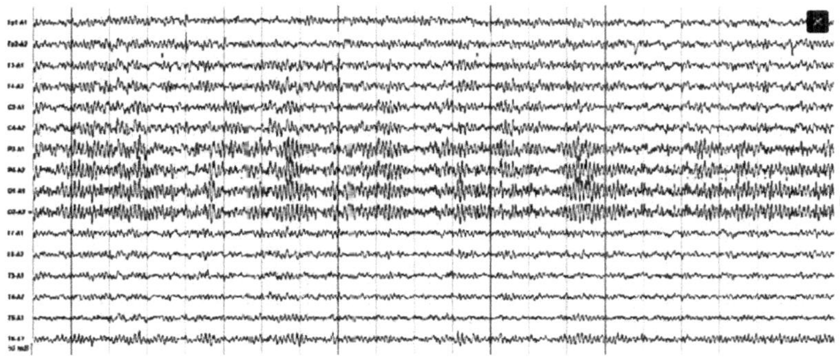

Fig. 75. *Normal human EEG.*

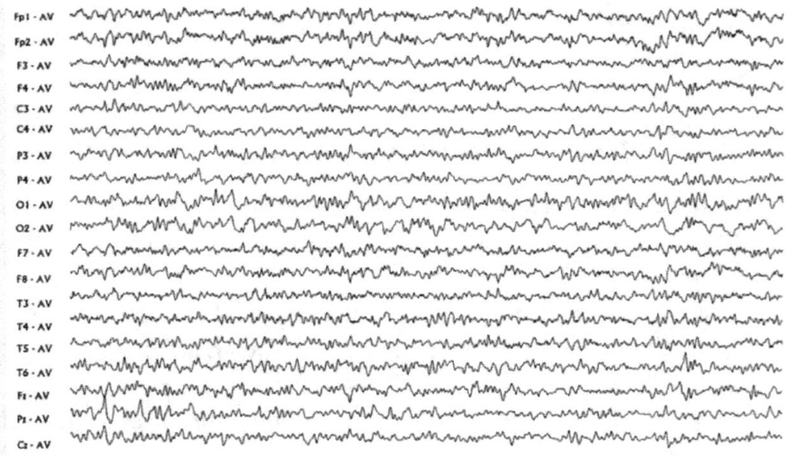

Fig. 76. *Diffuse changes in the brain's bioelectrical activity.*

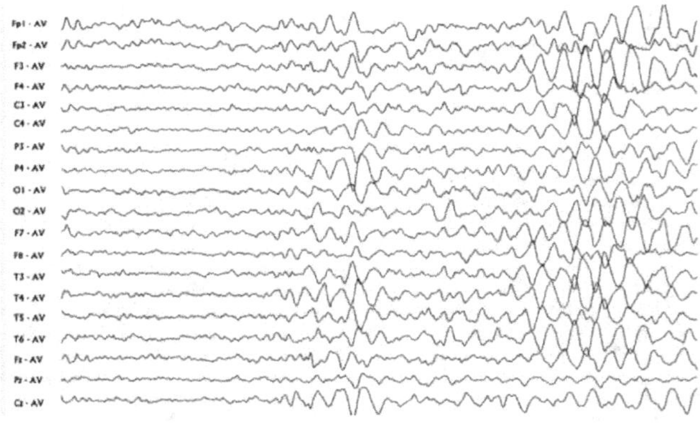

Fig. 77. *Signs of dysfunction of nonspecific midline structures: repeated delta wave bursts during a hyperventilation test.*

Concerning the conclusions "diffuse changes in the brain's bioelectrical activity" and "signs of dysfunction of nonspecific midline structures": these findings are nosologically nonspecific. That is, the same EEG changes described by these terms can be observed in patients with severe neurological disorders as well as in those with functional nervous system disturbances. The diagnostic informativeness of such conclusions is limited.

However, moderate to pronounced diffuse changes or moderate to pronounced dysfunction of nonspecific midline structures are typically recorded in patients with serious neurological conditions. In such cases, it is advisable to consult a neurologist and continue diagnostic evaluation.

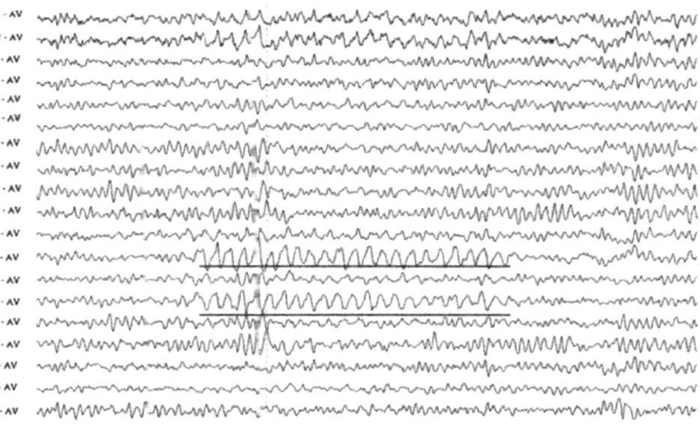

***Fig. 78.** Localized changes in the right temporal region*

The conclusion **"LOCAL CHANGES IN BRAIN BIOELECTRICAL ACTIVITY"** suggests the possible presence of a space-occupying lesion in the brain (e.g., tumor, cyst, etc.). With the advent of CT and MRI, EEG has lost its diagnostic significance for detecting such brain lesions.

If a physician reports local changes on an EEG, this is a valid reason to perform a CT or MRI of the brain.

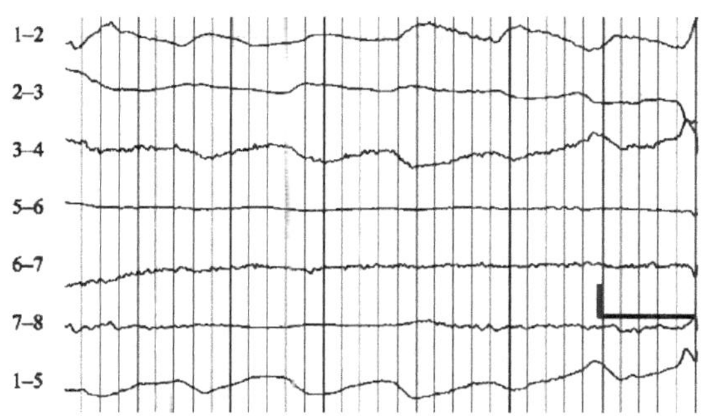

***Figure 79.** ECoG. "Reduced activity" over a glial tumor in the frontal cortex. Pronounced vascular artifact under electrode 1 (in leads 1–2 and 1–5 – bidirectional oscillations). Calibration signal: amplitude 1000 μV, duration 1 s. M.V. Alexandrov, A.Yu. Ulitin, 2012.*

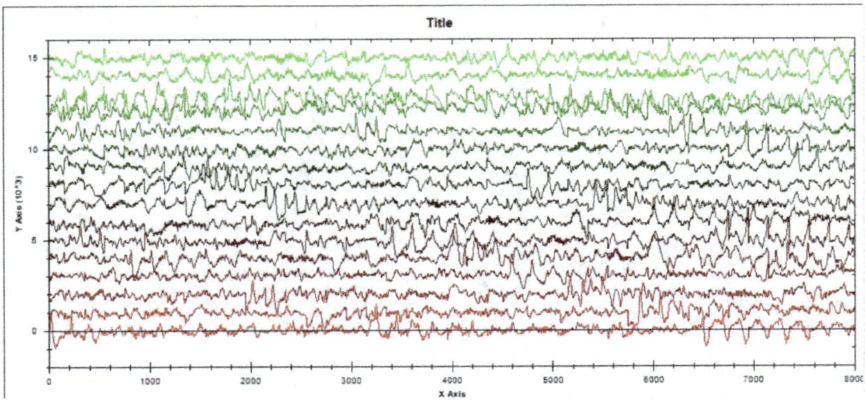

Figure 80. *Electroencephalogram following severe traumatic brain injury. Diffuse changes in the brain's bioelectrical activity.*

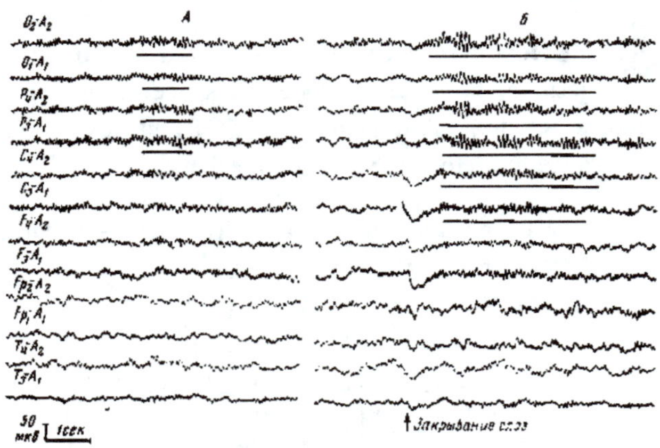

Figure 81. *EEG of patient B. with cystic arachnoiditis.*

A — background recording: synchronized beta activity predominates; the alpha rhythm is reduced. B — upon eye closure, a brief burst of high-amplitude alpha oscillations appears.

In patients with severe forms of basal arachnoiditis, spike-like oscillations are observed in all cortical regions against a background of reduced alpha rhythm. This indicates diffuse irritation of the brain involving both basal and convexital regions. These spike-like EEG potentials in arachnoiditis differ from those seen in tumors of the basal brain regions, where such activity is recorded only when the tumor leads to the development of basal arachnoiditis.

In inflammatory diseases of the meninges, slow-wave activity is usually mildly expressed, predominantly in the form of isolated, non-prominent delta waves.

All the listed pathological EEG changes in patients with arachnoiditis are diffuse in nature, without signs of stable interhemispheric asymmetry or persistent focal cortical abnormalities. Only in some cases of cystic arachnoiditis can unstable focal changes be observed on EEG.

For example, as shown in studies by S. M. Movsisyan (1967), arachnoiditis of the cerebellopontine angle may be associated with bursts of slow-wave activity on the side of the lesion.

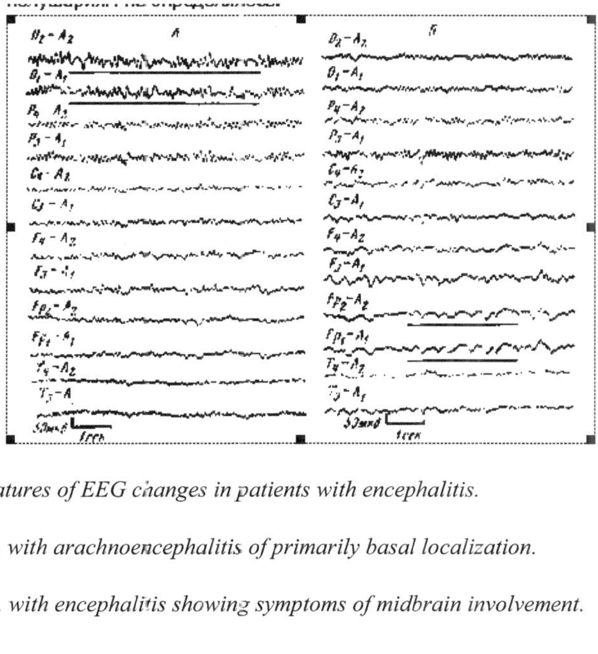

Figure 82. *Features of EEG changes in patients with encephalitis.*

A — Patient P. with arachnoencephalitis of primarily basal localization.

B — Patient C. with encephalitis showing symptoms of midbrain involvement.

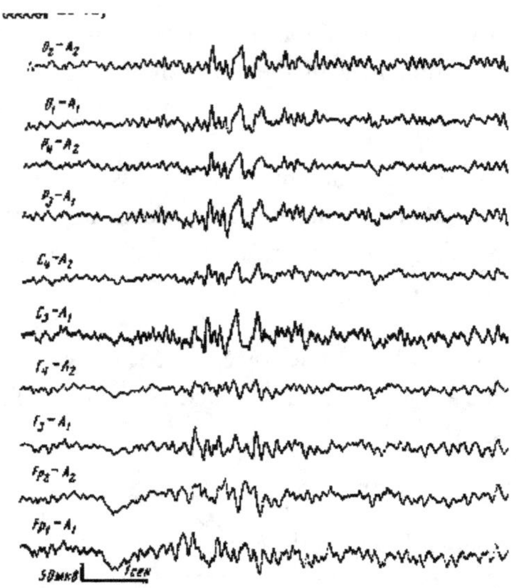

Figure 83. *EEG of patient M. with occlusive hydrocephalus; obstruction at the level of the third ventricle. Bursts of generalized theta and delta waves. (G. Walter, 1940; Cobb, 1944; D.G. Zhuchepko, 1955; van der Drift Magnus, 1961; Schwab & Carter, 1962; A.Sh. Velibekov, 1966, et al.). According to these studies, in 50–70% of patients with brain abscesses, EEG reveals a focal area of pathological activity in the form of delta waves and slower oscillations localized to the region of the abscess*

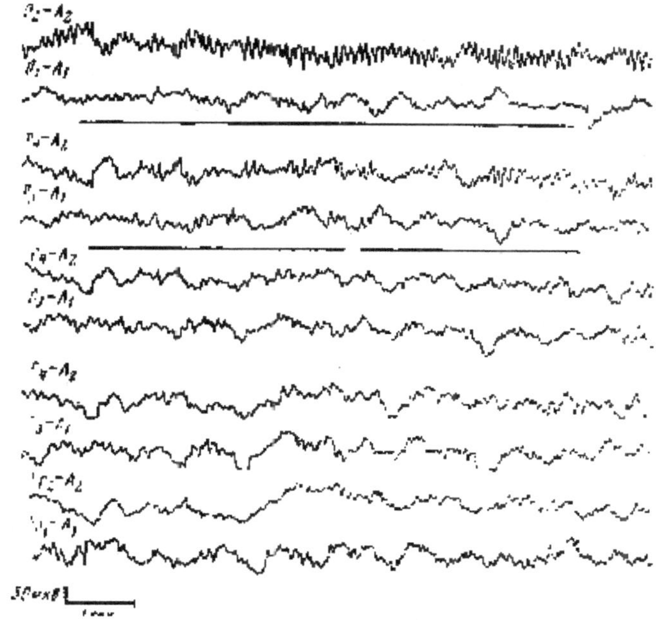

Figure 84. *EEG of patient K. with an echinococcus in the left posterior parietal region. Marked interhemispheric asymmetry in the occipito-parietal leads with reduction of alpha waves and the presence of delta waves on the left.*

As an example, Fig. 84 presents the EEG of patient K., in whom a large echinococcus localized in the left posterior parietal region was discovered during surgery. A clear interhemispheric asymmetry of the basic rhythm is recorded due to a significant reduction of alpha oscillations in the posterior regions of the left hemisphere. Delta waves are observed in all areas. In the parietal regions, interhemispheric asymmetry is revealed in the form of greater stability of delta activity on the left.

7.1. The Effect of Ethanol on Electrogenesis

According to pharmacological classification, ethanol belongs to narcotic substances with a depressant type of action. However, stimulating properties of ethanol are also known. Thus, in clinical alcohol intoxication, euphoria, elevated mood, disinhibition, hypomanic state, cheerfulness, and uninhibited behavior are observed (Waldman A.V., 1996).

Ethanol may act as a neurochemical surrogate of environmental reinforcing stimuli such as food and sex (Melnik E.V., 1998). This assumption is supported by studies demonstrating ethanol-induced activation of neurotransmitter turnover, such as dopamine, GABA, and opioids, which are also activated by environmental reinforcing stimuli (Di Chiara et al., 1996).

It has been shown that disturbances of interhemispheric interaction represent one of the important pathogenetic mechanisms of mental disorders (Otto et al., 1987; Carter et al., 1996). For example, functional disturbances in the right hemisphere occur in depression, while in schizophrenia they occur in the left hemisphere. There are also data (Bruder et al., 1992) on the differentiation of various types of depression according to the pattern of interhemispheric asymmetry.

Alcohol dependence is based on psychophysiological mechanisms associated with nonspecific modulation of the tone of motivational systems of positive and negative reinforcement (Waldman A.V., Maisky A.I., Kampov-Polevoy A.B., Treskov V.G., 1988), обусловленные изменениями функциональной межполушарной асимметрии (ФМПА) ритмов ЭКоГ. Clinical studies indicate that manifestations of alcohol intoxication such as elevated mood, silliness, and underestimation of one's condition are associated with impaired right hemisphere activity under the influence of ethanol (Melnik E.V., 1998). It has been shown that euphoria occurring during acute ethanol exposure is associated with activation of the right prefrontal cortex and is linked to the endogenous opioid system (Tiihonen J., Kuikka J., Hakola P., 1994). EEG studies in patients with alcoholism have demonstrated suppression of the total power of brain bioelectrical activity predominantly in the right hemisphere. The reduction in EEG rhythm power is explained by the authors as a result of the spread of nonspecific activation and enhancement of desynchronization processes in the cerebral cortex (Koekina O.I., Gaidamakina A.M., Koroleva M.V., 1991). Reshikova T.N. (1980) also established that under the influence of alcohol, cortical activity is suppressed more strongly in the right hemisphere.

Therefore, the search for methods to correct the asymmetric effects of ethanol is of interest.

The aim of these series of studies was to investigate the combined effect of VER on rat ECoG.

7.1.1. Study of the Effect of VER on ECoG Parameters

For this purpose, the effect of intraperitoneal administration of VER on rat ECoG was studied in 4 animals at a dose of 2 g per 100 g of body weight.

Before administration of the solution, the ECoG exhibited a synchronized–desynchronized pattern (Fig. 85A). Two minutes after administration, an increase in delta activity in the ECoG was observed (Fig. 85B). By 12 minutes after administration, the representation of slow-wave activity in the ECoG had increased (Fig. 85). By 25 minutes after VER administration, a decrease in the level of slow-wave activity in the ECoG and restoration of pronounced fast rhythms were noted (Fig. 85D).

Digital analysis of left and right hemisphere ECoG before and after VER administration showed that after intraperitoneal injection of VER (Figs. 86–87), the amplitude of beta-2 rhythms in both hemispheres was statistically significantly reduced.

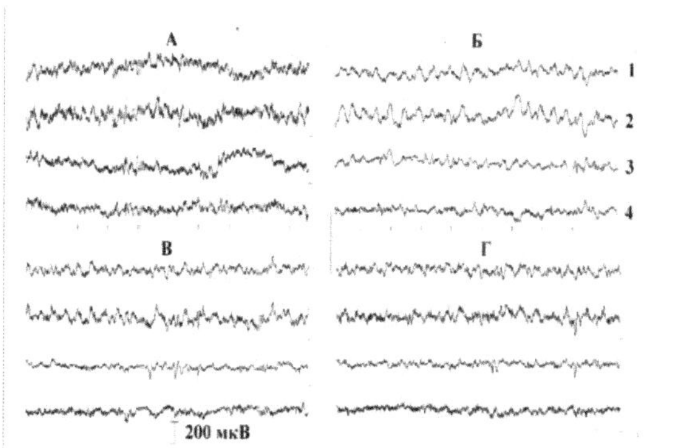

Figure 85. *Effect of intraperitoneal administration of VER on rat ECoG.*

Legend: A – before ethanol administration; B – 2 minutes after VER administration; C – 12 minutes after VER administration; D – 25 minutes after VER administration.

A decrease in the amplitude of beta-1 and alpha rhythms was observed in both hemispheres during the first 20 minutes of observation, and during the last 10-minute interval only in the right hemisphere. A statistically significant decrease in theta rhythm amplitude in both hemispheres was observed during the first 15 minutes after VER administration. A reduction in delta rhythm amplitude in both hemispheres was observed only by the 15th minute of observation; however, at 25 and 30 minutes after VER administration, the delta rhythm amplitude increased in the left hemisphere, while remaining unchanged in the right hemisphere.

The duration indices of the beta-2 rhythm were reduced in both hemispheres throughout the 30-minute observation period after VER administration. The duration index of the beta-1 rhythm in the left hemisphere was decreased for 20 minutes, and in the right hemisphere for 15 minutes. A decrease in the alpha rhythm duration index in the right hemisphere was noted throughout the entire observation period, whereas in the left hemisphere it was observed only during the first 20 minutes after VER administration.

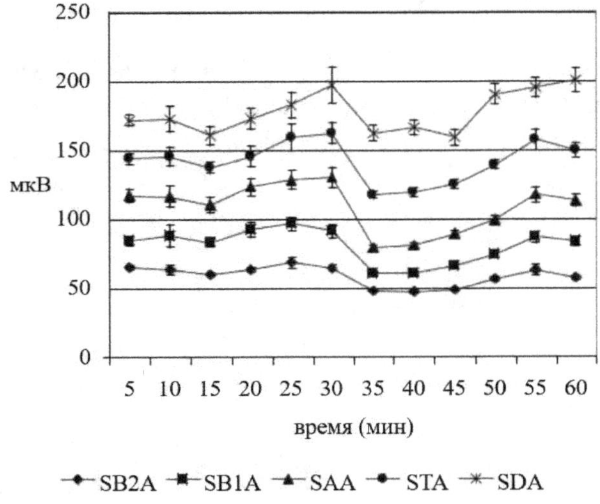

Figure 86. *Dynamics of ECoG rhythm amplitudes in the left hemisphere before (5–30 min) and after (35–60 min) VER administration.*

The theta index in the right hemisphere was reduced throughout the entire observation period, whereas in the left hemisphere its changes at 15 and 25 minutes were not statistically significant. The values of the delta rhythm duration indices during all observation periods in both hemispheres were statistically significantly increased.

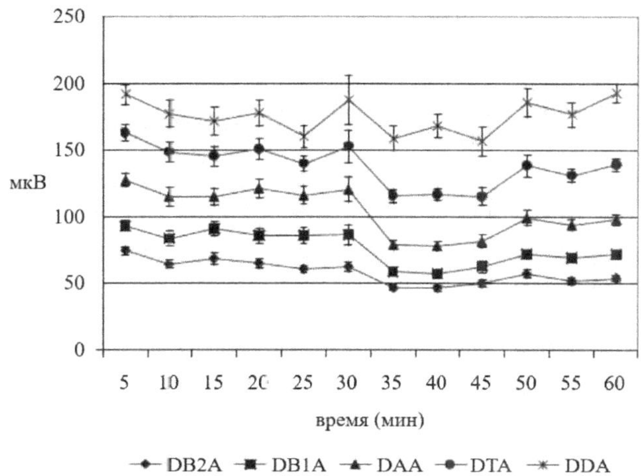

Figure 87. Dynamics of ECoG rhythm amplitudes in the right hemisphere before (5–30 min) and after (35–60 min) VER administration.

7.1.2. Changes in functional interhemispheric asymmetry (FIHA) indices of the ECoG following VER administration

Before VER administration (Table 10), averaged over the 30-minute observation period, FIHA indices of ECoG rhythm amplitudes were statistically non-significant. After VER administration, also averaged over a 30-minute observation period, FIHA indices of beta-2, beta-1, and alpha rhythm amplitudes were statistically significantly changed and positive.

Changes in FIHA indices of theta and delta activity amplitudes were not statistically significant.

FIHA indices for ECoG rhythm frequencies were statistically non-significant before VER administration and remained statistically unchanged after administration.

FIHA indices of the duration indices of beta-1, theta, and delta rhythms were statistically non-significant before VER administration, whereas the FIHA duration index of the beta-2 rhythm was positive and statistically significant. After VER administration, the FIHA duration index of the beta-2 rhythm showed a statistically significant inversion and was expressed as a negative value (–6.75 ± 2.20%).

Table 10. Indices of interhemispheric asymmetry of ECoG rhythms before and after VER administration.

Rhythm	Parameter	Before (VER) Administration	After Administration (VER)
Beta-2	A	−0.87 ± 2.01	10.25 ± 3.67*
	F	−0.15 ± 0.17	−0.49 ± 0.18*
	I	12.19 ± 4.59	−6.75 ± 5.04*
Beta-1	A	0.93 ± 1.78	10.33 ± 3.56*
	F	−0.71 ± 0.34	−0.44 ± 0.41*
	I	2.3 ± 1.29	2.47 ± 1.43
Alpha	A	0.79 ± 1.44	10.92 ± 3.6*
	F	−0.29 ± 0.3	−0.74 ± 0.31*
	I	1.2 ± 1.25	7.14 ± 2.6*
Theta	A	−0.26 ± 1.82	5.52 ± 3.18*
	F	0.07 ± 0.43	−0.28 ± 0.15*
	I	−0.02 ± 1.23	4.7 ± 1.1*
Delta	A	−0.36 ± 1.75	−0.26 ± 2.65
	F	−0.49 ± 0.34	−0.16 ± 0.48*
	I	−1.12 ± 1.42	−8.65 ± 2.09*

Note: ** $P < 0.05$*

A statistically significant negative value was observed for the FMPA index of delta rhythm duration (−8.65 ± 1.61%). The FMPA indices of alpha and theta rhythm duration were statistically significantly positive, amounting to 7.14 ± 1.16% and 4.70 ± 1.63%, respectively.

7.1.3. Relationships Between ECoG Rhythm Amplitudes in the Left and Right Hemispheres Before and After VER Administration

Before VER administration, 4 relationships were identified in the left hemisphere (Fig. 88A), including 3 positive and 1 negative. In the right hemisphere (Fig. 88), 16 relationships were detected, of which 10 were positive and 6 negative.

After VER administration, 16 relationships were identified in the left hemisphere (Fig. 88B), including 9 positive and 7 negative. In the right hemisphere after VER administration (Fig. 89C), 11 relationships were detected, including 7 positive and 4 negative.

Thus, after VER administration, the number of relationships increased in the left hemisphere and decreased in the right hemisphere. Accordingly, before VER administration, the number of relationships predominated in the right hemisphere, whereas after VER administration, they predominated in the left hemisphere.

When calculating two-dimensional correlation coefficients between ECoG rhythm amplitudes in the left hemisphere, 4 correlation coefficients were identified before VER administration and 10 after administration; in the right hemisphere, 3 and 9 coefficients were identified, respectively.

Therefore, after VER administration, the number of correlation coefficients between ECoG rhythm amplitudes increased in both hemispheres.

The number of regression relationships between ECoG rhythm amplitudes after VER administration increased from 4 to 16 in the left hemisphere and decreased from 16 to 11 in the right hemisphere.

Correlation analysis revealed 4 statistically significant correlation coefficients in the left hemisphere before ethanol administration and 3 in the right hemisphere. After ethanol intake, the number of statistically significant correlation coefficients increased in both hemispheres, reaching 10 in the left hemisphere and 9 in the right hemisphere.

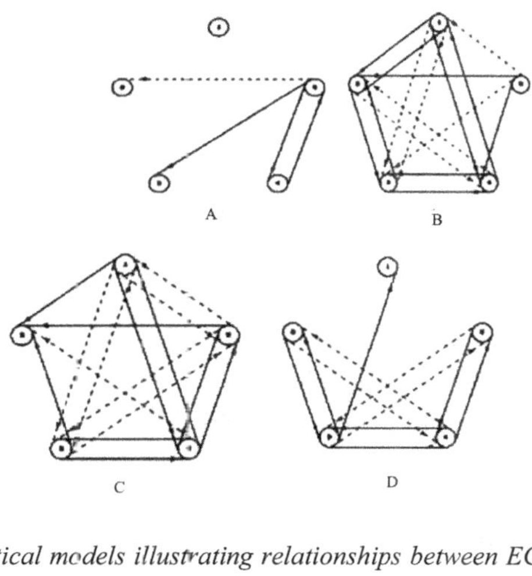

Figure 88. *Mathematical models illustrating relationships between ECoG rhythm amplitudes in the left (A, B) and right (C, D) hemispheres before (A, C) and after (B, D) VER administration.*

Our studies revealed that the effect of VER on the left hemisphere ECoG consisted of a reduction in rhythm amplitudes during the initial stage (5–20 minutes after ethanol administration) and an increase in the delta-band amplitude of the left hemisphere (25 and 30 minutes after VER administration). ECoG rhythm amplitudes in the right hemisphere remained decreased throughout the 30-minute observation period compared to baseline. Following VER administration, a reorganization of ECoG was observed in both hemispheres, characterized by decreased duration indices of beta-2, beta-1, alpha, and theta rhythms and an increased duration index of the delta rhythm.

After VER administration, the activation coefficient (AC) increased in both the left and right hemispheres during the first 15 minutes relative to pre-VER levels. By 20, 25, and 30 minutes post-administration, changes in AC were not statistically different from baseline.

It is known that ethanol consumption produces two stages: excitation and inhibition. The phenomenon of EEG rhythm desynchronization following ethanol intake has been reported by other authors, including human studies. For example, Melnik E.V. (1998) observed that healthy volunteers receiving a euphoric dose of ethanol (0.5–0.7 g/kg) showed decreased beta and alpha rhythm amplitudes, reduced alpha duration index, and increased beta duration index at peak euphoria. The activation coefficient increased from 0.79 ± 0.02 to 1.1 ± 0.02, which the author interpreted as evidence of marked EEG desynchronization. These changes occurred in all leads, suggesting involvement of the mesencephalic reticular formation. Alterations in brain electrical activity after ethanol intake are thought to result from changes in the tone of the brain's reticular formation (Bobrov A.E., 1987).

7.1.4. EEG in Alcoholism

Coutin-Churchman P. et al. (2006) investigated qEEG changes in 191 male patients with alcoholism during detoxification. This large cohort showed reduced power of slow rhythms (δ, θ), correlating with cortical atrophy due to chronic alcoholism. Increased β-band power was associated with pharmacological load (e.g., benzodiazepines), sensory-perceptual disturbances, clinical seizures, and family history of alcoholism. δ/θ changes were specifically linked to chronic cortical damage rather than age or other psychiatric variables.

Conclusion: chronic alcoholism is accompanied by significant EEG spectral changes reflecting structural and functional brain impairments.

Robledo P. et al. (1993) found that ethanol administration in non-preference rats increased 16–32 Hz waves in brain bioelectrical activity.

Thus, both clinical and experimental studies, including our own, indicate that ethanol intake produces electrophysiological signs of brain activation.

Kozhechkin S.N. et al. (2004) studied ethanol effects on ECoG in a multiparametric analysis (840 parameters across 24 points) of dorsal cortical ECoG in outbred rats. Ethanol was administered intraperitoneally at low (0.75 g/kg), medium (2.0 g/kg), and high pre-narcotic (4.5 g/kg) doses. Acute low-dose intoxication increased spectral power and connectivity in the dominant theta rhythm band (5.75–7.25 Hz), reflecting activation of the septo-hippocampal system, which regulates attention, memory, and exploratory behavior. Connectivity also increased in high-frequency alpha and beta bands. Medium and high doses shifted the dominant theta peak downward (4.5–5.75 Hz), indicating reduced septo-hippocampal activity and CNS functions. These doses also reduced spectral power and connectivity in high-frequency alpha and beta bands, reflecting decreased cortical energy and synaptic activity, leading to sedative and narcotic effects. Using reliable parameter sets and algorithms, EEG fragments may be identified to verify ethanol dose (Kozhechkin S.N. et al., 2004).

Human studies have shown that within the first 35 minutes of ethanol consumption (blood concentration ~0.3%), significant EEG increases occur in frontal regions in theta (4–7.75 Hz), alpha 1 (8–9.75 Hz), and beta 1 (13.25–19.75 Hz) rhythms, with alpha 1 also increased in central and posterior regions. No significant changes were observed in theta and beta frequencies in central and posterior regions or in the alpha 2 band (10–13 Hz) across all regions (Tran Y. et al., 2004).

Studies of EEG dimensionality (D2) showed that alcoholics exposed to alcohol-related images displayed significant increases in D2 in frontal, right posterior temporal, and occipital regions compared to non-alcohol-related images. The authors suggested these brain structures are key in forming alcohol consumption motivation. Nonlinear D2 EEG assessment may also aid chronic alcoholism diagnosis (Kim D.J. et al., 2003).

Increased ECoG associations detected via linear correlation and nonlinear D2 measures likely reflect brain activation (desynchronization), while regression coefficients may additionally assess the functional asymmetric influence of the mesencephalic reticular formation on ECoG. In our experiments, correlation analysis used amplitude values within a single ECoG lead, whereas cited studies used coherence across leads; nevertheless, the results are consistent.

The post-VER left-hemisphere ECoG amplitude lateralization may indicate differential ethanol effects on the left and right mesencephalic reticular formation and asymmetric activation of cerebral hemispheres. Brain activation level is thought to correlate with catecholamine levels (Chernositov A.V. et al., 1980; Anichkov S.V., 1982). Acute ethanol administration triggers catecholamine release in the midbrain and limbic structures, producing psychomotor and autonomic excitation underlying ethanol's euphoric effect (Anokhin I.P., 1987–1989). Catecholamines participate in avoidance, self-stimulation, sleep-wake balance, and emotional and motivational regulation, and are linked to psychopathological states (Morozov G.V. et al., 1983).

Norepinephrine and dopamine are considered key reinforcement mediators. Self-stimulation behavior may result from activation of either catecholaminergic pathway: the dorsal system from the locus coeruleus (noradrenergic) or the ventral system from the area surrounding the interpeduncular nucleus (dopaminergic) (Olds J., 1972, 1977; Crow T.J., Spear P.J., 1972; Routtenberg A. et al., 1971).

Norepinephrine is considered a mediator in brain areas that reinforce positive self-stimulation (Budantsev A.Yu., 1976).

The role of the dopaminergic system in brain reward mechanisms and the development of substance addiction is well established. Existing studies in animals and humans indicate that the density and function of the DA D2 receptor are reduced in alcoholics. These results suggest that drugs that enhance dopaminergic activity, such as partial DA agonists, may restore suboptimal levels of dopaminergic activity, reduce ethanol craving, and promote abstinence and euphoria by stimulating ethanol-induced dopamine production in the nucleus accumbens. According to the authors, this mechanism may provide negative reinforcement to prevent relapse (Tupala E., Tiihonen J., 2004).

The effects of ethanol (2 or 4 g/kg, 20% aqueous solution) on concentrations of norepinephrine, dopamine, serotonin, and their metabolites in the hippocampus and striatum of rats were studied. Ethanol was administered daily for 30 days. Monoamines were measured 30 minutes or 48 hours after the last ethanol administration. The study revealed increased serotonin levels in the hippocampus at 4 g/kg ethanol and decreased dopamine and 3,4-dihydroxyphenylacetic acid levels. Higher ethanol doses also reduced norepinephrine and 5-hydroxy-3-indoleacetic acid levels in the striatum 48 hours after the last dose compared to controls. Measurements taken 30 minutes after the last ethanol dose showed decreased striatal norepinephrine and dopamine and increased 3,4-dihydroxyphenylacetic acid and serotonin levels. Ethanol at 2 g/kg increased homovanillic acid levels and the homovanillic acid/dopamine ratio. The authors suggest that these changes in monoamine levels, mainly in the striatum, are associated with ethanol dose and timing after the last administration (Vasconcelos S.M., Cavalcante R.A., Aguiar L.M., Sousa F.C., Fonteles M.M., Viana G.S., 2004).

Plasma norepinephrine levels were studied in two groups of male chronic alcoholics: those actively drinking (bingeing) and those in remission (abstinent for at least three months). Healthy males served as controls. Plasma norepinephrine levels were highest in chronic alcoholics during active drinking, compared with remission and control groups. No differences were observed between stages one and two of alcoholism. These results indicate that chronic ethanol consumption increases plasma norepinephrine, which also manifests during withdrawal. However, norepinephrine activity normalizes after prolonged abstinence (Patkar A.A., Marsden C.A., Naik P.C., Kendall D.A., Gopalakrishnan R., Vergare M.J., Weinstein S.P., 2004).

Four weeks after ceasing repeated daily ethanol consumption, rats exhibited anxiolytic-like behavior similar to that observed in abstinent chronic alcoholics. This behavior is linked to sympathoadrenal activation. In control rats, plasma adrenaline and norepinephrine increased 150–300% within five minutes of being placed in a new cage. Rats exposed to ethanol for nine weeks showed a 195% increase in plasma adrenaline after five weeks of abstinence compared to controls. When moved to a new environment, no changes were observed in the ethanol-exposed rats. These results suggest that daily ethanol consumption can cause persistent increases in sympathoadrenal activation during subsequent abstinence, contributing to relative resistance to further stimulation (Rasmussen D.D., Wilkinson C.W., Raskind M.A., 2006).

The response to immobilization stress was studied in rats given 5% ethanol for one week. Tail arteries were cannulated for blood collection before, during, and after stress. Ethanol-exposed rats had higher plasma adrenaline and norepinephrine than controls. Stress increased adrenaline and norepinephrine more than twofold in ethanol-exposed animals compared with controls. Corticosterone levels were also higher in ethanol-exposed rats. Ethanol further increased levels of tyrosine hydroxylase, dopamine β-hydroxylase, and phenylethanolamine N-methyltransferase, enzymes involved in catecholamine biosynthesis. Tyrosine hydroxylase increased only in ethanol-exposed, non-immobilized rats. The authors suggest that ethanol administration itself acts as a stressor that can enhance immobilization effects, highlighting the importance of minimizing additional stressors when studying ethanol's physiological effects (Patterson-Buckendahl P., Kubovcakova L., Krizanova O., Pohorecky L.A., Kvetnansky R., 2005).

According to Kiyatkin E.A. (1990), dopamine metabolism increases most during nociceptive or other aversive stimuli that induce a stress state, rather than during reinforcing stimuli.

Dopamine and norepinephrine mechanisms, together with the brain's opioid system, are involved in alcohol's reinforcing effects via activation of the positive reinforcement system, while the serotonergic system modulates negative reinforcement (Nevo I., Hamon M., 1995). The noradrenergic system is closely linked to the dopaminergic system (Budantsev A.Yu., 1976).

In a study by Carlson J.N. and Drew Stevens K. (2006), rats given 6% ethanol for 14 days showed an increased homovanillic acid/dopamine ratio in the medial prefrontal cortex and depletion of dopamine and serotonin in the medial prefrontal cortex and serotonin in the amygdala. These effects were more pronounced on the right in right-turning rats, which also consumed more ethanol than left-turning rats. This suggests that one mechanism increasing motivation to consume ethanol during abstinence is asymmetric activation of neurons in the medial prefrontal cortex and amygdala, disrupting brain neurochemistry. Rats without rotational preference also exhibited ethanol-induced right-sided neurochemical activation of the medial prefrontal cortex. This study indicates that individual rats differ in brain neurochemistry after ethanol cessation, and these differences relate to functional brain asymmetry (Carlson J.N., Drew Stevens K., 2006).

These findings suggest asymmetric effects of ethanol on neuronal structures of the left and right hemispheres, driven by neurochemical (pharmacological) brain asymmetry. They may also indicate that changes in functional midline potentials (FMPA) in alcoholism are an important pathogenetic link of the disease.

Alcohol dependence is based on psychophysiological mechanisms related to non-specific modulation of motivational systems for positive and negative reinforcement.

Low doses of ethanol (1–2 g/kg) in a single administration have activating effects on brain bio-potentials and increase GABA levels in the cerebral hemispheres and cerebellum (Sytinsky I.A., et al., 1986).

According to current understanding, the synapse is the most sensitive CNS element for mediating ethanol's effects. Most research focuses on postsynaptic interactions of ethanol with glutamatergic and GABAergic receptors. Nevertheless, some evidence suggests presynaptic receptor membranes play a critical, possibly primary role. Acute ethanol administration can both increase and decrease neurotransmission in GABAergic, glutamatergic, and peptidergic vesicles (Siggins G.R., Roberto M., Nie Z., 2005).

Ethanol enhances GABAergic synaptic inhibition, largely determining its behavioral effects. The prevailing hypothesis is that ethanol increases GABAergic neurotransmission via allosteric potentiation of postsynaptic GABA receptors. Presynaptic GABA receptors may also regulate behavioral sensitivity to ethanol (Ariwodola O.J., Weiner J.L., 2004).

Recent studies show ethanol's effects on GABA receptors depend on the γ2 subtype, and genetically determined sensitivity to ethanol-induced motor impairment results from a single-nucleotide mutation in a cerebellar GABA receptor subtype (Korpi E.R., 1994). Some evidence also suggests the GABA system's response to ethanol is secondary and mediated by biogenic amine levels (Morozov G.V., et al., 1983).

It can be assumed that the biphasic changes in ECoG after VER administration are due to activation of different neurotransmitter systems: the first stage involves catecholaminergic systems, manifested by decreased ECoG rhythm amplitudes and increased activation coefficients (KA); the second stage involves GABAergic systems, expressed as increased delta rhythm amplitudes in the left hemisphere at 25–30 minutes post-VER. By this time, KA decreases to baseline.

Changes in brain electrical activity after ethanol intake are believed to result from altered reticular formation tone (Bobrov A.E., 1987). Alcohol consumption involves two stages: excitation and inhibition.

Studies of KA during human alcohol exposure revealed activation responses across all EEG leads, suggesting generalized activation and involvement of the mesencephalic reticular system (Melnik E.V., 1998).

Thus, clinical and experimental studies, including ours, indicate that ethanol produces electrophysiological signs of brain activation.

EEG changes in alcoholism represent characteristic brain bioelectrical activity patterns reflecting neurofunctional disturbances but are not, by themselves, specific diagnostic markers of the disease.

Bauer L.O. & Hesselbrock V.M. (1993) examined the relationship between EEG coherence and clinical manifestations of alcohol dependence. Changes in EEG spectra, such as reduced power in certain bands, were associated with symptom severity and impaired mental functioning.

Pizzagalli D.A., et al. (2003) described reduced theta-band EEG coherence in individuals with alcohol dependence. This reduction was linked to more severe forms of the disorder, suggesting that theta activity may serve as a marker of disease severity.

Hillyard S.A. & Picton T.W. (2000) discussed cognitive and neurophysiological aspects of alcohol dependence, including EEG changes, emphasizing their impact on cognitive function and potential use in patient monitoring.

Overall, EEG is a valuable tool for studying brain activity changes in alcohol dependence. Changes in EEG coherence and spectra can be used to assess disease severity and treatment efficacy, with particular attention to theta-band activity.

Coutin-Churchman P., Moreno R., Añez Y., Vergara F. (2006) evaluated the frequency and clinical correlates of abnormal QEEG parameters in 191 male patients hospitalized for detoxification. QEEG analysis (frequency analysis, absolute and relative power in four classical wavebands) was performed. Psychiatric, medical, and neurological assessments were conducted to correlate clinical and paraclinical signs with QEEG data. Only seven patients had normal QEEG.

The most frequent abnormalities were: reduced slow-wave power (delta/theta) with increased beta activity (81 cases), isolated slow-wave reduction

(33), increased beta only (29), reduced slow and alpha waves without beta changes (28), and reduced alpha only (6).

Clinical correlations: reduced slow waves (delta/theta) significantly correlated with cortical atrophy on MRI (especially in early-onset alcoholism) and duration of alcohol abuse in younger patients. Some association with arterial hypertension was noted; no correlation with age or other psychiatric signs was found.

Increased beta activity was primarily linked to benzodiazepine use during detoxification, sensory/perceptual disturbances (hallucinations, illusions), clinical seizures, and family history of alcoholism, indicating cortical hyperexcitability.

Holker R., Susan S. (2024) proposed developing new quantitative EEG (QEEG) features for automated alcoholism diagnosis. Their hypothesis: altered inter-electrode functional brain connectivity in alcohol-dependent individuals can be quantitatively measured through linear EEG signal associations.

The authors' methodology involved EEG decomposition: the original multichannel EEG signals were decomposed into five standard frequency bands: delta (0.5–4 Hz), theta (4–7 Hz), alpha (7–13 Hz), beta (13–30 Hz), and gamma (30–100 Hz). Decomposition was performed using the direct/inverse Fast Fourier Transform (FFT/IFFT). Within each band, absolute Pearson correlation values were calculated between all possible pairs of 64 electrodes, reflecting the linear monotonic association of signals. A 64×64 correlation matrix was constructed for each band, from which 2,016 unique features were extracted. To reduce dimensionality, ensemble feature selection was applied, combining filter methods (ANOVA and χ^2 criterion) with a wrapper method (greedy forward selection). As a result, 492 most significant features were selected for classification.

Classification: Four machine learning models were tested: SVM (support vector machines), RF (random forest), ANN (artificial neural network), and KNN (k-nearest neighbors).

SVM achieved the highest performance: 100% accuracy on the test set and 99.58% in cross-validation.

The authors concluded that inter-electrode EEG correlations serve as powerful QEEG features for distinguishing between alcoholic and healthy control states. Beta and gamma bands carry the most diagnostically informative information distinguishing the groups. Regional analysis indicated that frontal, central, and parietal brain areas are particularly involved in changes in functional connectivity in alcoholism. The proposed ensemble feature selection effectively reduces dimensionality and helps identify the most significant features.

This study offers a concrete computer-aided diagnostic approach based on quantitative EEG parameters and machine learning, achieving high accuracy in assessing the risk of alcohol dependence.

Tcheslavski G. V. and Gonen F. F. (2012) quantitatively evaluated changes in power spectrum, coherence, and phase synchrony of brain electrical activity (EEG) in individuals with alcohol dependence compared to healthy participants. The primary aim was to identify neurophysiological markers that distinguish alcohol dependence at the cortical electrical activity level.

EEG data were collected from 77 hospitalized male alcoholics and 45 male healthy controls during active wakefulness with eyes open. Standard preprocessing methods were applied (artifact removal, average spatial filtering), followed by analyses of:

Spectral analysis: assessing power values in classical frequency bands (delta, theta, alpha1, alpha2, beta1, beta2, gamma1);

Coherence: evaluating functional connectivity between electrode pairs across frequency bands;

Phase synchrony: measuring phase relationship consistency between EEG signal generators.

Statistical differences between groups were assessed using the Kruskal–Wallis nonparametric test with post-hoc analysis.

Key results:

Alcohol-dependent patients showed reduced spectral power across a wide frequency range (delta, theta, alpha1, alpha2, and beta1) compared to controls in key cortical regions, indicating reduced expression of primary oscillatory rhythms at rest.

Coherence values between electrode pairs were lower in alcoholics, especially in low-frequency rhythms, reflecting impaired functional connectivity between cortical regions.

Phase synchrony between rhythms (particularly in alpha2 and beta1 bands) was also reduced in alcoholics, indicating disrupted coordination of oscillatory dynamics across brain regions.

Interpretation and significance:

Reduced spectral power in alcoholics may reflect impaired neurophysiological rhythm generators, potentially due to chronic alcohol effects on neural tissue. Reduced coherence and phase synchrony indicate dysfunction in interregional cortical communication, reflecting loss of network integration necessary for cognitive coordination and control.

This work demonstrates that EEG spectral and coherence parameters can serve as objective markers of neurophysiological changes associated with alcohol dependence. These markers may be useful for qEEG-based diagnosis, disease progression monitoring, and treatment response assessment.

Fein G. and Allen J. (2005) studied EEG spectral characteristics in treatment-naive active alcoholics (TxNA) at rest, comparing them with healthy controls. Emphasis was placed on theta to high beta frequency ranges to determine whether spectral power differed in alcohol-dependent individuals without comorbid psychiatric diagnoses.

The study included 51 TxNA participants (actively drinking alcoholics without other psychiatric or substance disorders) and an age- and sex-matched control group. EEGs were recorded with eyes closed, followed by spectral power analysis in theta to high beta ranges at midline electrodes. Participant selection excluded any comorbid disorders to ensure that observed spectral features reflected alcohol dependence rather than other psychopathologies.

Key Results.

Increased Spectral Power Across Frequency Bands: TxNA participants exhibited significantly higher EEG power in frequency ranges from theta to high beta compared to controls, distinguishing actively drinking alcoholics in the absence of comorbid psychiatric diagnoses.

Frequency Band Differences: The magnitude and topographical distribution of differences varied across frequency bands, suggesting that different spectral generators are affected differently in alcoholic subjects.

Correlation with Alcohol Consumption: Within the TxNA group, EEG spectral power was inversely proportional to the duration and quantity of alcohol consumption (average/peak drinking measures). This indicates that heavier and longer-term alcohol use may reduce spectral power, despite initially elevated levels in active drinkers.

Interpretation and Conclusions:

Elevated EEG spectral power in the theta–beta ranges in TxNA participants may reflect a predisposition to alcoholism, potentially related to disinhibited behavioral traits with a genetic component. Negative correlations of spectral power with alcohol consumption measures suggest that prolonged heavy intoxication may lead to decreased EEG power, possibly due to degenerative or adaptive neurophysiological changes. The study model proposes that in early stages, or in relatively young active drinkers, spectral activity increases as a risk trait, but with chronic abuse, this effect may diminish or reverse.

Scientific and Clinical Significance:

The study highlights EEG spectral analysis as an informative biomarker of neurophysiological changes associated with alcoholism, even prior to treatment. These findings help distinguish toxic effects of alcohol from phenotypic risk traits, which is important for diagnosis, prognosis, and potential early interventions.

Colrain I. M., Turlington S., Baker F. C. (2009) conducted a comprehensive evaluation of chronic alcoholism's effects on sleep architecture and EEG spectral characteristics during sleep in men and women without major medical or psychiatric comorbidities. Special attention was given to slow-frequency EEG changes during sleep, which reflect sleep depth and quality.

Study Sample: 42 alcoholic patients (27 men) and 42 healthy controls (19 men). All participants underwent polysomnography (PSG), including an adaptation night followed by a main night with multi-channel scalp EEG recording. Analyses included spectral EEG analysis and sleep architecture assessment, with age as a covariate.

Key Results:

1. **Sleep Architecture Changes:** Alcoholic participants showed reduced slow-wave sleep (SWS) duration, indicating shallower sleep. There were increased

proportions of Stage 1 and REM sleep, reflecting lighter and more fragmented sleep compared to controls.

2. **EEG Spectral Changes:** During NREM sleep, alcoholics had significantly reduced slow-wave activity (0.3–4 Hz) and theta power (4–6 Hz) compared to controls. Spectral power reductions spanned the slow spectrum down to delta frequencies, particularly in frontal cortical regions. No differences were observed during REM sleep, indicating some REM spectral characteristics remain resilient to alcoholism.
3. **Gender Differences:** Women generally had higher slow-wave and theta activity than men; however, no significant gender × diagnosis interactions were found, indicating similar effects of alcoholism across sexes.

Interpretation: Reduced SWS and theta power during sleep in chronic alcoholics reflect impaired deep sleep stages, likely due to cortical and subcortical alterations from prolonged alcohol exposure. Altered sleep architecture and spectral changes serve as objective neurophysiological markers of CNS effects of alcoholism, persisting even during long-term remission or abstinence.

Scientific and Clinical Significance: Sleep EEG spectral analysis is a sensitive tool for detecting persistent brain function changes in alcoholism. Altered slow-wave parameters may predict recovery quality and relapse risk, as deep sleep disruption impacts cognition, emotional regulation, and overall recovery.

Winterer G., Enoch M.A., White K.V., et al. (2003) aimed to identify characteristic EEG phenotypes of alcoholism, specifically changes in EEG coherence, and evaluate whether these reflect endophenotypic features associated with depressive traits or symptoms. EEG coherence reflects functional synchronization of cortical networks and serves as a potential neurophysiological marker of alcoholism vulnerability.

Participants: 10 non-abstinent alcoholics, 16 long-term abstinent alcoholics (mean remission 7.7 ± 5.8 years), and 25 healthy controls. EEG was recorded at rest. Anxiety and depression levels were assessed using standardized questionnaires. Analysis included spectral power and coherence between EEG channels across frequency bands, focusing on alpha (8–12 Hz) and beta (13–30 Hz) ranges.

Key Results:

EEG Spectral Power: No statistically significant intergroup differences were found, though numerical differences aligned with previous data.

EEG Coherence: Alcoholics exhibited significantly increased coherence between bilateral and intrahemispheric posterior regions in alpha and beta bands, particularly when depressive symptoms were included as a covariate. Increased coherence was present in both actively drinking and long-term abstinent patients, suggesting a stable endophenotype independent of current alcohol consumption.

Relationship with Depression: Higher depressive symptom levels amplified coherence differences between alcoholics and controls, indicating that depressive traits enhance cortical rhythm synchronization in alcoholics.

Interpretation: EEG coherence reflects functional synchronization across cortical regions. Increased alpha- and beta-band coherence may indicate heightened cortical interconnectivity in alcoholics, potentially linked to endophenotypic features increasing vulnerability to alcoholism. Including depressive symptoms as a covariate suggests interaction between depressive traits and EEG phenotypes, reflecting involvement of GABAergic and/or glutamatergic neurotransmission in alcoholism and depression.

Scientific and Clinical Significance: Elevated EEG coherence can serve as an objective endophenotypic marker for alcoholism, especially when combined with depressive traits. Findings deepen understanding of neurophysiological correlates of alcoholism and depression, and may aid in developing biological risk markers, predicting treatment outcomes, and guiding research on mechanisms of dependence and comorbidity with affective disorders.

Table 11. Summary of Key EEG Features in Alcoholism

Feature	Observation in Alcoholics	Frequency/Region	Clinical/Scientific Significance
Spectral Power	Reduced in chronic alcoholics; elevated in TxNA	Theta–Beta (active drinkers); Delta–Theta (sleep)	Risk marker vs. toxic effect; reflects neural dysregulation
Coherence	Increased in posterior alpha/beta; persists in abstinence	Bilateral/intrahemispheric posterior	Endophenotype; linked with depressive traits; network synchronization
Phase Synchrony	Reduced in alpha2/beta1	Frontal/Central/Parietal	Reflects disrupted interregional coordination
Sleep Architecture	Reduced SWS; increased Stage 1 & REM	Frontal/Global	Marker of deep sleep disruption; prognostic for recovery

7.2. Electroencephalographic Changes in Schizophrenia

Electroencephalographic (EEG) alterations in schizophrenia represent an important research target, as they can be utilized for diagnosis, assessment of patient status, and monitoring of treatment efficacy. Studies indicate that patients with schizophrenia exhibit various abnormalities in brain activity, including changes in coherence, reduced alpha- and beta-band activity, and disrupted interactions among different brain regions.

Schizophrenia remains one of the most significant challenges in psychiatry. Despite over a century of study, the nature of the disorder remains unclear, and its classification and modern diagnostic frameworks are largely conventional. Currently, psychiatrists lack objective methods to detect brain abnormalities responsible for psychiatric symptoms, complicating timely and accurate diagnosis.

Accordingly, the search for biomarkers of schizophrenia, particularly those related to central nervous system activity, is of high relevance. Neurophysiological diagnostic methods, especially EEG, most fully reflect the morphofunctional state of the CNS underlying the mechanisms of mental activity.

Key Studies on EEG in Schizophrenia

Roschke & Cohen (1997) investigated EEG anomalies in schizophrenia and their relationship to clinical manifestations. Findings included reduced alpha activity

and alterations in the theta band, correlating with impaired cognitive and psychosocial functioning.

Jandl et al. (2010) studied EEG coherence in schizophrenia, reporting decreased coherence in high-frequency bands, reflecting disrupted interhemispheric and interregional interactions.

Moran et al. (2010) reviewed typical EEG changes in schizophrenia, including alpha deficits and increased theta activity, discussing potential clinical applications of EEG for diagnostic and monitoring purposes.

Perry et al. (2001) analyzed theta- and alpha-band activity in relation to cognitive deficits, concluding that dysfunction in these bands may underlie attention and memory impairments in schizophrenia.

Clementz et al. (2006) examined the effects of antipsychotic medications on EEG, showing that antidepressants and antipsychotics can modulate alpha- and beta-band activity, providing a potential measure of treatment efficacy.

Muthukumaraswamy et al. (2013) explored changes in oscillatory neural networks, explaining how imbalances across alpha, beta, and theta frequencies affect cognition, perception, and other mental functions in schizophrenia.

Chavez et al. (2009) correlated EEG alterations, particularly reduced alpha and increased theta activity, with cognitive deficits, highlighting EEG's utility in monitoring treatment response.

Uhlhaas et al. (2006) demonstrated impaired neuronal synchrony in the visual cortex, linking disrupted oscillatory coordination to perceptual and cognitive deficits.

General Conclusions from the Literature

1. EEG abnormalities in schizophrenia typically include reduced alpha activity and increased theta activity, associated with cognitive and psychosocial impairments.

2. Decreased EEG coherence between brain regions is an important marker, reflecting disrupted interregional connectivity.
3. Cognitive functions such as attention, memory, and perception are closely linked to EEG c
4. hanges, which can predict functional deficits.
5. EEG alterations reflect neuronal and cortical rhythm dysregulation but are not diagnostic in isolation; clinical assessment remains primary.

Main EEG Features in Schizophrenia

1. Frequency Spectrum Changes

Increased slow rhythms (δ and θ): Commonly observed in resting-state schizophrenia, indicating generalized cortical network dysfunction.

Reduced α- and β-activity: Particularly in frontal and temporo-parietal regions, correlating with cognitive deficits and attentional impairments.

γ-band anomalies: High-frequency activity changes are reported, but findings vary depending on methodology and medication status.

These alterations reflect impaired functional integration of the cerebral cortex.

2. Reactivity and Coherence

Reduced EEG reactivity: Patients show diminished rhythm changes in response to external stimuli (e.g., visual stimulation, attention tasks).

Impaired interregional coherence: Reduced synchronization across cortical regions indicates deficits in inter-cortical connectivity.

These effects are present even at the first psychotic episode, reflecting network integration deficits.

3. Sleep EEG Patterns

Schizophrenia is associated with reduced slow-wave activity and disrupted sleep architecture, which correlate with cognitive deficits and symptom severity.

Recent Comprehensive Analysis – "EEG Multiverse"

Gordillo et al. (2022) conducted a detailed study applying multiple analytical approaches to EEG in schizophrenia, termed the "EEG multiverse." The goal was to determine which EEG aspects truly reflect the neurophysiological characteristics of schizophrenia and how these features relate to one another.

Traditional EEG studies rely on a limited set of measures (e.g., power in specific frequency bands or microstate dynamics), which show differences between patients and controls. However, it is unclear to what extent these measures capture overlapping versus distinct aspects of pathophysiology.

The study aimed to:

1. Analyze a broad spectrum of EEG features rather than isolated parameters.
2. Examine interrelations among these features.
3. Identify features that meaningfully characterize EEG in schizophrenia.

Methods and Sample:

Resting-state EEG from 121 patients with schizophrenia and 75 healthy controls.

Feature extraction employed multiple signal processing methods (time-domain, frequency-domain, nonlinear, connectivity, etc.), resulting in **194 EEG features**, including temporal parameters, spectral measures, connectivity indices, and nonlinear dynamic characteristics.

As a result of the study, it was found that **69 out of 194 EEG features (~36%) showed statistically significant differences between patients and controls**, indicating that most of these features capture characteristics associated with the disorder.

However, correlations between these significant features were very low, meaning that different measures reflect distinct, possibly independent aspects of schizophrenia neurophysiology.

The authors discuss that these results indicate **high heterogeneity of EEG patterns in schizophrenia**, and that different analytical methods capture different aspects of the pathology.

They propose a **reconsideration of EEG analysis approaches**: instead of seeking a single universal biomarker for schizophrenia, it is more appropriate to consider the observed EEG "multiverse," where different signal properties reflect different mechanisms of dysfunction. Combining **"deep" and "shallow" analytical methods** may provide a more comprehensive understanding of the disorder's pathophysiology.

This study demonstrates that EEG analysis is **complex and multidimensional**; it emphasizes that different EEG aspects do not necessarily correlate, even if they distinguish patients from healthy controls, and it suggests new directions for developing diagnostic algorithms and neurophysiological models of schizophrenia.

Frequency and Spatial Characteristics of EEG in Paranoid Schizophrenia

Bochkaryov, V. K., Kirenskaya, A. V., Tkachenko, A. A., et al. (2015) studied the frequency and spatial characteristics of EEG in patients with paranoid schizophrenia, aiming to identify relationships between spectral EEG parameters and clinical manifestations (positive vs. negative symptoms) in resting-state conditions.

Sample: 35 unmedicated patients with paranoid schizophrenia and 19 healthy male controls of comparable age.

EEG recordings: eyes-closed wakefulness, 19 electrodes according to the international 10–20 system.

Spectral analysis: fast Fourier transform in the 1–70 Hz range, divided into 12 independent frequency bands (δ, θ, α, β, and γ).

Statistical analysis: ANOVA and correlations between EEG frequency characteristics and clinical scales (PANSS — Positive and Negative Syndrome Scale).

Frequency Changes:

Patients exhibited **increased power in high-frequency bands (β3, β4, γ1, γ2)**, especially those with predominant negative symptoms.

Reduced power in mid-frequency rhythms (θ, α) in convexital regions compared to controls.

Spatial Features:

δ-rhythm increase: mainly in frontal, occipital, and posterior-temporal regions.

β- and γ-rhythm increase: diffuse, but with hemispheric lateralization, especially in the negative symptom group.

Clinical Correlations:

Negative symptoms correlated with generalized enhancement of δ-, β-, and γ-activity, suggesting severe cortical dysfunction.

Positive/psychotic symptoms (e.g., delusions with thought insertion) were associated with localized β-range changes in the left frontal cortex, while paranoid syndrome correlated with β alterations in right hemisphere cortical zones.

This work highlights the importance of **spectral EEG parameters, including high frequencies (>20 Hz),** as reflections of neurophysiological changes in schizophrenia. It demonstrates the significance of **spatial distribution of spectral changes** (frontal, central, temporal regions) in linking neural activity to specific psychopathological features and confirms that EEG frequency and spatial characteristics depend on the clinical symptom profile, carrying both diagnostic and pathophysiological relevance.

EEG Coherence and Reactivity in First-Episode Schizophrenia

Alfimova, M. V., Melnikova, T. S., Lapin, I. A. (2010) examined EEG coherence and reactivity during psychophysiological tasks in first-episode schizophrenia. The main aim was to determine the characteristics of **synchronization and functional connectivity between cortical areas**, as well as their dynamics when transitioning from passive states to active tasks.

Concepts:

EEG coherence: quantitative measure of synchrony between two cortical regions, reflecting the degree of functional connectivity in specific frequency bands. High coherence indicates strong synchronization; low coherence indicates reduced connectivity.

EEG reactivity: the brain's ability to modulate spectral characteristics and coherent connections in response to external stimuli or psychophysiological tasks (e.g., photostimulation, cognitive load).

Key Findings:

Resting-state coherence: First-episode patients exhibited **increased coherence** in certain frequency bands (especially slow waves), suggesting excessive neural network synchronization and impaired integrative brain function.

Intrahemispheric coherence was increased, particularly in posterior regions.

Interhemispheric coherence was also elevated, indicating reduced lateralization.

Reactivity to stimulation: During photic stimulation with flickering light, patients showed **blunted increases in coherence and evoked activity**, particularly in β- and γ-bands, compared to controls. This suggests impaired functional cortical reorganization in response to active tasks.

Interpretation:

Elevated resting coherence may reflect abnormally tight functional links between cortical zones, consistent with impaired neuronal integration in schizophrenia.

Reduced adaptive reactivity indicates decreased flexibility of neural networks and their ability to reorganize in response to external stimuli.

These findings demonstrate **differentiated dynamics of neural connectivity even at early disease stages**, with potential diagnostic and pathophysiological significance.

This study underscores the role of **functional synchronization** in schizophrenia pathogenesis and suggests that coherence and reactivity abnormalities may serve as **biophysical markers for diagnosis and monitoring of disease progression**.

EEG and Sleep in Schizophrenia

Schizophrenia is accompanied by disturbances in perception, cognitive function, and emotional regulation. One particularly relevant aspect is **sleep disruption**, reflected in EEG patterns.

Studies indicate abnormalities in **sleep stages**, including REM sleep disturbances, reduced sleep depth, and alterations in **alpha and theta rhythms**, which may serve as **disease indicators or progression markers**.

1. Sleep Phase Disturbances

Studies show that individuals with schizophrenia often experience **increased time in REM sleep** and **reduced sleep depth (NREM)**, which may be associated with impairments in memory, perception, and cognitive functioning. For example, a large study found a **decrease in low-frequency wave power during deep sleep**, which serves as a marker of cognitive deficits in schizophrenia patients (Cajochen et al., 2000).

2. Alpha and Theta Rhythm Abnormalities

These changes are particularly noticeable during **transitional sleep phases**. During drowsiness or the transition from wakefulness to sleep, patients with schizophrenia frequently show **alterations in alpha and theta rhythms**, which may indicate difficulties in regulating wake-sleep states. These abnormalities can also be associated with psychotic symptoms and perceptual disturbances (Mohn et al., 2005).

3. Impact of Schizophrenia on Sleep Structure and Function

An important aspect is understanding how **sleep disruption affects schizophrenia symptoms**. Research indicates that poor sleep quality can significantly impair cognitive function and emotional regulation, potentially exacerbating symptoms such as hallucinations and delusions (Tam et al., 2012).

4. Potential Biomarkers

Some studies suggest that **sleep EEG patterns may serve as biomarkers** for diagnosing or monitoring schizophrenia. Particular attention is given to correlations between EEG patterns and psychopathological manifestations. For example, **theta-range changes during REM and NREM sleep** may relate to specific aspects of cognitive deficits and emotional lability in schizophrenia (Keshavan et al., 2011).

5. Treatment and Symptom Modulation

Understanding how **sleep disturbances interact with psychopathological symptoms** is important for developing effective interventions. Restoring normal sleep patterns and using medications aimed at improving sleep structure can be part of a comprehensive treatment plan to enhance cognitive functioning and reduce psychotic symptoms.

7.2.1. Quantitative EEG (qEEG) in Psychiatry

Quantitative EEG (qEEG) is a method for analyzing and interpreting brain activity based on electrical signal measurements. In recent decades, qEEG has increasingly been used in psychiatry to study disorders such as **schizophrenia and depression**, which share some neurophysiological features while also displaying distinct patterns. qEEG research plays a crucial role in **diagnosis, monitoring, and treatment** of these disorders.

1. Schizophrenia and qEEG

Schizophrenia is characterized by **significant disturbances in perception, thinking, and emotion**. In schizophrenia, qEEG is used to detect abnormalities in brain rhythms that may reflect cognitive deficits, changes in consciousness, and altered responsiveness to external stimuli. Common findings in schizophrenia patients include:

Altered alpha and theta activity: particularly increased theta power in brain regions responsible for attention and perception.

Reduced beta activity: associated with cognitive and attentional deficits.

Hemis

pheric asymmetry: especially in frontal and parietal regions, suggesting disruptions in neural networks involved in information processing.

2. Depression and qEEG

Depression is a common psychiatric disorder accompanied by changes in brain activity. qEEG in depression often shows:

Reduced alpha activity (particularly in frontal regions), linked to mood disturbances and decreased activity in networks supporting positive affect.

Increased theta power, reflecting depressive symptoms such as apathy and slowed cognitive processing.

Enhanced slow-wave (delta and theta) power in posterior regions, indicative of decreased motivation and depressive dysfunction.

3. Comparative Analysis of Schizophrenia and Depression via qEEG

A key aspect is the **differentiation of EEG patterns** between schizophrenia and depression. Despite some shared features, such as increased theta activity, **distinct localization and frequency characteristics** allow differentiation:

Schizophrenia: more pronounced beta abnormalities and hemispheric asymmetry.

Depression: greater alpha reduction, especially in frontal regions.

4. Clinical Applications of qEEG

qEEG can be a valuable tool for **diagnosis, treatment monitoring, and patient management**, including:

Assessing neurophysiological changes associated with symptoms.

Predicting responses to pharmacological or psychotherapeutic interventions.

Developing personalized treatments, including neurofeedback.

5. Research Potential

Beyond clinical applications, qEEG is actively used to **study neurobiological mechanisms** of schizophrenia and depression. It allows precise detection of neuronal activity changes, contributing to a better understanding of pathogenesis and to the development of novel therapeutic approaches.

Table 12a Brief Table of EEG Changes in Schizophrenia

Indicator	Features in Schizophrenia
δ rhythm (Delta)	Increased power
θ rhythm (Theta)	Increased at rest
α rhythm (Alpha)	Decreased power
β/γ rhythms (Beta/Gamma)	Altered power and reactivity
Coherence	Reduced between brain regions
Reactivity	Impaired response to external stimuli
Sleep patterns	Altered slow-wave spectrum

Summary

EEG in schizophrenia is characterized by a wide range of abnormalities—from changes in power across different frequency bands to disrupted synchrony and impaired response to stimuli. These features reflect disturbances in the functional organization of the brain associated with the clinical symptoms of the disorder.
Antipsychotic medications influence EEG patterns, which can also be used to monitor treatment efficacy.

These studies highlight the importance of EEG as a tool for diagnosis, understanding the neurophysiological mechanisms of schizophrenia, and monitoring therapy.

7.2.2. Study of EEG Features in Schizophrenia Using Computerized Electroencephalography

EEG research has shown promise in detecting brain lesions, automatically identifying epileptic seizures, early diagnosis of mild cognitive impairments in Alzheimer's disease, and schizophrenia. Spectral analysis of EEG in schizophrenia demonstrates increased delta activity, elevated fast beta rhythms, and reduced alpha activity.

However, the neurodynamic mechanisms of schizophrenia have rarely been studied using periodometric EEG mapping analysis, despite this computerized EEG method being one of the most informative and promising approaches for identifying pathognomonic EEG features of the disorder.

Interhemispheric relationships in endogenous psychoses are of particular interest, as studies report contradictory findings. Schizophrenia pathogenesis is believed to involve multiple genes affecting brain structure development and interregional cortical connectivity. EEG remains a key method for assessing these connections.

Spectral analysis shows increased delta activity, high fast beta activity, and reduced alpha frequency (Kirdan, 1996; Kudlaev, 2000; Nosov, 1995; Strelets et al., 2004, 2006; Yuryeva & Nosov, 1995; Karson et al., 1988).

Studies report reduced interhemispheric asymmetry in schizophrenia, especially in slow-frequency bands, compared to healthy controls (Nikiforov & Bochkarev, 1991). Other findings suggest minimal motor asymmetry in healthy individuals and maximal in schizophrenia patients (Davtyan & Ostretsov, 1996).

EEG allows the assessment of functional relationships between cortical areas, and periodometric analysis can evaluate the amplitude, frequency, and duration indices of EEG rhythms. Early studies in healthy subjects have shown regression relationships between homologous EEG rhythm parameters across different leads (Lobasyuk & Bodelan, 2016). Comparing the architecture of these interactions in healthy and schizophrenia subjects is of interest.

Study Objective:

To investigate EEG rhythm amplitude, frequency, interhemispheric asymmetry, and relationships between rhythm parameters using periodometric and multiple regression analyses.

Materials and Methods:

Main group: 58 schizophrenia patients (ICD-10 F20.8), age 20–69, mean 39 years

Control group: 34 healthy participants, age 16–66, mean 34 years

EEG recorded at rest with eyes closed, using 16 cortical zones (10–20 system)

Bipolar ring montage; bandwidth 0.5–35 Hz, sampling rate 500 Hz

Periodometric analysis performed in five frequency bands: δ 0.5–4 Hz, θ 4–8 Hz, α 8–13 Hz, β1 13–20 Hz, β2 20–32 Hz

Own Research Results:

Due to heterogeneity in schizophrenia, cluster analysis of EEG amplitudes was performed. The control group did not cluster; the main group split into two subgroups (42 and 17 participants). The smaller subgroup (17) showed higher synchronization and EEG amplitudes (~1.3× higher). Mahalanobis distance = 20.47 ($P < 0.000001$). The 42-person subgroup was selected for further analysis.

Statistical analysis of EEG rhythm amplitudes (Table 13) showed that schizophrenia patients had lower amplitudes than healthy controls (1.13–1.28× lower). The greatest decrease was in low beta rhythms in parieto-occipital leads of both hemispheres.

Table 13. *Statistically Significant Amplitude Ratio Coefficients of EEG Rhythms in Patients with Schizophrenia Compared to the Control Group*

Leads	Delta (0.5–4 Hz)	Theta (4–8 Hz)	Alpha (8–13 Hz)	Beta-Low (13–20 Hz)	Beta-High (20–32 Hz)
F3–C3	-1.10	-1.16	-1.16	-1.18	—
F4–C4	—	—	-1.19	-1.14	-1.14
F7–T3	—	-1.12	-1.21	-1.21	-1.24
F8–T4	-1.11	-1.16	-1.25	-1.28	-1.19
P3–O1	—	-1.30	-1.38	-1.41	-1.39
P4–O2	—	-1.32	-1.43	-1.46	-1.45
T4–T6	—	-1.22	—	-1.13	-1.25
C3–P3	—	-1.17	-1.20	—	—
C4–P4	-1.13	-1.19	-1.24	-1.18	-1.13
T5–O1	—	-1.33	-1.27	-1.22	-1.18
T6–O2	—	-1.33	-1.27	-1.22	-1.18
Average	-1.13	-1.28	-1.26	-1.21	-1.16

Changes in EEG Rhythm Frequencies The reductions in EEG rhythm frequencies were observed mainly in the theta range (Table 14).

Table 14. *Statistically Significant Frequency Ratio Coefficients of EEG Rhythms in Patients with Schizophrenia Compared to the Control Group*

Electrode Pair	Delta Rhythm	Theta Rhythm	Alpha Rhythm	Beta-LF Rhythm	Beta-HF Rhythm
F8-T4		-1.02			
P3-O1		-1.04			
P4-O2		-1.05			
T3-T5		-1.04			
T5-O1		-1.03	-1.02		-1.04
T6-O2		-1.04			

Table 15. *Statistically Significant Duration Index Ratios of EEG Rhythms in Patients with Schizophrenia Compared to the Control Group*

Electrode Pair	Delta Rhythm	Theta Rhythm	Alpha Rhythm	Beta-LF Rhythm	Beta-HF Rhythm
FP2-F8	1.29				
F3-C3				-1.33	
F4-C4					-1.65
F7-T3					
F8-T4	1.65		-1.25	-1.40	
P3-O1	2.33		-1.17	-1.39	
P4-O2	1.83		-1.25	-1.32	
T4-T6	1.67		-1.22		
C3-P3					
C4-P4		1.20			
T5-O1					
T6-O2	1.73	1.27			

*Notes: Values >1 indicate **increased amplitude** compared to controls.*

*Values <1 (negative ratios) indicate **decreased amplitude** compared to controls.*

Average FMAP values across all EEG leads in healthy subjects were negative in the delta, theta, and alpha ranges, and positive in the beta ranges (Table 16, Fig. 89). The average FMAP values in patients with schizophrenia differed from those in healthy controls.

In the delta range, the negativity of FMAP in patients was reduced compared to controls.

In the theta and alpha ranges, FMAP values in patients were inverted and became positive.

In the beta ranges, the positivity of FMAP in patients was higher than in controls.

Table 16. *FMAP coefficients in control and schizophrenia groups*

ead	Delta Rhythm	Theta Rhythm	Alpha Rhythm	Beta-Low Rhythm	Beta-High Rhythm
	Control	**Schizophrenia**	**Control**	**Schizophrenia**	**Control**
FP-F	-2.50	-1.21	-0.32	0.12	-2.30
FP-F	-3.14	0.16	-3.63	-0.21	-4.08
F-C	-1.88	-5.53	0.87	-2.37	-0.78
F-T	-0.41	1.97	-1.56	0.32	1.09
P-O	6.90	4.35	1.97	2.66	-1.87
T-T	-10.38	-1.38	-6.84	1.42	-2.44
C-R	-3.17	-0.49	-2.40	-0.63	-2.88
T-O	0.00	0.00	0.00	0.00	0.00
Average	-1.82	-0.27	-1.49	0.16	-1.66

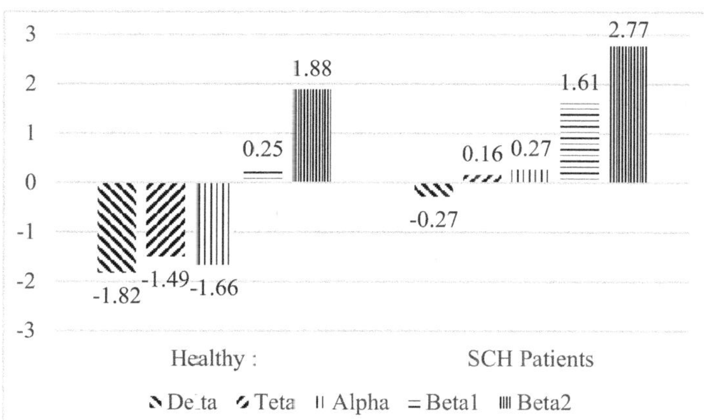

Figure 89. *FMPA Values in Healthy and SCH Patients*

In the multiple regression and correlation analysis of interactions between EEG r hythm amplitudes, the total number of statistically significant regression coefficients in the **Healthy** and **SCH Patients** groups differed slightly: 254 and 251, respectively (Table 17).

In the delta and theta ranges, the number of regression coefficients was higher in the **Healthy** group than in the **SCH Patients** group, while in the alpha, beta-low, and beta-high ranges, it was lower.

The number of two-dimensional correlation coefficients between amplitudes of corresponding rhythms was also higher in the **Healthy** group than in the **SCH Patients** group. Additionally, the magnitude of these coefficients in the **Healthy** group was greater than in the **SCH Patients** group (Table 17).

Table 17. *Statistically Significant Regression and Correlation Coefficients Between EEG Rhythm Amplitudes*

EEG Rhythms	**Regressions**		**Correlations**		**Correlation Coefficient Values**	
	Healthy (H)	SCH Patients (SCH)	Healthy (H)	SCH Patients (SCH)	Healthy (H)	SCH Patients (SCH)
Delta	75	38	93	19	0.59	0.44
Theta	61	42	102	47	0.64	0.48
Alpha	56	79	95	34	0.68	0.47
Beta-Low	31	56	75	48	0.57	0.45
Beta-High	31	36	58	53	0.56	0.46
Total	254	251	423	201	—	—

During multiple regression and correlation analysis of the interrelations of EEG rhythm frequencies, the total number of statistically significant regression coefficients and two-dimensional correlation coefficients was higher in the control group compared to the patient group.

Table 18. Statistically Significant Regression and Correlation Coefficients Between EEG Rhythm Frequency Measures

EEG Rhythms	Regressions		Correlations		Correlation Values	
	Healthy (H)	SCH Patients (SCH)	Healthy (H)	SCH Patients (SCH)	Healthy (H)	SCH Patients (SCH)
Delta	32	40	44	28	0.50	0.52
Theta	34	44	84	88	0.46	0.64
Alpha	29	10	29	71	0.54	0.58
Beta-Low	32	6	22	9	0.57	0.40
Beta-High	38	48	49	5	0.54	0.59
Total	165	148	228	201	—	—

Discussion

The observed decrease in EEG rhythm amplitudes in patients with schizophrenia, i.e., increased desynchronization compared to the control group, was accompanied by a reduction in the number of multiple regression coefficients in the delta and theta bands between the amplitudes of homologous rhythms, and an increase in the alpha and both beta bands. The number of two-dimensional correlation coefficients between EEG rhythm amplitudes in patients with schizophrenia was lower than in the control group. According to the views of the Rusinov school (19), an increase in the number of correlations between different EEG components reflects an overall increase in cortical tone, while a decrease indicates a reduction in this tone.

A seemingly unusual situation arises in which the reduction in EEG rhythm amplitudes, indicating increased desynchronization and, consequently, CNS activation, is accompanied by a decrease in two-dimensional correlation coefficients between different EEG components. The only type of relationship measured by the correlation coefficient is linear (direct), while multiple regression coefficients account for both linear and nonlinear relationships.

The observed reduction in correlation coefficients between EEG rhythm amplitudes corresponds to the coherence reduction reported by several researchers in schizophrenia compared to normal controls (Strelets V.B., Garakh Zh.V., Norman R.M., Malla A.K., 1997; Tauscher J., Fischer P., 1998; Winterer G., Egan M.F., Rödler T., Hyde T., Coppola R., Weinberger D.R., 2001).

However, a decrease in the number of two-dimensional correlation and multiple regression coefficients was observed only in the delta and theta bands. Therefore, it can be confidently stated that EEG coherence in the delta and theta bands in patients with schizophrenia is lower than in healthy individuals.

In the alpha and both beta bands, the number of correlation links between EEG rhythm amplitude indicators in patients with schizophrenia was lower than in the control group, whereas the number of multiple regression coefficients was higher. This may indicate that coherence in the alpha and beta bands is increased in schizophrenia compared to normal, but the relationships between alpha and beta components are realized through nonlinear functions. Evidence for increased coherence in schizophrenia compared to controls is presented in several studies (Mann K., Maier W., Franke P., Röschke J., Gänsicke M., 1997; Merrin E.L., Floyd T.C., Fein G., 1989; Nagase Y., Okubo Y., Matsuura M., Kojima T., Torua M., 1992).

These results suggest that using the correlation coefficient alone to assess EEG synchrony may be insufficient. Combining two-dimensional correlation calculations with multiple regression analysis provides a more accurate assessment of the oriented interactions between CNS neuronal elements based on EEG data.

The negativity of FMPA in the delta rhythm band in patients with schizophrenia was reduced compared to controls, while in the theta and alpha bands, FMPA inverted and became positive. In the beta bands, FMPA positivity in patients was greater than in healthy subjects (Nosov S.G., 1995). These results indicate activation of the right hemisphere relative to the left in patients with schizophrenia, possibly due to reduced activating influence from the reticular formation of the midbrain (Lobasyuk B.A., 2005).

Duration indices in the delta and theta bands in patients with schizophrenia were increased compared to healthy subjects, while duration indices of alpha and beta rhythms were decreased.

Previously, we conceptualized a unit of mental activity as a psychophysiological construct formed based on multiple regression analysis of EEG indicators and the anxiety index from the Luscher test (Bitensky V.S., Lobasyuk B.A., Bodelan M.I., *Neuropsychology and Neuropsychiatry*). It was shown that in mentally healthy individuals, regression relationships exist between psychological test scores (Benton Test, pictogram, and the Minnesota Multiphasic

Personality Inventory – MMPI), whereas in mentally ill individuals, such relationships are either minimal or absent (Lobasyuk B.A., Primachek I.O , Savostin A.P., Aimedov K.V.). This result can be interpreted as evidence that in mentally ill patients, due to both illness and psychotropic treatment, the chains of mental acts and states are disrupted, leading to psychological disintegration.

We hypothesize that the decrease in EEG rhythm amplitudes, coherence disturbances, increased duration indices in the delta and theta bands, and decreased duration indices in the alpha and beta bands observed in patients with schizophrenia are the neurophysiological basis of higher nervous (mental) activity impairments in these patients.

Key EEG Changes in Schizophrenia:

1. **Alpha activity deficit:** Patients with schizophrenia often show reduced alpha activity, indicating impaired normal brain relaxation and increased baseline cortical activity.
2. **Increased theta activity:** Elevated theta activity in some patients is associated with cognitive and attention deficits.
3. **Reduced coherence:** Lower EEG coherence between brain regions may reflect impaired connectivity and integration.
4. **Beta rhythm disturbances:** Increased or decreased beta activity may correlate with cognitive dysfunction and motor disturbances.
5. **Frontal dysfunction:** Changes in the frontal cortex, associated with planning, attention, and executive functions, are often detected on EEG.

Spectral and Spatial Features of EEG in Schizophrenic Disorders:

Spectral Features:

Increased theta power (Schulman J.J., Cancro R., Lowe S., Lu F., Walton K.D., Llinas R.R., 2011)

Low alpha rhythm (Schulman J.J., Cancro R., Lowe S., Lu F., Walton K.D., Llinas R.R., 2011)

Decreased beta power (Strelets V.B., Magomedov R.A., Garakh Zh.V., Novototsky-Vlasov V.Y., 2004)

Spatial Features:

Localization in medial ventral prefrontal cortex and temporal lobe (Schulman J.J., Cancro R., Lowe S., Lu F., Walton K.D., Llinas R.R., 2011; Basar-Eroglu C., Schmiedt-Fehr C., Marbach S., Brand A., Mathes B., 2008)

Sources in various brain areas (Schulman J.J., Cancro R., Lowe S., Lu F., Walton K.D., Llinas R.R., 2011)

Alpha and beta power reduction prominent in frontal regions (Knyazeva M.G., Jalili M., Meuli R., Hasler M., De Feo O., Do K.Q., 2008)

Coherence:

High intra- and inter-hemispheric coherence (Melnikova T.S., Lapin I.A., Sarkisyan V.V., 2009)

Reduced frontal coherence and impaired synchronization (Strelets V.B., Magomedov R.A., Garakh Zh.V., Novototsky-Vlasov V.Y., 2004)

Decreased gamma activity and weakened or absent interhemispheric gamma connections (Schulman J.J., Cancro R., Lowe S., Lu F., Walton K.D., Llinas R.R., 2011; Kirenskaya A.V., 2006)

7.3. Analysis of Changes in Electrogenesis in Intellectual Disability Using Computer Electroencephalography

Intellectual disability is a group of various hereditary, congenital, or early-acquired conditions characterized by general mental underdevelopment. According to ICD-10, intellectual disability is a condition of arrested or incomplete development of the psyche, primarily characterized by impairments of abilities manifested during the developmental period and contributing to the overall level of intelligence, including cognitive, speech, motor, and social abilities. In ICD-10, intellectual disability is coded under section F7 (F70–F79).

The term “intellectual disability” refers to a persistent reduction in cognitive activity caused by organic damage to the central nervous system (Bely, 1989; Bryzgalova & Naidanova, 2014).

Neurophysiological diagnostics, particularly electroencephalography (EEG), most adequately reflects the morpho-functional state of the central nervous system, which underlies the mechanisms of mental activity. The specific features of brain bioelectrical activity can be considered a key indicator determining the reduction in intellectual development and thus characterizing this condition (Isaev, 2003; Kostina, 2002; Smirnov, 2000; Farber & Alferova, 1972). This highlights the importance of identifying highly informative indicators of brain bioelectrical activity in children with intellectual impairments.

Electrophysiological examination of children with psychiatric disorders, although included in mandatory diagnostic procedures, is often limited to detecting epileptic activity. However, EEG contains far more information that is extremely useful for assessing a child's condition, determining age-appropriate EEG patterns, and diagnosing syndromic forms of mental disorders. This information is largely ignored in practice (Gorbachevskaya et al., 1996).

Significant advances in understanding the neurobiology of mental disorders require improvement in diagnostic methods, where quantitative EEG (QEEG) plays an important role. Age-based quantitative assessment of EEG parameters allows the establishment of normative values at any age, which can serve as benchmarks when children demonstrate developmental delays or other atypical and maladaptive behaviors.

A review of current literature on QEEG methods, used as an adjunct tool to identify children who differ from typical development—and in some cases from other clinical groups—demonstrates sufficient sensitivity and specificity to warrant consideration as a diagnostic instrument in developmental assessment (Cantr & Chabot, 2000). Moreover, QEEG indicators may help determine treatment effectiveness for underlying brain dysfunctions in pediatric disorders.

EEG research has shown promise in cases of brain injury, automatic detection of epileptic seizures, and early identification of mild cognitive impairment in Alzheimer's disease and schizophrenia patients.

Numerous studies report that resting-state EEG with closed eyes in subjects with learning disabilities most often shows excessive slow-wave activity, mainly in the theta frequency range (Alvarez et al., 1992; Colon et al., 1979; Fein et al., 1986; Fernández et al., 2002), and reduced alpha activity (Byring et al., 1991; Chabot et al., 2001; Colon et al., 1979) compared to typically developing children. Excessive delta activity has been reported in cases of severe disability (Harmony et al., 1990).

Spectral EEG analysis in intellectual disability reveals greater expression of slow frequencies at rest and immature activation patterns (Kiroy et al., 2002). Children with learning difficulties show higher absolute power in delta and theta frequencies in the left frontotemporal region and lower gamma power (Roca-Stappung & Fernández, 2017). The temporal cortex has been shown to play an important role in pervasive developmental disorders (Ünal et al., 2012). Frontal lobes, particularly prefrontal regions, are affected regardless of etiology in individuals with intellectual disability (Martín-Loeches et al., 2001).

Children aged 8.5–10 years with learning difficulties demonstrate pronounced slow-wave activity in anterior (especially left frontal) cortical regions. These findings are interpreted as reflecting delayed functional maturation of brain structures. A relationship has been found between reduced cognitive performance in younger schoolchildren with speech disorders and insufficient alpha activity formation (Peresleni & Rozhkova, 1996).

Cortico-subcortical immaturity is also suggested by increased theta power in occipital and central cortical areas in children with memory and attention deficits. In dementia, EEG background frequency shifts toward delta and theta ranges, with reduction or disappearance of central alpha frequency. Decreased alpha and beta activity has been reported in studies over the past decade. Alpha rhythm may serve as a diagnostic marker, as alpha frequency decreases to 6.0–8.0 Hz in mild dementia.

Another QEEG tool is coherence analysis (Coh), which assesses covariance of spectral measures between electrode pairs. Coherence reflects structural and functional connections between cortical regions and is used to quantify interhemispheric connectivity via the corpus callosum.

Leuchter et al. reported decreased coherence in dementia patients compared to controls. Besthorn et al. found reduced coherence in theta, alpha, and beta bands in central and frontal regions. Locatelli et al. observed reduced alpha coherence in the left temporoparietal-occipital area in dementia.

Low coherence positively correlates with IQ and serves as an IQ predictor. This suggests that the more complex and spatially differentiated the neural network, the lower the coherence between different neural pathways (Kanda et al., 2009).

Studies of EEG power and coherence at rest and during working memory tasks in patients with mild cognitive impairment revealed higher EEG power values compared to controls both at rest and during task performance, suggesting compensatory processes and disrupted normal cortical connectivity (Jiang, 2005).

In children with mild intellectual disability, resting-state coherence was higher than in controls (Gasser et al., 1987).

Patients with mental infantilism syndrome demonstrated EEG characteristics typical of earlier ontogenetic stages, including increased spectral power in delta, theta1, theta2, and alpha1 bands, and decreased interhemispheric coherence in frontal and temporal regions. During cognitive tasks, these patients showed insufficient differentiation of functional responses across frequency bands, topography, and lateralization, with predominance of theta2 shifts related to nonspecific activation processes. Auditory stimulation increased slow-wave power and interhemispheric coherence in frontal-temporal areas only in patients. These findings indicate delayed hemispheric specialization and impaired maturation of left-hemisphere neural networks, along with frontal-temporal dysfunction (Kirenskaya-Berus et al.).

However, neurodynamic mechanisms in intellectual disability have not been studied using periodometric EEG mapping analysis. This computer EEG method is considered highly informative (Nikiforov & Bochkarev, 1991) and promising for identifying pathognomonic EEG features in intellectual disability (Makushkin, 2001).

Sleep spindles, a hallmark of stage 2 sleep synchronization, are rhythmic, monomorphic waves between 10–14 Hz with maximal amplitude at the vertex. Abnormal sleep spindle phenomena are frequently observed in intellectually disabled children under five years of age (Spinosa & Garzo, 2007).

Studies examining the relationship between mean EEG frequency and IQ scores indicate a strong association between IQ and mean frequency asymmetries in homologous left and right brain regions, particularly in posterior areas (Giannitrapani, 1969).The issue of interhemispheric relationships in the clinical presentation of organic lesions of the central nervous system (CNS) is of considerable interest. However, conclusions drawn by different researchers on this matter are often contradictory.

At present, physiologists identify a direct relationship between the degree of hemispheric asymmetry and an individual's intellectual abilities. Motor skills, speech, thinking, memory, attention, and imagination have developed so intensively in humans largely due to the plasticity of the brain and the innate predisposition of the hemispheres toward functional specialization.

As a rule, the process of lateralization is not yet completed in preschool age. Studies on functional hemispheric asymmetry allow specialists to better understand the objective causes and mechanisms underlying cognitive impairments and deviations in children with developmental delay (Buduk-ool). Physiologists, neuropsychologists, and morphologists have obtained evidence indicating later maturation of left frontal lobe functions in children with developmental delay. Compared with typically developing peers, these children demonstrate delayed structural and functional maturation of the left hemisphere, particularly its higher cortical regions (Bely, 1982; Simernitskaya, 1982; Farber, 1979; Shevchenko, 1972).

In children with developmental delay, according to characteristics of evoked potentials, activation of the left hemisphere during right hemisphere stimulation is significantly weakened compared to normal values. This likely reflects reduced reactivity of the left hemisphere to information transmitted via callosal pathways from the right hemisphere. Analysis of interhemispheric transfer time during perception indicates delayed development of evoked potentials in right hemisphere structures when the left hemisphere is stimulated, reflecting slowed transmission of information from the left hemisphere to the right (Buduk-ool).

Dyslexia is a developmental disorder of unknown etiology characterized by primary cognitive impairments in the linguistic system. In children with dyslexia, a significant reduction of EEG power in the left hemisphere has been identified, and no left-hemisphere dominance was observed during phonological working memory tasks (Xu et al., 2014).

The term "intellectual disability" refers to a persistent reduction in cognitive activity due to organic damage to the central nervous system. Neurophysiological diagnostics, particularly electroencephalography (EEG), most adequately reflects the morpho-functional state of the CNS, which underlies the mechanisms of mental activity. The specific features of brain bioelectrical activity may be considered key indicators determining reduced intellectual development and thereby characterizing this condition.

Therefore, the search for markers of this condition—primarily those associated with CNS functioning—is highly relevant.

Aim

A comparative study using periodometric analysis of EEG parameters (amplitude, frequency, duration index) and interhemispheric asymmetry of EEG rhythm amplitudes.

Materials and Methods

Sixty-five patients diagnosed with intellectual disability (ICD-10 category F70) aged 16–18 years comprised the main group. These patients were undergoing inpatient examination and treatment at the Municipal Non-Commercial Enterprise "Odesa Regional Mental Health Center" of the Odesa Regional Council.

The control group consisted of 34 individuals aged 16–24 years.

EEG recording was performed in a state of relaxed wakefulness with eyes closed using a "Neuron-Spectrum-2" electroencephalograph with a sampling rate of 500 Hz and a 16-channel bipolar circular montage.

Electrodes were positioned according to the international 10–20% system in 16 cortical areas. EEG was recorded from frontal (F3, F4), central (C3, C4), parietal (P3, P4), occipital (O1, O2), anterior temporal (F7, F8), mid-temporal (T3, T4), and posterior temporal (T5, T6) regions. Odd numbers denote left hemisphere areas; even numbers denote right hemisphere areas.

The band-pass filter was set at 0.5–35 Hz with a sampling rate of 500 Hz.

Periodometric analysis was performed in five standard frequency bands:

Delta (0.5–4 Hz)

Theta (4–8 Hz)

Alpha (8–13 Hz)

Beta-1 (13–20 Hz)

Beta-2 (20–32 Hz)

The coefficient of functional EEG asymmetry by amplitude was calculated using the formula:

Uas = (L – R) / (L + R) × 100,

where L represents the left hemisphere value and R represents the right hemisphere value.

Thus, positive values indicated left-hemisphere amplitude predominance, and negative values indicated right-hemisphere predominance.

Differences between indicators were assessed using ratio coefficients (RC), calculated by dividing the larger value by the smaller one.

Results of the Study

Statistical analysis of EEG rhythm amplitude differences (Table 19) revealed that in intellectual disability, rhythm amplitudes were 1.16–1.78 times higher than in healthy controls.

The greatest increase was observed in theta rhythm amplitude in FP1–F7 and T3–T5 derivations of the left hemisphere. The largest increase in low-frequency beta activity was found in the T4–T6 derivation, while high-frequency beta rhythm showed the greatest increase in the F3–C3 derivation.

Table 19. Statistically significant ratio coefficients of EEG rhythm amplitudes in intellectual disability compared with the control group.

Derivations	Delta Rhythm	Theta Rhythm	Alpha Rhythm	Beta-LF Rhythm	Beta-HF Rhythm
C3–P3					
C4–P4					
F3–C3		1.48			1.52
F4–C4		1.39			
F7–T3	1.33	1.60		1.27	
F8–T4		1.42*		1.24*	1.34*
FP1–F3		1.37			1.24
FP1–F7		1.78*		1.34	
FP2–F4		1.40			
FP2–F8		1.41			
P3–O1		1.38*		1.22	1.44
P4–O2		1.33*			
T3–T5		1.53*	1.44*	1.36*	1.26*
T4–T6		1.41*	1.46*	1.44*	1.60*
T5–O1				1.17	1.16
T5–O2					
Mean		1.37	1.46	1.45	1.29

* *Statistically significant differences ($p < 0.05$)*

Decreases in EEG rhythm frequencies were observed in the delta range at the C3–P3 derivation; in the theta range at P4–O2, T4–T6, and T5–O1 derivations; and in the high-frequency beta range at C3–P3, F7–T3, and P3–O1 derivations.

An increase in delta rhythm frequency was observed at F8–T4, P3–O1, and T4–T6 derivations.

An increase in low-frequency beta rhythm was observed at F7–T3 and F8–T4 derivations.

Table 20. *Statistically significant ratio coefficients of EEG rhythm frequencies in intellectual disability compared with the control group.*

Derivations	Delta Rhythm	Theta Rhythm	Alpha Rhythm	Beta-LF Rhythm	Beta-HF Rhythm
C3–P3	-1.02			-1.06*	-1.24
C4–P4					
F3–C3					
F4–C4			1.02		
F7–T3				1.02*	-1.13
F8–T4	3.92		1.02*		
FP1–F3					
FP1–F7					
FP2–F4					
FP2–F8				1.01*	-1.03*
P3–O1	1.09*				
P4–O2		-1.02			
T3–T5				1.02*	
T4–T6	1.13*	-1.02		1.01*	
T5–O1		-1.03		1.01	
T5–O2					
Mean					

* *Statistically significant differences ($p < 0.05$)*

Duration indices in the delta, theta, and alpha EEG frequency bands in intellectual disability, compared with the control group, were increased, whereas the duration indices of beta rhythms were decreased (Table 21).

Table 21. *Statistically significant ratio coefficients of EEG rhythm duration indices in intellectual disability compared with the control group.*

Derivations	Delta Rhythm	Theta Rhythm	Alpha Rhythm	Beta-LF Rhythm	Beta-HF Rhythm
C3–P3	5.44*	3.32*	3.49*		-2.64*
C4–P4	5.13*	3.33*			3.82*
				-3.30*	
F3–C3	5.50*	3.46*	3.17*		1.86*
F4–C4	5.41*	3.65*	3.17*		-1.88*
F7–T3	2.35*	3.38*	2.40*	-1.19*	
F8–T4	3.99*	2.85*	2.41*	-1.22*	
FP1–F3	5.43*	3.71*	2.52*	-1.46*	
FP1–F7	1.96	3.51*	2.51*	-1.15	
FP2–F4	6.52*	3.83*	2.61*	-1.32*	-1.39*
FP2–F8		3.18*			3.01*
P3–O1	3.24*	3.11*	4.04*		-2.66*
P4–O2		2.93*	4.02*		-2.64*
T3–T5	3.25*	2.58*	2.76*		
T4–T6	3.82*	2.72*	2.94*		
T5–O1		2.33*	3.64*	1.14*	
T5–O2		2.53*	3.87*		-1.38*

* *Statistically significant differences ($p < 0.05$)*

The mean values of the Functional Interhemispheric Asymmetry Coefficient (FIA) across all derivations in healthy subjects were negative in the delta, theta, and alpha ranges, and positive in the beta ranges (Table 22, Fig. 91).

The mean FIA values across all derivations in intellectual disability differed from those observed in healthy individuals. In intellectual disability, the negativity of FIA in the delta, theta, and alpha ranges was reduced compared with the control group. In contrast, in the beta ranges, the positivity of FIA in patients was greater than that observed in healthy subjects (Table 22, Fig. 90).

Table 22. *Functional Interhemispheric Asymmetry (FIA) coefficients in the control group and in intellectual disability.*

Derivations	Delta Rhythm (Control)	Delta Rhythm (Main)	Theta Rhythm (Control)	Theta Rhythm (Main)	Alpha Rhythm (Control)	Alpha Rhythm (Main)	Beta-LF Rhythm (Control)	Beta-LF Rhythm (Main)	Beta-HF Rhythm (Control)	Beta-HF Rhythm (Main)
FP–F	-2.5	0.35	-0.32	-1.09	-2.3	-0.72	-2.92	2.88	3.54	9.44
FP–F	-3.14	-3.08	-3.63	0.58	-4.08	-0.26	-3.8	2.43	1.2	3.93
F–C	-1.88	-0.07	0.87	2.31	-0.78	0.91	2.3	1.33	-1.79	6.98
F–T	-0.41	4.39	-1.56	-0.10	1.09	-2.70	2.08	3.60	7.63	0.36
P–O	6.9	-0.11	1.97	3.48	-1.87	3.50	0.14	4.45	-6.15	10.00
T–T	-10.38	-0.27	-6.84	-2.01	-2.44	-1.01	1.79	0.85	3.98	-0.87
C–P	-3.17	-2.02	-2.4	-3.68	-2.88	-3.50	2.39	1.16	6.61	8.44
Mean	-1.82	-0.11	-1.49	-0.07	-1.66	-0.54	0.25	2.39	1.88	5.47

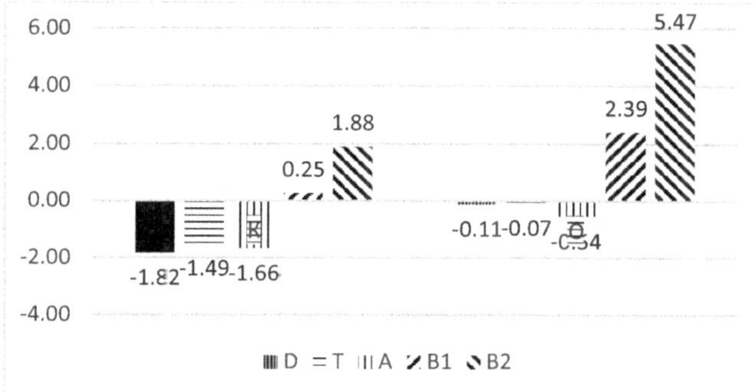

Healthy **Intellectually Disabled**

Figure 90. *FIA values in healthy subjects and in intellectual disability Legend: D – Delta rhythm, T – Theta rhythm, A – Alpha rhythm, B1 – Beta-LF rhythm, B2 – Beta-HF rhythm.*

Discussion. In intellectual disability, EEG rhythm amplitudes were higher than in healthy subjects. Duration indices in the delta, theta, and alpha EEG bands were increased compared with the control group, whereas duration indices of beta rhythms were decreased. This may indicate reduced functional activity of the ascending reticular activating system of the brainstem, or alternatively, increased functionnal activity of thalamic structures.

7.4. Major EEG Changes in Alzheimer's Disease

EEG is a recording of the brain's electrical activity, reflecting cortical and subcortical function with high temporal precision. EEG changes in Alzheimer's disease (AD) reflect progressive neurodegeneration and disruption of functional connectivity between different brain regions.

In the study by Burd S.G., Lebedeva A.V., Rublyova Y.V. et al. (2025), quantitative EEG changes characteristic of AD patients are analyzed, and their diagnostic value is discussed. Alzheimer's disease is the leading cause of dementia in the elderly, and its pathophysiological process begins several years before clinical symptoms appear. Therefore, finding accessible methods for early diagnosis remains a key challenge in modern neurology. EEG is highlighted as a non-invasive, safe, and inexpensive method that can be applied in outpatient settings and repeated as needed.

The study included patients with a confirmed diagnosis of AD and a control group. EEG recordings were analyzed using spectral and coherence analyses, allowing evaluation of both absolute frequency spectra and functional connectivity between cortical regions.

Results showed slowing of EEG activity in AD patients: relative power of slow delta and theta rhythms was increased, while faster rhythms (alpha and beta) were reduced compared to healthy controls. EEG coherence, an indicator of functional connectivity between cortical regions, was significantly decreased, particularly in the beta band, reflecting impaired integrative function of brain networks.

Researchers emphasize that these patterns—reduced alpha frequency, increased slow-wave proportion, and decreased coherence—reflect the neural network disruptions characteristic of the degenerative process in AD. This aligns with data on cortical dysfunction and impaired interregional connectivity in dementia.

The authors conclude that EEG shows promise as a screening tool for detecting AD at early stages of cognitive decline, though they caution that current findings are preliminary and require further studies with larger samples and consideration of disease stages.

Kozhokaru A.B., Azhigova A.M., Larkina E.S. (2023) examined EEG as a non-invasive method for identifying functional brain changes in cognitive impairment, including prodromal states, mild cognitive impairment (MCI), and dementia, particularly Alzheimer's disease.

With increasing life expectancy, the prevalence of cognitive impairment and dementia is rising, creating significant social and economic burdens on healthcare systems. Current biomarkers for early AD diagnosis (e.g., cerebrospinal fluid markers or neuroimaging) are often expensive, require specialized equipment, and are not always accessible in clinical practice. EEG is therefore considered a promising, accessible, safe, and reproducible method suitable for routine screening and repeated measurements.

The authors review the literature and show that EEG parameters—including spectral analysis, functional connectivity, and coherence—can identify characteristic brain activity changes in patients with cognitive deficits. Spectral measures (e.g., the ratio of slow to fast rhythm power) and network-level EEG metrics demonstrate high sensitivity to disruptions in neural network integration.

Key findings and conclusions:

Spectral EEG features, such as increased slow-wave power (delta/theta) and decreased fast-wave power (alpha/beta), correlate with cognitive impairment severity and prolongation of cognitive processing latency.

Functional connectivity (coherence) reflects disruption of interregional neural network interactions, consistent with the "disconnection syndrome" concept in dementia.

EEG parameters can differentiate patients with early cognitive impairment from cognitively healthy individuals, demonstrating potential diagnostic value.

Proper selection of EEG markers and standardization of methodology can enhance diagnostic sensitivity and specificity, and may be useful for monitoring disease progression and therapy effectiveness.

The study demonstrates that EEG can serve as a complementary tool for early detection of cognitive impairment, supplementing traditional clinical and neuropsychological assessments. The authors advocate further development of quantitative EEG analysis methods and their inclusion in diagnostic algorithms for suspected AD and other dementias.

For quantitative assessment, Sergeev A.V., Medvedeva A.V., Voznesenskaya T.G. (2011) investigated EEG changes in Alzheimer's disease. Patients with mild to moderate dementia were compared with cognitively healthy elderly individuals. Special attention was given to EEG responses to functional tasks, which help identify early neural activity disturbances not evident at rest.

The main EEG parameters analyzed were:

Spectral power of primary rhythms (delta, theta, alpha), reflecting cortical neural network activity;

Intra- and interhemispheric coherence, indicating synchronization across brain regions;

EEG reactivity to functional tasks, measuring changes in electrical activity under cognitive load (e.g., attention, memory).

The study included 22 AD patients (mild to moderate dementia) and 25 cognitively healthy elderly controls. Standard EEG recordings were performed at rest and during functional tasks. Quantitative spectral analysis and coherence evaluation between derivations were subsequently conducted.

In patients with Alzheimer's disease (AD), there was a significant increase in slow rhythms (delta and theta) and a reduction in alpha activity, especially in the frontal, central, and temporal regions. These changes reflect disrupted activation processes and impaired integration of neural networks in the cortical structures of the brain in dementia.

Intra- and interhemispheric coherence was significantly reduced in AD patients compared to controls, indicating weakened functional connectivity between different cortical regions. This reflects the so-called "disconnection syndrome" characteristic of neurodegenerative processes.

Under functional cognitive loads, EEG change patterns became more pronounced, highlighting the sensitivity of quantitative EEG methods for early detection of cognitive deficits.

The study demonstrates that quantitative EEG parameters—spectral power and coherence—serve as sensitive markers of altered brain activity in AD, reflecting not only the presence but also the severity of cognitive impairment. EEG change patterns correlate with dementia stage and are amplified under cognitive load, making these parameters promising for early diagnosis and monitoring disease progression.

The results support the use of quantitative EEG as an accessible complement to neuropsychological and clinical assessment in patients suspected of AD. Spectral analysis and coherence evaluation methods can be implemented in clinical practice to assess therapy efficacy, track disease dynamics, and detect pathological changes at early stages.

Chetty C.A., Bhardwaj H., Kumar G.P. (2024) conducted a comprehensive study of EEG markers in AD and prodromal AD (early stages with mild cognitive impairment) to identify EEG features capable of reliably distinguishing AD or prodromal AD patients from cognitively healthy individuals. This is critical for early diagnosis, disease monitoring, and treatment evaluation, as EEG is non-invasive, accessible, and relatively inexpensive.

EEG data were collected at rest with eyes closed from three groups: AD patients, prodromal AD patients, and age-matched healthy controls. Two independent preprocessing pipelines were applied to enhance result reliability.

From each EEG signal, 41 features were extracted, including spectral measures, power ratios across frequency bands, complexity measures, entropy metrics, and functional connectivity characteristics.

Key findings:

Spectral changes: AD patients showed a significant increase in theta power (4–8 Hz) and elevated theta/alpha and theta/beta ratios, reflecting slowed brain rhythms characteristic of dementia.

Functional connectivity: AD patients exhibited reduced connectivity in the theta band compared to controls, indicating impaired coordination of neural networks.

Prodromal AD: Participants with prodromal AD showed increased gamma power and enhanced gamma connectivity, distinguishing early-stage disease from full AD and normal aging.

Complexity and entropy: After correction for multiple comparisons, complexity and entropy measures did not show significant differences in AD or prodromal AD, indicating limited diagnostic value of these measures in this sample.

The authors developed a comprehensive Feature Analyzer tool that extracts 41 EEG markers, providing a multidomain view of brain functional activity. This includes spectral ratios, time-series parameters, and network integration measures.

The study demonstrates that spectral measures and EEG functional connectivity—especially in the theta and gamma bands—have potential as biomarkers for early detection of AD and prodromal AD. Specific patterns were identified for disease stages: slowed rhythms and reduced connectivity indicate AD, while enhanced gamma activity may indicate prodromal changes. These patterns can be used for diagnosis, staging, and monitoring treatment effects.

The authors note that this was a cross-sectional study, and longitudinal research is needed to fully understand the trajectory from prodromal AD to AD. Additionally, the relationship between EEG markers and other biomarkers (e.g., beta-amyloid and tau protein levels) requires further investigation.

Horváth A., Szűcs A., Csukly G., et al. (2018) critically reviewed studies using EEG and event-related potentials (ERP) as potential biomarkers for AD. The main goal was to assess the strengths, limitations, and potential of EEG and ERP metrics for diagnosis, monitoring, and understanding the neurobiological mechanisms of AD.

The authors systematically examined several key areas:

1. **Classical EEG measures:** Initial analyses focused on visual inspection of EEG and simple spectral analysis (power of frequency bands), confirming known patterns: increased slow-wave proportion (delta/theta) and decreased fast-wave activity (alpha/beta) in AD patients compared to cognitively healthy controls.
2. **Dynamic systems and network analysis:** More advanced methods, including dynamical systems approaches and functional connectivity analysis, were discussed. These approaches assess complex interregional interactions in the brain, reflecting synchrony and network integration disruptions typical of neurodegeneration in AD.
3. **ERP components in dementia:** A significant part of the review focused on ERP components, which measure brain responses to stimuli (e.g., sensory or cognitive tasks). The authors evaluated the utility of early and late ERP components (e.g., P300) in dementia research, linking them to impairments in memory, attention, and other cognitive functions.

Mismatch Negativity (MMN) and Prospects of Computational Neurology

Special attention is given to studies of **Mismatch Negativity (MMN)**—an event-related potential (ERP) component reflecting the automatic detection of changes in a stream of stimuli. Its findings, limitations, and possibilities for integration with modern approaches in computational neurology are discussed.

Sleep and EEG Markers

The authors also review studies involving EEG recording during sleep, which is particularly relevant because sleep disturbances may accompany cognitive decline and reflect additional neurophysiological alterations in Alzheimer's disease (AD).

Differential Diagnosis

The publication addresses the use of EEG in the differential diagnosis of cognitive disorders, enabling differentiation of AD from other neurodegenerative conditions based on specific EEG/ERP patterns.

Main Conclusions

EEG and ERP measures reflect disturbances in synaptic transmission and network integration in the brain characteristic of AD.

Many EEG markers have potential as biomarkers; however, their clinical application remains limited due to methodological heterogeneity and insufficient standardization.

ERP components, especially late components associated with cognitive processing, may complement spectral EEG measures, increasing diagnostic sensitivity and specificity.

To enhance the clinical utility of EEG/ERP, inter-laboratory standards, advanced analytical methods, and long-term clinical studies are required.

Key Practical Recommendations

Combined analytical approaches (spectral analysis, connectivity measures, ERP components) provide a more comprehensive understanding of AD neurophysiology than isolated methods.

A promising future direction is the integration of EEG/ERP data with other biomarkers (neuroimaging, fluid biomarkers) for comprehensive diagnosis and prognosis of the disease.

Given the rapid growth of the elderly population and the increasing prevalence of Alzheimer's disease, early detection of neurodegenerative changes occurring before

clinical symptom onset remains a critical challenge in neurology. A reliable biomarker capable of detecting alterations in brain activity prior to clinical manifestation would enable timely treatment and therapeutic intervention. EEG is a non-invasive, accessible, and relatively inexpensive method that can reflect alterations in information-processing mechanisms in AD, making it a promising tool for early diagnosis.

Al-Nuaimi A.H., Jammeh E., Sun L., Ifeachor E. (2016) aimed to develop a reliable EEG biomarker suitable for early detection of AD based on quantitative assessment of EEG amplitude changes—a key feature of brain slowing commonly observed in dementia.

This study, presented at the IEEE EMBC 2016 conference, introduced a novel EEG amplitude marker (ΔEEGA), which measures the temporal dynamics of EEG amplitude changes, reflecting the degree of slowing in brain electrical activity. The authors compared this marker with Lempel–Ziv Complexity (LZC) to evaluate its effectiveness in classifying AD patients and healthy controls.

The proposed ΔEEGA marker demonstrated high sensitivity (100%) and high specificity (approximately 88.9%) in distinguishing AD patients from healthy participants. ΔEEGA outperformed the traditional complexity-based LZC marker in diagnostic performance, suggesting its promise for early detection.

These findings confirm that alterations in EEG amplitude characteristics are sensitive indicators of neurodegeneration, reflecting functional impairments in cortical network connectivity and activation characteristic of AD. The authors interpret ΔEEGA as reflecting reduced speed and variability of brain electrical activit

y, potentially associated with impaired neuronal synchrony during early cognitive decline.

Slowing of brain rhythms—a well-known phenomenon in dementia—affects EEG amplitude characteristics, and quantitative assessment of these changes may enable sensitive detection of pathological alterations even before clear clinical manifestations.

Clinical Significance and Prospects

The development and validation of ΔEEGA support the role of EEG amplitude parameters as potential early biomarkers of AD, complementing traditional neuropsychological testing and neuroimaging. Such a biomarker could be valuable in clinical screening programs, particularly in settings with limited access to expensive diagnostic methods, and in therapeutic research for monitoring disease progression.

Conclusions: EEG as a Tool in Alzheimer's Disease

EEG shows systematic alterations in Alzheimer's disease, including:

Slowing of rhythms

Increased slow-wave activity

Decreased coherence

Characteristic spectral features

EEG holds significant potential as an adjunct biomarker for diagnosis and monitoring of AD—especially at early stages—due to its accessibility and non-invasiveness.

7.5. EEG in Parkinsonism

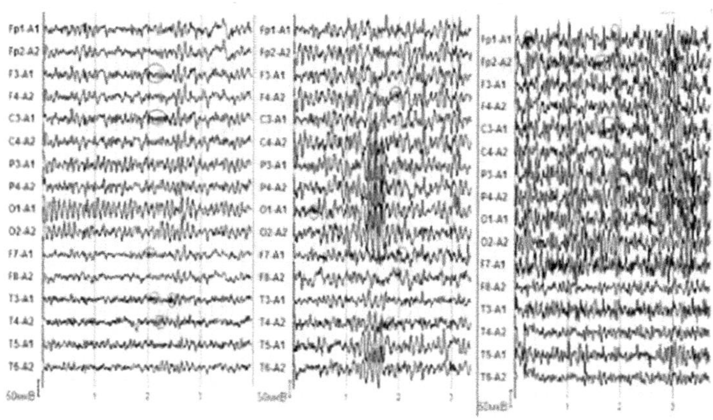

Figure 92. *EEG patterns in patients with Parkinsonism.*

EEG Changes in Parkinsonism / Parkinson's Disease

1. General Characteristic Changes

In parkinsonism, nonspecific but fairly characteristic electroencephalographic changes are observed:

- **Slowing of background activity** — a reduction in the dominant frequency with an increase in slow rhythms (δ and θ) and a decrease in fast rhythms (α and β). Such changes occur in approximately 30–50% of patients and become more pronounced as the disease progresses.

- **Increased δ- and θ-activity** — particularly in patients with cognitive impairment and Parkinson's disease dementia, reflecting more pronounced slowing.
- **Decreased α- and β-activity**, especially at more advanced stages of the disease, along with reduced reactivity to stimuli (photic stimulation and hyperventilation).
- **Reduced interhemispheric synchronization** and decreased amplitude of fast oscillations, reflecting disruption of cortical network functioning.
- **Altered coherence and spectral parameters** — increased β-synchronization between cortical regions has been associated with the severity of motor symptoms.

Review studies confirm that EEG in patients with Parkinson's disease often demonstrates diffuse slowing, reduced reactivity, and disruption of spectral frequency balance compared with healthy elderly individuals.

Table 23. *Spectral changes across frequency bands in parkinsonism.*

Frequency Band	Typical Change in Parkinsonism
δ (0.5–4 Hz)	Increased power (slow-wave activity)
θ (4–8 Hz)	Increased activity
α (8–13 Hz)	Decreased power
β (13–30 Hz)	Decreased power and reduced synchronization
γ (>30 Hz)	Occasionally altered; may have diagnostic significance in certain studies

Such spectral shifts generally reflect nonspecific cortical dysfunction associated with the progression of the neurodegenerative process.

Functional and Cognitive Correlates

Changes in spectral characteristics correlate with both motor and cognitive symptoms of parkinsonism.

Event-related potentials (ERPs) may also be altered, reflecting impairments in attention and cognitive processing.

Aperiodic EEG spectrum parameters may differ during cognitive control tasks.

Practical Significance of EEG

Although EEG is not a specific diagnostic test for Parkinson's disease, it may be used:

To monitor disease progression

In combination with other markers (clinical and biochemical)

To assess treatment efficacy

For research purposes and in the development of machine learning methods

Soikkeli R., Partanen J., Soininen H. et al. (1991) investigated spectral EEG characteristics in patients with Parkinson's disease (PD), including those with and without dementia, compared with age-matched controls.

Study Design

Three groups were included:

18 patients with PD and dementia

18 patients with PD without dementia

20 healthy elderly volunteers (controls)

EEG was recorded in a resting state with eyes closed using a standardized T6–O2 (parieto-occipital) derivation.

The analysis included spectral decomposition of the signals and calculation of absolute and relative amplitudes for classical frequency bands:

δ (0.5–4 Hz)

θ (4–8 Hz)

α (8–13 Hz)

β (13–30 Hz)

Peak frequency and mean spectral frequency were also evaluated.

Main Results

1. **General EEG slowing in PD**

    Patients with PD showed significantly lower brain rhythm frequencies compared with healthy elderly controls. This was most clearly reflected by increased power of slow δ and θ waves.

2. **Dementia and EEG slowing**

    Patients with PD and dementia exhibited more pronounced EEG slowing than those without dementia—particularly evident in increased δ activity and reduced α and β activity.

3. **Group differences**

    In the dementia group, all spectral parameters differed significantly from controls (including slow-wave amplitudes and mean frequency).

    In patients without dementia, EEG slowing was also present but less pronounced and mainly characterized by increased θ activity.

4. **Authors' conclusions**

    Different subgroups of patients with parkinsonian syndrome demonstrate distinct EEG spectral patterns:

PD with dementia — marked predominance of slow rhythms and reduction of fast rhythms, correlating with severe cognitive dysfunction.

PD without dementia — moderate slowing, with θ activity exceeding normal values.

This indicates that EEG slowing is a common neurophysiological feature of parkinsonism and becomes more pronounced with cognitive deterioration.

Clinical Significance

EEG may serve as a noninvasive marker of cortical alterations in PD, particularly for assessing cognitive impairment, although it is not a standalone diagnostic test.

EEG slowing in PD patients correlates over time with disease progression and the degree of cognitive deficit.

Notes and Important Details

The data confirm that increased δ and θ activity, reduced α and β activity, and decreased overall spectral frequency are consistent features in PD compared with healthy elderly individuals.

Spectral EEG parameters—such as mean frequency and the fast/slow power ratio—correlate with clinical manifestations and cognitive status.

Shirahige L., Berenguer-Rocha M., Mendonça S. et al. (2020) systematically summarized quantitative EEG (qEEG) characteristics in patients with Parkinson's disease and identified potential cortical biomarkers associated with motor symptoms at rest and during movement.

The authors conducted a comprehensive systematic search in MEDLINE, LILACS, CINAHL, Web of Science, and CENTRAL databases following PRISMA guidelines. Studies including clinically confirmed PD patients were analyzed, comparing qEEG findings either with healthy controls or across different conditions (e.g., rest vs. movement).

Nineteen studies (18 cross-sectional and 1 crossover) were included, comprising 312 PD patients and 277 healthy participants.

Main qEEG Findings

Decreased fast-frequency components (alpha and beta bands)

Increased slow-wave activity (delta and theta bands)

These changes were observed both at rest and during complex motor task performance.

Alterations were particularly prominent in central and frontal cortical regions, possibly reflecting impaired cortical motor control and cognitive components of motor tasks.

Despite consistent trends toward EEG "slowing" in PD patients, no specific qEEG biomarker for motor symptoms has been definitively established. This is largely due to heterogeneity of study protocols, small sample sizes, and methodological limitations.

Conclusion (EEG in Parkinson's Disease and Organic Mental Disorders)

The accumulated evidence indicates that patients with Parkinson's disease exhibit characteristic alterations in the spectral composition of EEG, reflecting shifts in cortical activity and impaired dopaminergic neurotransmission. Despite the reproducibility of several quantitative EEG (qEEG) measures and their correlation with clinical severity (including the Unified Parkinson's Disease Rating Scale) and DAT PET findings, there is currently no clearly validated and standardized qEEG biomarker suitable for routine assessment of motor impairment in Parkinson's disease.

The study by Waninger et al. (2020) demonstrated that:

EEG measures show satisfactory test–retest reliability;

source localization methods (sLORETA) reveal cortical differences (anterior cingulate cortex, temporal regions) consistent with known disease pathophysiology;

increased beta-band synchronization between cortical regions correlates with clinical severity and the degree of dopaminergic synaptic loss;

machine learning approaches can generate discriminant models reflecting the extent of dopaminergic denervation.

Thus, qEEG shows potential as:

an objective tool for monitoring disease progression;

a pharmacodynamic marker in clinical trials;

a functional biomarker for developing personalized therapeutic strategies.

However, the authors emphasize the need for larger, methodologically rigorous studies with standardized EEG acquisition and analysis protocols to definitively establish the diagnostic and prognostic value of qEEG in Parkinson's disease.

EEG in Organic Mental Disorders

Organic mental disorders are characterized by persistent disturbances of brain function resulting from structural or metabolic damage (e.g., traumatic brain injury, epilepsy, toxic exposure). EEG in these conditions reflects dysfunction primarily in frontal and temporal cortical regions.

Typical EEG findings include:

increased slow-wave activity (delta and theta bands);

reduced alpha rhythm power;

disorganization of rhythmic structure;

altered interhemispheric asymmetry and coherence.

In patients with aggression and autoaggression, frontal lobe dysfunction—more often in the left hemisphere—is frequently observed, accompanied by increased delta power in frontal leads. In children with developmental delay, slowing of baseline rhythmic activity, frontal dysfunction, and immature cortical specialization with increased coherence are commonly noted.

Sexual disorders (particularly paraphilias) are often associated with right temporal epileptiform activity and involvement of limbic structures, accompanied by increased interhemispheric coherence between temporal regions.

Differentiation Between Organic and Functional Psychopathology

EEG has significant diagnostic value in distinguishing organic from functional psychiatric disorders:

In organic disturbances of consciousness (e.g., delirium), a normal EEG pattern is rare.

In functional psychoses, a normal EEG is considerably more common.

This distinction is particularly important in cases of acute cognitive deterioration and diagnostically uncertain presentations.

Psychoorganic Syndrome and Dementia

Psychoorganic syndrome is typically associated with:

diffuse EEG abnormalities and rhythm disorganization;

increased theta and delta activity;

reduced alpha activity;

diminished regional differentiation.

In patients who have experienced a stroke and exhibit psychoorganic features, EEG often demonstrates marked slowing of background activity.

In degenerative disorders such as Alzheimer's disease, EEG typically shows:

increased slow-wave activity (theta/delta);

reduced alpha rhythm;

bilateral synchronous slow oscillations reflecting disruption of cortical and thalamocortical networks.

General Conclusion

EEG remains an accessible, noninvasive, and informative method for assessing brain functional status. In Parkinson's disease and organic mental disorders, it reveals characteristic patterns of cortical dysfunction, helps evaluate severity, and supports differential diagnosis.

However, further large-scale studies with methodological standardization are required to transition EEG from a research tool to a fully validated clinical biomarker.

EEG and Epilepsy as a Cause of Psychopathology

In patients with unstable or phenomenologically variable psychopathology (e.g., brief depressive episodes with psychotic features), pathological EEG activity and epileptiform discharges are observed more frequently than in patients with pure depression.

These findings are clinically important because they may indicate an underlying epileptic (organic) component contributing to the symptomatology, which may require adjustment of pharmacological treatment.

3) Sensitivity and Limitations of the Method

Sensitivity and Specificity

Classical EEG abnormalities in organic conditions are relatively sensitive but not specific. Many slow-wave changes may also occur in depression, toxic states, medication effects, and other conditions.

EEG Changes in the Elderly Population

Abnormal EEG findings are common in patients with cognitive impairment; however, similar abnormalities may also be present in psychiatric patients without dementia (e.g., in major depression).

Routine vs. Advanced Quantitative Analysis

Routine visual EEG assessment provides limited information. Modern quantitative methods of spectral and coherence analysis (qEEG) significantly enhance diagnostic informativeness and may help identify endophenotypes of organic brain dysfunction.

Practical Application of EEG in Psychiatry

EEG is recommended:

When an organic basis of psychopathology is suspected (delirium, dementia, psychoorganic syndrome);

In diagnostically unclear psychotic states with a possible organic component;

In cases of epileptiform activity or unexplained paroxysmal events.

Important considerations:

EEG is an adjunctive tool and must be interpreted within a comprehensive clinical assessment;

EEG abnormalities do not always indicate structural brain damage—they may reflect medication side effects, psychogenic phenomena, or age-related changes.

Study by Primavera A. et al. (1983)

In their study, Primavera A., Folis E., and Abbruzzese M. (1983) examined the diagnostic value of EEG in acute and subacute organic brain conditions, particularly for differential diagnosis from functional psychiatric disorders.

The authors aimed to demonstrate that EEG is a rapid, accessible, and informative method that can help distinguish organic brain syndromes (e.g., delirious states, organic mental syndrome) from functional psychiatric symptoms, especially in emergency settings.

The study analyzed 114 consecutive patients referred for evaluation of acute or subacute confusional states. All patients underwent clinical assessment and standard EEG examination. EEG findings were then compared with the final clinical diagnosis (organic vs. functional psychiatric disorder).

Key findings:

83% of patients with functional psychiatric disorders had normal EEGs;

Only 8% of patients with organic conditions had normal EEGs.

Thus, pathological EEG changes were significantly more frequent in organic conditions than in purely functional psychiatric disorders.

The authors emphasized that:

EEG can be a valuable diagnostic tool, particularly for excluding organic causes of symptoms (e.g., delirium, encephalopathy);

EEG is not always specific, as abnormalities may occur in other conditions;

Due to its high sensitivity, EEG is useful as a screening test, especially when the clinical presentation is unclear and there is a risk of misdiagnosing functional psychosis.

Study by Jin Y. et al. (1993). Jin Y., Coyle D., Francis B., et al. (1993) investigated the prevalence of EEG abnormalities in adults with suspected organic mental syndrome and assessed the diagnostic value of EEG in relation to cognitive imprment.

ai The study included 350 adults aged ≥50 years:

312 patients evaluated for suspected organic mental disorder;

38 healthy controls.

All participants underwent standard EEG and cognitive assessment using the Mini-Mental State Examination (MMSE) at the time of EEG recording. EEGs were evaluated for abnormalities (slowing, disorganization, epileptiform discharges, etc.). Clinical diagnoses and treatment data were analyzed retrospectively by an investigator blinded to EEG results.

Key findings:

Abnormal EEGs were observed in 67% of patients with suspected organic disorders versus 11% in controls;

The frequency of EEG abnormalities increased with the severity of cognitive impairment:

~42% in individuals with questionable cognitive deficit;

up to ~65% in those with mild-to-moderate impairment.

However, abnormal EEG findings were not specific for dementia, as a significant proportion of patients with depression also showed pathological EEG changes.

Clinical Significance

EEG is a moderately sensitive but nonspecific marker of organic brain dysfunction in elderly patients.

The frequency of EEG abnormalities is closely related to the severity of cognitive impairment but does not reliably distinguish dementia from psychogenic depression.

Importantly, a normal EEG was rare in patients with confirmed organic disorders, whereas it predominated in control subjects.

Conclusions

EEG frequently shows abnormalities in patients with suspected organic mental disorders, particularly in the presence of significant cognitive impairment.

However, EEG is not a diagnostic "gold standard" for dementia or organic psychosis, as nonspecific abnormalities may also occur in other conditions such as depression.

Review by Boutros N.N. (1992)

The review by Boutros N.N. (1992) analyzed the clinical indications for routine (non-computerized) EEG in psychiatric practice. The primary objective was to determine in which clinical situations EEG provides meaningful diagnostic benefit and when its use may be unwarranted.

The author emphasizes that EEG is an accessible, noninvasive, and relatively inexpensive neurodiagnostic tool widely used in psychiatric settings. Its principal value lies in identifying possible organic causes of psychiatric symptoms and clarifying diagnosis in cases where the clinical picture is uncertain.

Indications for Routine EEG Noted in the Review

In the review by Boutros N.N. (1992), the author outlines specific clinical situations in which routine (non-computerized) EEG is justified and informative:

Assessment of an organic component in psychiatric disorders, particularly when altered consciousness, confusion, delirium, or suspected structural brain involvement is present.

Dementia and other neurocognitive disorders, when additional confirmation of underlying pathophysiological brain changes is required.

Suspected delirium, where EEG may demonstrate diffuse cortical slowing typical of delirium or help exclude alternative causes.

Lithium toxicity and other drug-induced encephalopathies, in which EEG is useful both diagnostically and for monitoring severity.

Pre-electroconvulsive therapy (ECT) evaluation, to exclude epileptiform activity or other abnormalities that may affect procedural safety.

The author emphasizes that **routine screening EEG for all psychiatric patients without clear clinical indications is not recommended**, given its relatively low diagnostic yield when a thorough neurological examination has already been performed.

Overall, EEG is considered a valuable tool when there is suspicion of an organic basis for psychopathology. It is particularly helpful in delirium, dementia, toxic encephalopathies, epileptic phenomena, and before ECT. However, indiscriminate use in all psychiatric patients is inefficient and clinically unjustified.

Neuropsychiatric "Border Zone" Syndromes

(Study by Chandra S.R. et al., 2017) Chandra S.R., Asheeb A., Dash S., et al. (2017) analyzed the diagnostic and therapeutic role of EEG in conditions where neurological and psychiatric symptoms overlap—so-called neuropsychiatric "border zone" syndromes. These include disorders in which organic neurological diseases (e.g., epilepsy, encephalitis, dementia) present with prominent psychiatric manifestations, complicating diagnosis and treatment selection.

The authors conducted a retrospective review of challenging clinical cases over five years. Clinical diagnoses were correlated with EEG findings and compared with the available literature on "border zone" syndromes.

Key Conclusions

1. Diagnostic Utility of EEG

EEG helps differentiate organic from primary psychiatric causes of symptoms. However, in neuropsychiatric border syndromes, EEG may be either normal or abnormal, and a "pathological EEG" alone does not necessarily confirm organic pathology.

2. Non specific Changes

Nonspecific ("soft") EEG abnormalities are frequently observed in patients with psychiatric diagnoses and do not automatically indicate structural brain damage.

Clinically, such mild changes should not be interpreted as proof of organic psychopathology without corroborating evidence.

3. Typical EEG Patterns

Distinct pathological findings (e.g., epileptiform discharges, marked background slowing) may suggest specific diagnoses such as epilepsy or encephalitis.

However, the absence of pronounced abnormalities does not exclude an organic component, underscoring the need for comprehensive assessment.

4. Monitoring of Therapy

EEG can be used to monitor therapeutic efficacy and medication toxicity, particularly when psychotropic drugs influence brain activity (e.g., clozapine and the risk of epileptiform activity).

EEG monitoring is also useful in suspected drug toxicity or overdose.

5. Biofeedback (Neurofeedback)

The authors discuss EEG biofeedback (neurofeedback) as an adjunctive therapeutic tool in psychiatry. This technique trains patients to modulate specific EEG rhythms to improve attention regulation, emotional control, and related functions.

Clinical Significance

EEG is not a panacea but remains an important tool at the interface of neurology and psychiatry. It assists in diagnostic clarification, therapeutic monitoring, and assessment of medication-related risks, complementing neurological and psychiatric evaluation.

EEG findings must always be interpreted within the broader clinical context. On its own, EEG cannot always definitively determine whether pathology is organic or psychiatric in origin.

The authors note that:

Epileptiform abnormalities may be absent between seizures;

Mild EEG changes are often nonspecific;

EEG should not be used as a sole diagnostic marker but rather in combination with neurological examination, clinical assessment, and, when indicated, neuroimaging.

Main EEG Features in Organic Mental Disorders

A. Diffuse and Nonspecific Slowing of Activity

In organic brain disorders (e.g., encephalopathy, dementia, delirium):

Alpha activity (approximately 8–13 Hz) is reduced;

Slow waves (theta/delta) predominate;

The degree of slowing correlates with the severity of cognitive dysfunction.

These changes reflect impaired functional cortical activity and may be observed in organic mental syndromes.

EEG is typically markedly slowed during the acute phase of delirium and in severe encephalopathy, making electroencephalography particularly useful in differentiating these conditions from functional psychoses, which often present with a normal EEG pattern.

B. Focal Changes

In structural brain lesions (tumors, strokes, post-traumatic scars):

Localized areas of slowing or desynchronization may be observed;

Asymmetry and focal abnormalities are possible.

These findings reflect focal organic pathology that may accompany psychiatric symptoms in patients with structural brain damage.

C. Epileptiform Features and Paroxysmal Discharges

Organic brain damage (including chronic trauma, scar tissue, or vascular changes) increases the risk of epileptiform discharges, sharp waves, and spike-and-wave complexes.

This is clinically significant because psychiatric symptoms (e.g., altered consciousness, confusion, psychotic episodes) may be associated with underlying epileptic activity.

D. Cognitive Disorders and EEG Pattern Characteristics

In elderly patients with organic psychiatric disorders (e.g., dementia), marked changes in EEG spectral power and disruption of functional brain network integration are observed.

These patterns are associated with cognitive decline and provide information about the severity of the pathological process.

3. Application of EEG in Psychiatric Diagnosis

Clinical Situations Where EEG Is Particularly Useful

Delirium and acute organic states: EEG often shows diffuse slowing, helping differentiate delirium from primary psychotic disorders.

Uncertain organic etiology of psychosis or confusion: EEG assists in confirming or excluding an organic basis.

Suspicion of nonconvulsive status epilepticus or subclinical seizures: EEG is a key diagnostic tool.

4. Limitations of EEG in Organic Psychiatric Disorders

Low Specificity

EEG changes occur in many conditions—not only in organic psychiatric disorders but also in intoxications, medication effects, and primary psychiatric illnesses without structural brain damage.

Absence of Pathognomonic Patterns

There are no clearly specific "EEG signatures" for most psychiatric conditions (with the exception of epileptiform activity). This is considered a limitation of the method rather than evidence of ineffectiveness.

Need for Clinical Correlation

EEG alone does not establish a psychiatric diagnosis; it complements neurological and clinical evaluation.

5. Conclusion: Role and Interpretation of EEG in Organic Psychiatric Disorders

EEG is:

An informative tool for detecting organic brain dysfunction in psychiatric conditions;

A method for differentiating organic and functional psychiatric disorders (e.g., delirium vs. primary psychosis);

A useful modality for identifying epileptic activity underlying psychopathology.

However:

EEG abnormalities are nonspecific and require careful clinical interpretation.

Spectral and Spatial Characteristics of EEG in Organic Psychiatric Disorders

Aggression

Spectral Features

Increased delta power;

Decreased alpha power;

Decreased beta power.

Spatial Features

Frontal leads with left-sided asymmetry;

Abnormalities in frontal and occipital regions of both hemispheres;

Involvement of central, temporal, and parietal regions of the right hemisphere;

Frontal regions of both hemispheres and central and parietal regions of the right hemisphere.

Coherence

Reduced coherence between different brain structures.

Developmental Delay

Spectral Features

Slowing of baseline rhythmic activity.

Spatial Features

Frontal dysfunction.

Coherence

Increased coherence.

Sexual Disorders

Spectral Features

Increased delta and theta power;

Increased beta-band power (reported in some studies).

Spatial Features

Central, parietal, and occipital regions;

Fronto-central regions.

Coherence

Increased coherence between posterior temporal and temporal leads;

Decreased coherence in frontal and central leads across all frequency bands.

7.6. Affective Mental Disorders

Affective mental disorders, also referred to as mood disorders, are characterized by either excessive expression of natural emotions or a markedly apathetic attitude toward the surrounding world. These include depression, bipolar (manic–depressive) disorder, anxiety disorders, and panic attacks.

Theta and gamma frequency bands have been identified as particularly diagnostically relevant in affective psychopathology. Obsessive–compulsive disorder (OCD) is associated with alterations in low beta frequencies and the gamma range.

In the study by Schulman J.J. et al. (2011), current source localization of theta and alpha activity was presented. The authors demonstrated distinct spectral and source-localization features across different affective pathologies.

The diagnostic relevance of theta rhythm has also been emphasized in other studies (e.g., Pinner & Cavanagh, 2017; Jeste et al., 2015). According to Pinner and Cavanagh (2017), theta rhythm is generated in the medial prefrontal cortex and is associated with emotion generation and perception, working memory, episodic memory encoding, performance monitoring, and error processing.

In the work of Pashkov A.A., Dakhtin I.S., and Kharisova N.S. (2017), theta rhythm is proposed as a biomarker of both experimentally induced and chronic stress. These conditions are accompanied by increased theta power in the prefrontal cortex, where neurocognitive deficits are also observed. Simultaneously, increased high-frequency beta activity is recorded in posterior sensorimotor regions of the neocortex.

Regarding alpha activity, frontal alpha asymmetry and hypoactivation of the left frontal lobe have been reported under stress conditions, which are associated with an increased risk of developing psychiatric disorders. Koolhaas J.M. et al. (2011) similarly suggested that stress elevates the risk of depression, anxiety disorders, and other psychiatric conditions. Prolonged and/or intense stress exposure may lead to breakdown of adaptive regulatory systems, resulting in psychosomatic disorders.

Spectral and Spatial Features of EEG in Affective Mental Disorders

Stress

Spectral Features

Increased theta power;

Alpha rhythm: reduction in low-frequency alpha (8–10 Hz) and increased power in the 10–13 Hz range;

Increased beta activity.

Spatial Features

Prefrontal cortex involvement;

Frontal asymmetry;

Posterior sensorimotor cortical regions.

Coherence

Increased connectivity between the amygdala and dorsal striatum;

Decreased connectivity between the amygdala and hippocampus.

Depression

Spectral Features

Increased theta power;

Alpha peak shifted toward lower frequencies.

Spatial Features

Greater involvement of the right temporal lobe;

Medial occipital cortex;

Left temporal lobe.

Coherence

Reduced coherence between frontal regions.

Obsessive–Compulsive Disorder (OCD)

Spectral Features

Increased theta power;

Alterations in low beta and gamma frequency bands.

Spatial Features

Orbitofro

ntal cortex;

Bilateral temporal lobes.

Coherence

Altered frontotemporal connectivity (as reported in the literature).

7.7. EEG and Epilepsy

EEG is the primary and often the only outpatient neurological investigation performed in cases of epileptic seizures.

An electroencephalogram records the summed electrical activity of cortical neurons in the cerebral hemispheres. EEG recording for the detection of seizure activity is conducted both in experimental settings and in clinical practice.

Experimental studies of seizure activity contribute to understanding its mechanisms of initiation and maintenance, facilitating the development of therapeutic approaches. Seizure activity is fundamentally associated with impaired inhibitory mechanisms in the cerebral cortex—particularly deficits in glycinergic or GABAergic inhibition.

Cerebellar damage is frequently associated with the development of seizure activity, further highlighting the role of disrupted inhibitory control in epileptogenesis.

7.7.1. Modeling Epilepsy in Biological Models

To conceptualize the epileptic process as a coherent, continuous phenomenon, it is useful to study it in biological models of epilepsy. In humans, the development of epilepsy occurs over many years, which makes it difficult to perceive the process as a unified whole. Biological models allow researchers to examine the process as an integrated event and to explore its underlying mechanisms.

7.7.1.1. Application Model of Multifocal Cortical Epilepsy

Multifocal cortical focal epilepsy has been modeled by applying convulsants (such as strychnine and penicillin) to the sensorimotor cortex of cats (Lobasyuk B.A.). Additional approaches included cerebellar aspiration and intraperitoneal administration of penicillin.

These experimental models enable the study of epileptogenic mechanisms and the evaluation of pharmacological interventions under controlled conditions.

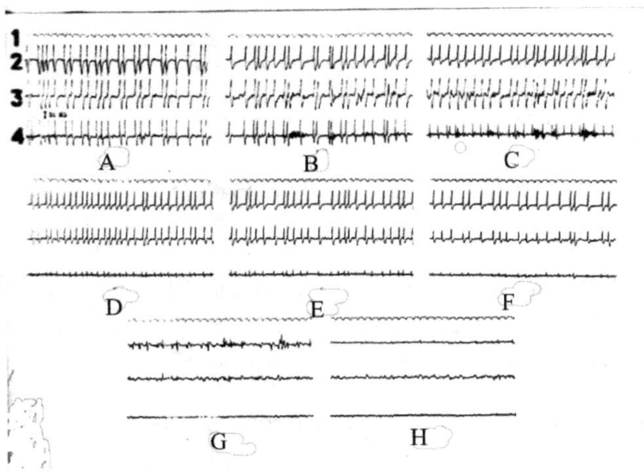

Figure 93. *Electrical Activity of a Strychnine-Induced Epileptic Complex Under Control Conditions*

Glycinergic inhibition in the cerebral cortex is disrupted.

***Legend: A** – Application of 0.1% strychnine to zones 3 and 4, and 3% strychnine to zone 2, producing an epileptic complex. **B, C, D, E, F, G, H** – Recordings at 10, 18, 46, 57, 68, and 72 minutes after **A**.*

***1** – Time mark (1 s), **calibration**: 500 μV*

***2** – Middle sigmoid gyrus*

***3** – Posterior sigmoid gyrus*

***4** – Anterior sigmoid gyrus*

Dependent seizure foci were located in the anterior and posterior sigmoid gyri, while the determinant focus was in the middle sigmoid gyrus of the cat brain.

Functional indicators of the multifocal cortical epileptic complex include:

1. Frequency of seizure potential generation by epileptic foci
2. Amplitude of seizure potentials at the foci

The biological model of the multifocal epileptic complex used in this study consisted of three foci:

Determinant focus – middle sigmoid gyrus

First dependent focus – posterior sigmoid gyrus

Second dependent focus – anterior sigmoid gyrus

This cortical epilepsy model can be conceptualized as a system of interacting foci, or a "complex of interacting components" (Bertalanffy L.).

As is well known, the cerebellum is, by Beritov's definition, the "central inhibitory ganglion of the nervous system," and all cerebellar outputs are GABAergic. Therefore, cerebellar vermis aspiration disrupts GABA-dependent cortical inhibition.

When modeling multifocal cortical focal epilepsy via strychnine application to the sensorimotor cortex in cats under cerebellar vermis aspiration, the duration of the epileptic complex was 2–3 times longer (216–288 minutes) than in an intact brain (70–80 minutes).

After 120 minutes in the vermis-aspirated condition, episodes of accelerated seizure potential generation were observed, reaching 90–100 potentials per minute, compared to 25–30 potentials per minute in the interictal period.

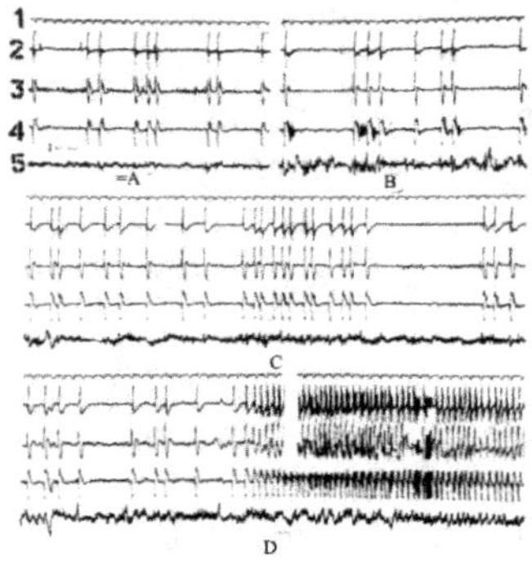

***Figure 94.** Electrical activity of the penicillin-induced epileptic complex in the absence of external influences (control). GABAergic inhibition in the cerebral cortex is impaired.*

***Legend:** A – An epileptic complex was induced by application of a 0.5% penicillin solution to areas 3 and 4, and a 3.5% penicillin solution to area 2.*

B, C, D – Recordings taken 20, 26, and 70 minutes after A.

1 – Time marker, 2 – Middle suprasylvian gyrus, 3 – Posterior suprasylvian gyrus, 4 – Anterior suprasylvian gyrus, 5 – Superior coronal gyrus, middle third,

Time calibration: 1 s. Amplitude calibration: 500 μV.

On the third day after aspiration of the cerebellar hemispheres in rats (Fig. 95), electrocorticography (ECoG) revealed hypersynchronous alpha-activity spindles, against which seizure activity of the spike-and-wave type was recorded, as well as unilateral isolated epileptiform potentials, groups of such potentials, and bilateral seizure activity.

It should be noted that in 3 out of 5 rats in this group, seizure activity predominated in amplitude on the right side.

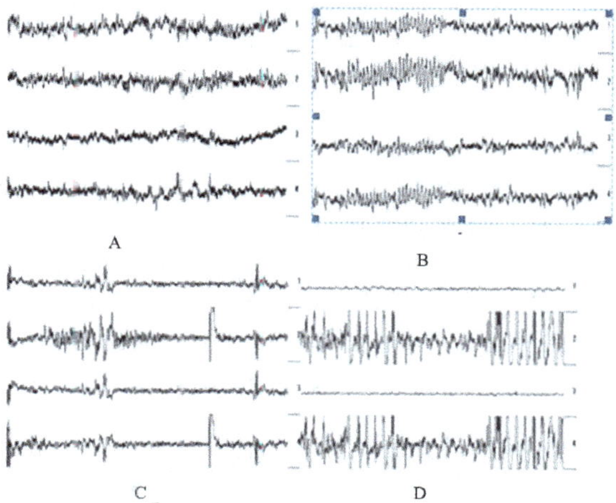

__Figure 95.__ ECoG of rats after aspiration of the cerebellar hemispheres.

***Legend:** A – intact rat;*

B–D – aspiration of the cerebellar hemispheres;

1 – left frontal cortex – left occipital cortex; 2 – right frontal cortex – right occipital cortex; 3 – left frontal cortex – right frontal cortex; 4 – left occipital cortex – right occipital cortex.

Calibration: for A and B – 409.6 μV; for C and D – 2048 μV.

Time marker: 2 s.

Under conditions of induction of an epileptic complex by application of 0.5% and 3.5% penicillin solutions to the cerebral cortex of cats (Fig. 94), an epileptic complex is formed in which ictal seizure activity periodically occurs.

7.7.1.2. Development of a biological model of multifocal cortical epilepsy by intraperitoneal administration of BP and analysis of seizure activity evolution

A previously developed biological model of a multifocal epileptic complex was formed by applying 2 × 2 mm pieces of filter paper soaked in strychnine or penicillin solutions to cortical areas of the cat brain (Shandra A.A., 1977). It was later shown that a similar biological model could also be created in the rat cerebral cortex (Makulin R.F., Shandra A.A., Lobasyuk B.A., 1979).

However, formation of this biological model required preparatory surgical procedures (craniotomy, placement of an indifferent electrode, tracheotomy), and the experiments themselves were conducted using muscle relaxants.

Therefore, we aimed to develop a biological model of a multifocal epileptic complex in which experiments could be performed under conditions of freely behaving animals. It was found that intraperitoneal administration of BP at a dose of 300,000 IU per 100 g of body weight resulted in the formation of a model of multifocal cortical epilepsy in the rat cerebral cortex, characterized by ictal and interictal periods (Method for modeling focal cortical epilepsy. Utility model declaration patent, 15.08.2005, Bulletin No. 8).

After BP administration, seizure activity first appeared 160–577 s after injection. Of nine rats, the first epileptiform discharges appeared in the right hemisphere in two animals and in the left hemisphere in six animals. In one rat, seizure potentials simultaneously appeared in both hemispheres.

Simultaneously with the onset of seizure activity in the hemispheres, regardless of lateralization, epileptiform activity (EpA) was also recorded in the occipital lead. EpA appeared last in the frontal cortex leads of both hemispheres, 569–1188 s (9.48–19.8 min) after BP administration.

In all experiments, the development of seizure activity in the frontal cortex lead began with spindle-shaped activity. During this observation period, synchronously occurring epileptiform potentials were recorded in all studied cortical regions, indicating the formation of interictal seizure activity.

Ictal seizure activity developed in all animals 16–85 minutes after BP administration.

Intervals between ictal discharges ranged from 2 to 50 minutes. During 3–3.5 hours of seizure activity evolution, the epileptic phenomenology remained relatively stable. In subsequent observation periods, the amplitudes of epileptiform potentials gradually decreased until they completely disappeared.

The mean duration of seizure activity was 313.25 ± 14.94 minutes.

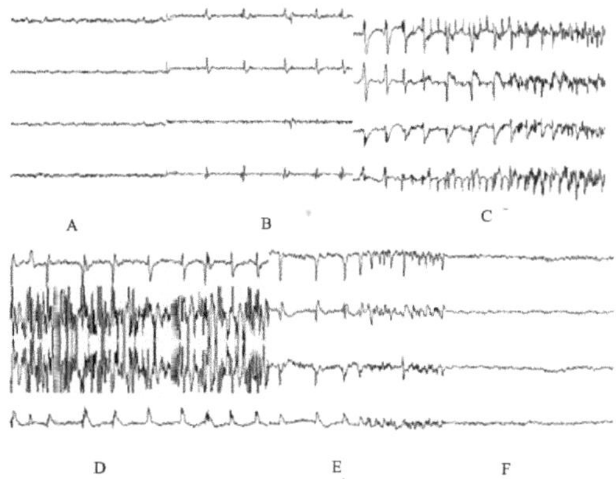

Figure 96. *Evolution of seizure activity induced by intraperitoneal administration of BP.*

A – before BP administration; B – first seizure potentials after BP administration (160–577 s from the time of injection); C – formation of interictal seizure activity;

D – development of ictal seizure activity; E and F – disappearance of seizure activity.

The amplitude dynamics were characterized by an increase in seizure potential values up to the 80th minute of observation after BP administration — from 579.11 ± 46.13 μV in the occipital cortex to 1567.27 ± 73.63 μV in the left hemisphere.

From the 100th to the 260th minute, a relatively stable period of seizure potential amplitude generation was observed.

By the 340th minute of observation, the amplitudes of seizure potentials approached zero.

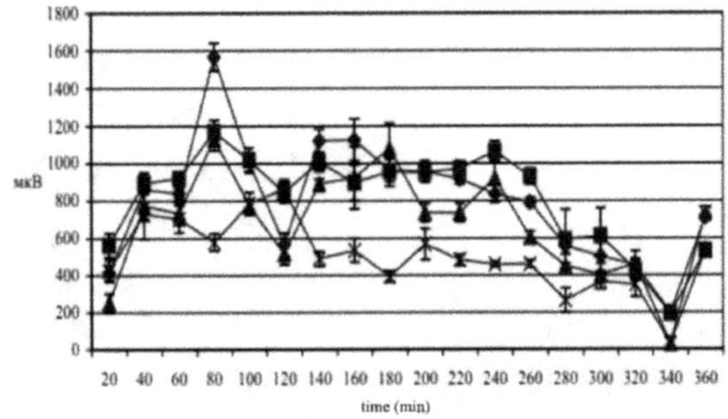

Figure 97. *Dynamics of seizure potential amplitudes during the evolution of the penicillin-induced epileptic complex.*

Changes in the frequency of seizure activity generation exhibited a wave-like pattern.

The maximum frequencies of seizure potential generation were recorded at the 180th minute after BP administration, ranging from 61.33 ± 17.39 seizure potentials per minute in the frontal cortex to 191.50 ± 25.55 seizure potentials per minute in the occipital cortex.

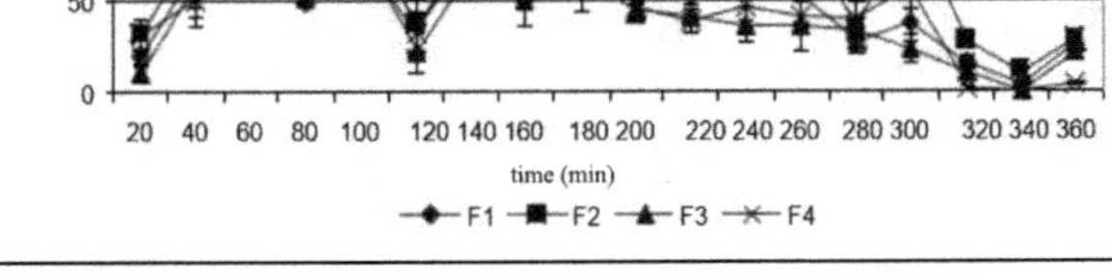

Figure 98. *Dynamics of seizure potential frequencies during the evolution of the penicillin-induced epileptic complex.*

Changes in ECoG parameters before and after the disappearance of seizure activity induced by intraperitoneal administration of BP

Table 24. *Statistically significant coefficients of left-to-right hemisphere ratios before and after the disappearance of seizure activity induced by intraperitoneal administration of BP*

ECoG Parameters	Condition	Left Hemisphere	Right Hemisphere
Beta-2	A	—	—
	F	—	—
	I	−1.11 ± 0.03	—
Beta-1	A	—	—
	F	—	—
	I	—	—
Alpha	A	1.40 ± 0.15	—
	F	—	—
	I	1.17 ± 0.10	—
Theta	A	—	—
	F	—	−1.02 ± 0.02
	I	1.12 ± 0.04	—
Delta	A	—	—
	F	—	1.03 ± 0.02
	I	−1.19 ± 0.08	1.15 ± 0.07

Legend: *A – Before BP administration, F – After disappearance of seizure activity, I – During seizure activity*

In the left hemisphere, after the disappearance of seizure activity compared with the period before penicillin administration, the frequency and duration index of the delta rhythm were increased by 1.03 ± 0.02 and 1.15 ± 0.07 times, respectively. The frequency of the theta rhythm was decreased by 1.02 ± 0.02 times.

In the right hemisphere, after the disappearance of seizure activity, a statistically significant increase in alpha rhythm amplitude was observed (1.40 ± 0.15-fold), as well as increases in the duration indices of the alpha and theta rhythms (1.17 ± 0.10 and 1.12 ± 0.04 times, respectively). A statistically significant decrease was noted in the duration indices of the beta-2 and delta rhythms (1.11 ± 0.03 and 1.19 ± 0.08 times, respectively).

Changes in Frontal Interhemispheric Asymmetry (FIAA) of ECoG Parameters After Disappearance of Seizure Activity

Before BP administration, FIAA values for the amplitudes of beta-2, beta-1, alpha, and theta rhythms were positive, ranging from 4.00 ± 0.93% to 9.81 ± 2.89%, indicating that the amplitudes of these rhythms were lateralized to the left hemisphere.

The FIAA value for delta rhythm amplitude was negative, indicating right-hemisphere lateralization of this rhythm by amplitude.

After cessation of seizure activity, FIAA values for the amplitudes of beta-2, beta-1, alpha, and theta rhythms became negative, ranging from 3.32 ± 0.81% to 6.55 ± 1.95%, indicating right-hemisphere lateralization of these rhythms.

The negativity of the FIAA value for delta rhythm amplitude increased after disappearance of seizure activity, from −0.17 ± 0.05% to −1.81 ± 0.44%.

Thus, the development of seizure activity in the cerebral cortex leads to inversion of ECoG rhythm amplitude lateralization toward the right hemisphere.

Table 25. Changes in FIAA ECcG parameters before BP administration and after disappearance of seizure activity induced by intraperitoneal BP administration.

ECoG Parameters	Index	Before BP Administration	After Disappearance of Seizure Potentials
Beta-2	A	4.00 ± 0.93	−3.32 ± 0.81*
	F	0.01 ± 0.00	−0.07 ± 0.01*
	I	−0.65 ± 0.10	3.53 ± 0.98*
Beta-1	A	6.76 ± 1.87	−6.55 ± 1.95*
	F	−0.05 ± 0.00	−0.03 ± 0.00*
	I	0.93 ± 0.13	1.12 ± 0.30
Alpha	A	9.81 ± 2.89	−6.76 ± 2.58*
	F	−0.11 ± 0.01	−0.37 ± 0.07*
	I	8.17 ± 1.49	−4.21 ± 1.56*
Theta	A	6.04 ± 1.82	−5.65 ± 1.46*
	F	0.55 ± 0.04	−0.77 ± 0.13*
	I	7.08 ± 1.04	−1.26 ± 0.40*
Delta	A	−0.17 ± 0.05	−1.81 ± 0.44*
	F	1.26 ± 0.11	1.64 ± 0.33
	I	−11.90 ± 2.27	3.65 ± 1.27*

Note: $^{*}p < 0.05$

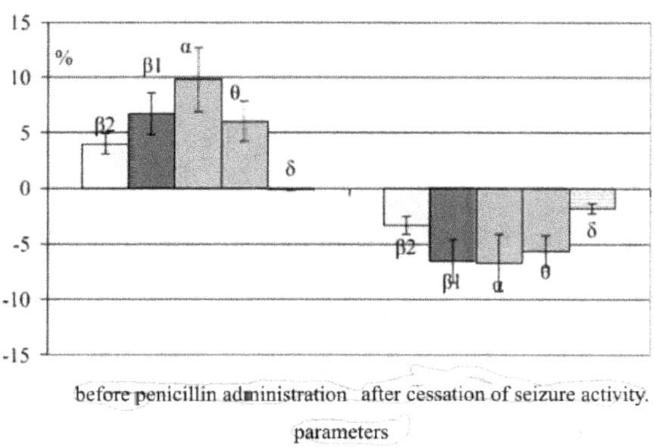

Figure 99. *Diagrams of functional interhemispheric asymmetry coefficients of ECoG rhythm amplitudes (β2, β1, α, θ, and δ) before and after BP administration.*

7.7.2. Epilepsy Diagnosis in the Clinic

Historical Background:

The earliest descriptions of epilepsy can be found in the works of Hippocrates, Galen, and Lucretius, who considered epilepsy a brain disease caused by natural, rather than supernatural, factors.

In the Middle Ages, there was continued progress toward scientific methods for diagnosing and treating epilepsy. The perception of the patient as being possessed by the devil gradually became less common in society, though it never completely disappeared. In fact, such beliefs may never entirely vanish.

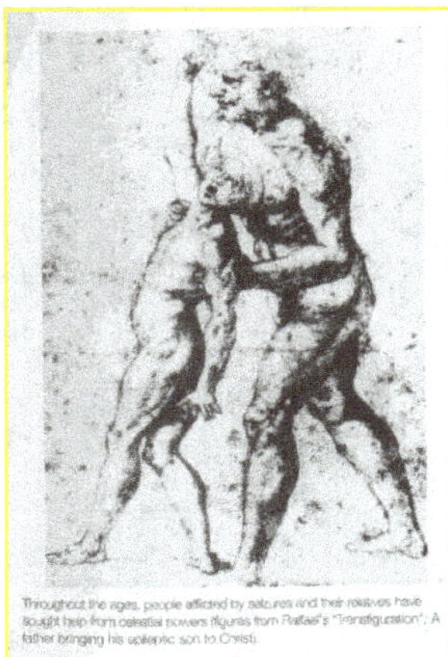

Figure 100. *For centuries, people suffering from seizure attacks, along with their relatives, sought help from divine forces (characters from Raphael's painting "Transfiguration": a father brings his epileptic son to Christ).*

The 20th century was marked by a transformation in the treatability of epilepsy—from an incurable disease to a condition in which sustained remission can be achieved in 80% of cases. Progress in epileptology has been driven by the development of diagnostic methods such as video-EEG monitoring, which allows for the assessment of seizure kinematics and the localization of epileptogenic foci in the brain.

Video-EEG monitoring (VEM) is the synchronous recording of the brain's bioelectrical activity (electroencephalography) and video images of the patient.

This technique has been used in clinical practice worldwide for more than 20 years.Progress in epileptology has been largely determined by the development of diagnostic methods, such as:

Neuroimaging, which allows identification of etiological factors in symptomatic epilepsies, including focal cortical dysplasias and others:

Magnetic Resonance Imaging (MRI)

Computed Tomography (CT)

Positron Emission Tomography (PET)

Functional MRI (fMRI)

Neurosonography

Advances in neuroimaging:

MRI

CT

PET

fMRI

Neurosonography

Progress in epileptology has also been determined by achievements in:

Molecular genetics – 90 genes responsible for various forms of epilepsy have been identified

Neurochemistry – mechanisms of ion channel function have been elucidated

Advances in classification and study of epilepsy include:

Development of new classifications

Detailed description and study of epilepsy forms and seizure types

Etiology of Epilepsy

Modern understanding holds that despite the diversity of etiological factors and syndrome heterogeneity, epilepsy remains a unified nosological entity, albeit a collective one (representing a group of different diseases). The main unifying criterion for epilepsy is the occurrence of **recurrent epileptic seizures** resulting from disturbances in neuronal excitation and inhibition in the brain.

Single or isolated seizures cannot be considered epilepsy; they represent a brain response under conditions of lowered seizure threshold and may occur in anyone under certain circumstances (Gusev E.U., Kryzhanovsky G.N., 2009).

Etiology can be influenced by multiple exogenous and endogenous factors. The main causes of epilepsy are considered to be:

Individual, constitutional, or hereditary predisposition

Presence of epileptogenic lesions

Localized or generalized electrical abnormalities in the brain

The stronger the influence of one factor, the less contribution is needed from other factors to trigger epilepsy.

The most significant etiological factors in all regions of the Russian Federation include: head trauma, stroke, brain tumors, perinatal pathology, and infectious diseases (Gekht A.B., 2004).

Depending on etiology, epilepsy is classified as:

Endogenous or idiopathic (from Latin *ideas* – "own")

Acquired or symptomatic (from Latin *symptoma* – "coincidence," indicating a specific cause)

Cryptogenic (from Greek *cryptos* – "hidden," *genesis* – "origin," indicating an unknown cause)

Currently, it is proven that symptomatic and cryptogenic epilepsies constitute the majority of cases.

Advances in genetics over the past 15 years have allowed identification of many new idiopathic forms, including the developmental programs responsible for the disease and specific prognoses for these forms.

The proportion of cryptogenic epilepsies is gradually decreasing due to the development of neuroradiology methods, brain imaging techniques, and classification of accumulated data compared with clinical manifestations of different epilepsies.

In recent years, the category of **epileptic encephalopathies** has been discussed – conditions in which epileptiform activity itself contributes to progressive brain dysfunction.

Epilepsy is a **polyetiological disease** with varying contributions of exogenous and endogenous factors in the development of its different forms.

Classification of Epileptic Seizures and Epilepsy (ILAE 2017)

The **International League Against Epilepsy (ILAE)**, 30 years after its last revision, approved the **2017 Working Classification of Seizure Types** and the **2017 Epilepsy Classification**.

According to the 2017 ILAE Seizure Classification:

Seizures may be **focal** or **generalized**, with the seizure onset being a decisive criterion.

Focal seizures are divided into:

Focal with retained awareness

Focal with impaired awareness

Several new types of generalized seizures were added.

Seizures are also classified based on the presence or absence of a motor component.

Seizures of unknown onset are categorized separately.

The 2017 ILAE Epilepsy Classification includes **three levels of categorization**:

1. **Seizure type** (per 2017 ILAE Seizure Classification)
2. **Epilepsy type** – focal, generalized, combined generalized and focal, or unknown
3. **Epileptic syndrome**

The etiological diagnosis should be refined as diagnostic data become available. Epileptic syndromes may have more than one etiological factor.

The term **"benign"** has been replaced by **"self-limited"** and **"pharmacoresponsive"**, depending on the case. The term **"age-related and epileptic encephalopathy"** can be applied partially or fully, depending on the clinical situation.

These classifications are useful in both daily clinical practice and research, helping to improve patient management and quality of life.

2017 ILAE Seizure Classification (Summary)

1. Seizure onset (key criterion):

Focal – begins in one hemisphere

Generalized – involves both hemispheres from the start

Unknown onset – onset cannot be determined

2. Focal seizures (details):

2.1 By level of awareness:

With retained awareness (formerly: simple partial)

With impaired awareness (formerly: complex partial)

2.2 By type of manifestations:

A. Motor:

Automatisms

Tonic

Clonic

Myoclonic

Atonic

Hyperkinetic

Epileptic spasms

B. Non-motor:

Sensory

Cognitive

Emotional

Autonomic

Behavioral arrest

A **focal seizure** may evolve into a **bilateral tonic-clonic seizure** (new term replacing "secondarily generalized").

3. Generalized Seizures

3.1. Motor

Tonic-clonic

Tonic

Clonic

Myoclonic

Myoclonic-tonic-clonic

Myoclonic-atonic

Atonic

Epileptic spasms

3.2. Non-motor (Absences)

Typical

Atypical

Myoclonic absences

Absences with eyelid myoclonia

4. Seizures of Unknown Onset

Motor

Non-motor

Unclassified (if insufficient data)

Changes from the old classification:

Terms “simple” and “complex partial” were removed

Concept of **awareness** introduced

More precise description of motor and non-motor manifestations

Universal and understandable language for both physicians and patients

Modern Classification of Antiseizure Medications (ASM / AEP)

Medications are classified based on **mechanism of action** and main pharmacological groups, which is most commonly used in clinical practice for treatment selection.

1) Mechanism-based classification

1.1 Modulation of ion channels

Drugs that block Na^+, Ca^{2+}, or other channels to stabilize neuronal membranes:

Na^+ channel blockers: carbamazepine, oxcarbazepine, lamotrigine, phenytoin, topiramate*

T-type Ca^{2+} channel blockers: ethosuximide, zonisamide*

Other ion modulators: lacosamide (slow Na^+ channel inactivation)

1.2 Enhancement of GABA-mediated inhibition

Drugs that increase inhibitory effect of γ-aminobutyric acid (GABA):

GABA-A receptor agonists: benzodiazepines (clonazepam, diazepam)

Barbiturates: phenobarbital

GABA transaminase/uptake inhibitors: vigabatrin, tiagabine

Valproates also enhance GABAergic effect

1.3 Reduction of excitatory glutamatergic transmission

Drugs that reduce the effect of excitatory neurotransmitter glutamate:

Topiramate (AMPA/kainate receptor antagonist)

Perampanel (selective non-competitive AMPA antagonist)

1.4 Modulation of presynaptic neurotransmitter release

Drugs affecting synaptic vesicle activity:

SV2A modulators: levetiracetam, brivaracetam

1.5 Multi-target / combined mechanisms

Drugs acting via multiple mechanisms simultaneously:

Valproates: Na^+ channel blockade + GABA enhancement + weak T-type Ca^{2+} channel blockade

Topiramate: Na^+ blockade + GABA enhancement + glutamate antagonism

Zonisamide: Na^+ and Ca^{2+} modulation + additional effects

2) Traditional pharmacological groups (chemical classes)

This classification is reflected in the **ATC system (N03)**, used in pharmacological references and drug registration.

Table 26. *ATC Classification of Antiseizure Medications (N03)*

Group	Example Drugs
Barbiturates and derivatives (N03AA)	Phenobarbital
Hydantoin derivatives (N03AB)	Phenytoin
Oxazolidine derivatives (N03AC)	Ethosuximide
Benzodiazepine derivatives (N03AE)	Clonazepam
Carbamazepine derivatives (N03AF)	Carbamazepine, Oxcarbazepine
Fatty acid derivatives (N03AG)	Valproates
Other antiseizure medications (N03AX)	Lamotrigine, Levetiracetam, Topiramate, Lacosamide, Gabapentin, Pregabalin, etc.

(ATC groups – an international system for classifying drugs by action/therapeutic use)

3) By Generation (historical, but often used in reviews)

This classification reflects the era of clinical introduction of the drugs:

First generation (classic):

Phenytoin, Carbamazepine, Valproates, Ethosuximide, Phenobarbital

Second generation:

Lamotrigine, Topiramate, Vigabatrin, Tiagabine, Gabapentin, Pregabalin

Third generation (new/enhanced):

Levetiracetam, Brivaracetam, Lacosamide, Perampanel, Ezogabine/Retigabine, etc.

4) By Clinical Use (conventional)

In practice, drugs are also distinguished according to the seizure types they are most often prescribed for:

Focal seizures: Carbamazepine, Oxcarbazepine, Lamotrigine, Levetiracetam, Lacosamide

Generalized seizures: Valproates, Ethosuximide, Lamotrigine, Topiramate, Clonazepam

Specific syndromes (e.g., absences): Ethosuximide

Key Points

Many modern antiseizure drugs have multiple mechanisms of action, providing broader therapeutic coverage.

When selecting therapy, clinicians consider seizure type, age, comorbidities, side effects, and potential drug interactions.

EEG remains the only available method for recording epileptiform activity, but it is not entirely specific. Some individuals may show epileptiform activity on EEG yet never have epilepsy, while some patients with epilepsy may not show epileptiform activity.

The diagnosis of epilepsy is clinical, meaning it does not require instrumental or laboratory confirmation, including EEG evidence of epileptiform activity.

EEG findings in epilepsy:

Increased seizure susceptibility is reflected by sharp waves and "spikes" superimposed on dysrhythmic background activity, often with hyper-synchronization of the dominant rhythm.

In **generalized tonic-clonic seizures**, EEG rhythms accelerate.

In **psychomotor seizures**, EEG activity slows.

In **absence seizures**, rapid and slow oscillations alternate, forming spike-and-wave complexes at 3 Hz.

Brain electrical potentials reach unusually high amplitudes (up to 1000 μV or more).

Clinical description of absence seizures:

Last 1–2 to 20–30 seconds, with sudden onset and rapid termination of consciousness impairment.

The person abruptly stops moving, appearing “frozen.”

After a few seconds, the interrupted movement resumes.

The gaze is fixed, facial expression remains unchanged, and memory is interrupted during the seizure.

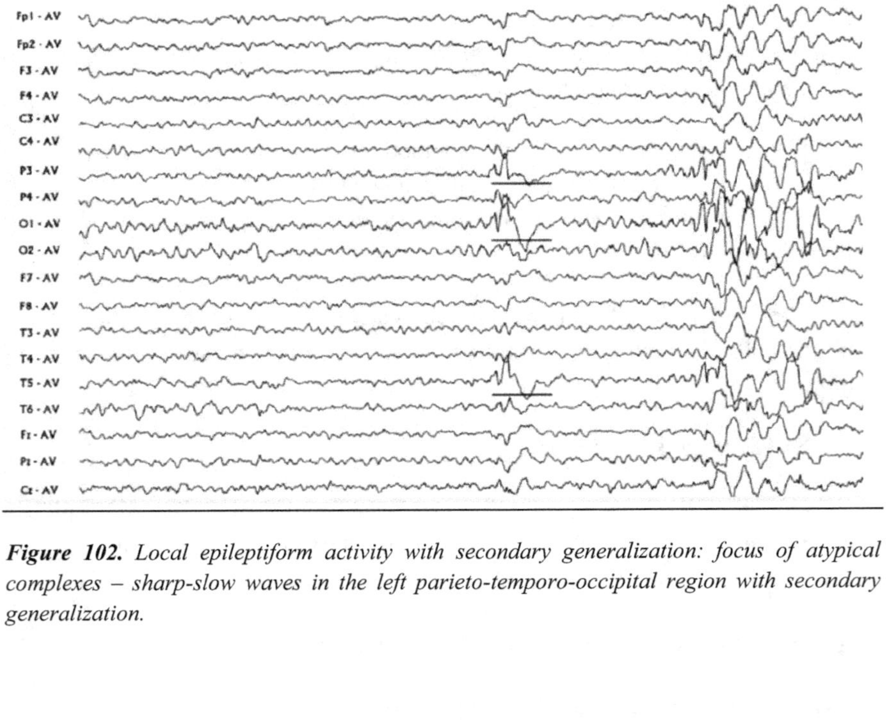

Figure 102. *Local epileptiform activity with secondary generalization: focus of atypical complexes – sharp-slow waves in the left parieto-temporo-occipital region with secondary generalization.*

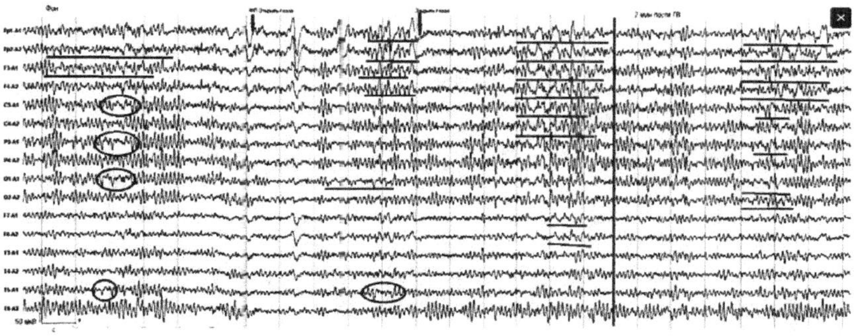

Figure 103. EEG of a 69-year-old patient. Two EEG segments recorded before and after hyperventilation.

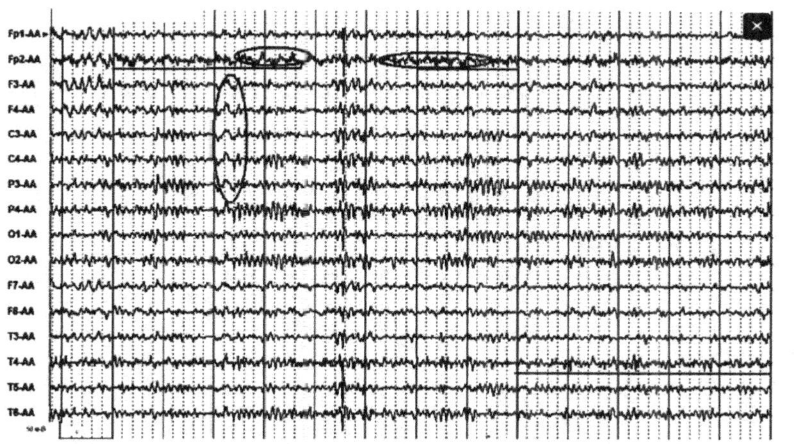

Figure 104. EEG of a 37-year-old patient. History includes a single generalized tonic-clonic seizure following exposure to lacquer fumes during floor painting.

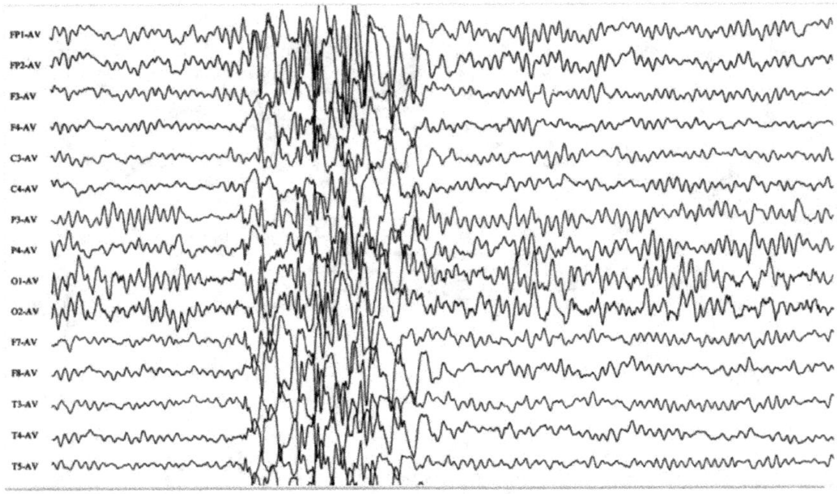

Figure 105. *Generalized epileptiform activity. A discharge consisting of a sharp–slow wave complex was recorded.*

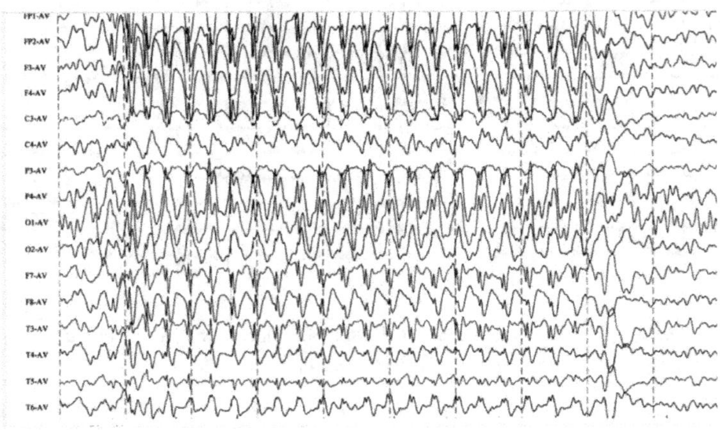

Figure 106. *Generalized epileptiform activity. Pattern of a typical absence seizure with a 3 Hz spike-and-slow-wave complex.*

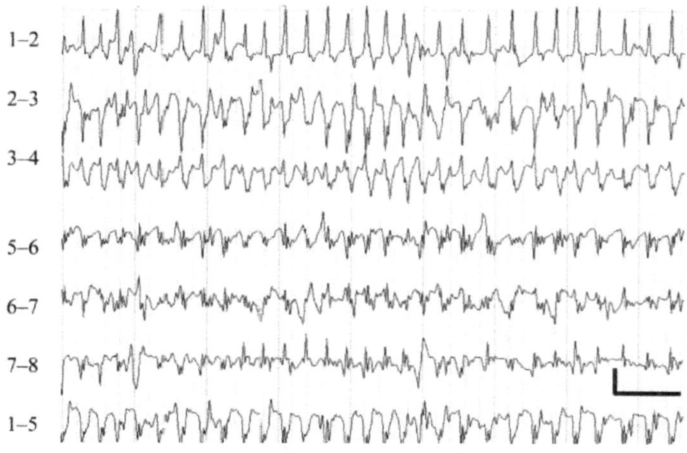

Figure 107. *ECoG. Pattern of continuous epileptiform activity. Primary focus is under electrodes 1–2; epileptiform discharges recorded under other electrodes indicate involvement of additional frontal cortex regions. Calibration signal: amplitude 500 μV, duration 1 s. M.V. Alexandrov, A.Yu. Ulitin, 2012.*

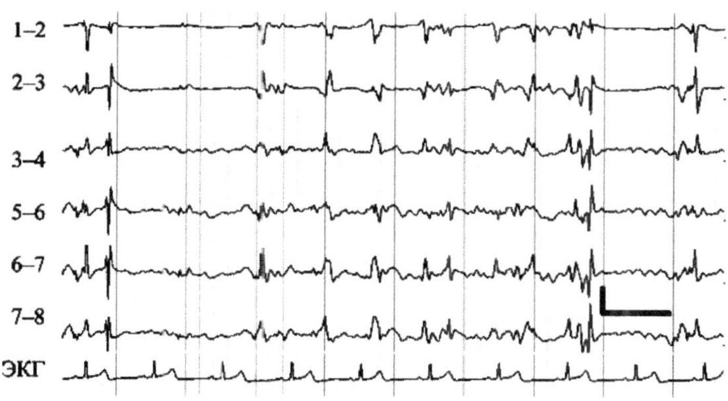

Figure 108. *ECoG. Cyclical bursts of epileptiform activity consisting of polyphasic spikes and spike–slow-wave complexes. To exclude masking of bursts by artifacts, an ECG recording is shown. Calibration signal. amplitude 500 μV, duration 1 s. M.V. Alexandrov, A.Yu. Ulitin, 2012.*

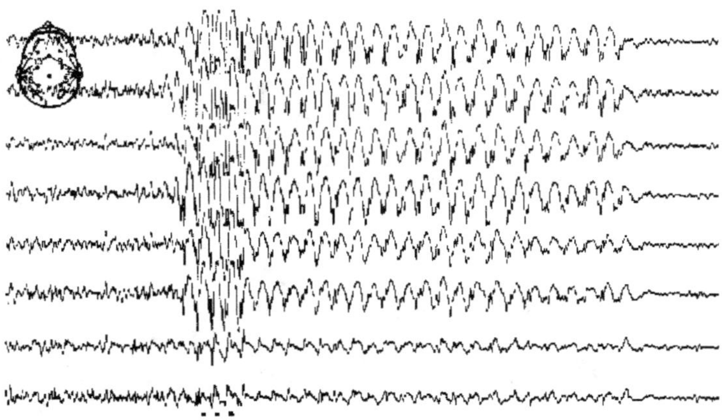

Figure 109. *Generalized epileptic activity*

Regarding epilepsy itself, despite centuries of study, many key aspects of the disorder remain incomplete, under development, or subject to debate. This includes the **etiology and pathogenesis of epilepsy**, clinical manifestations and classification, criteria for positive and differential diagnosis, treatment, and prevention. As a result, advances in modern epileptology have not yet fully met global expectations.

According to the literature, up to **10% of the population experience cerebral paroxysms (CP)**, with children representing the majority of affected individuals. By age eight, approximately **5% of children experience at least one epileptic seizure** (Gusev E.S., Burd G.S., 1994), and **18% of children and adolescents suffer from parasomnias** (Boldyrev A.I., 1987). Only **60% of patients achieve seizure control**, and an additional 10–20% may respond positively but experience some side effects. The proportion of **treatment-resistant cases can reach 40%**, and about **20% of children with epilepsy may become disabled or lose learning ability** due to frequent severe seizures and significant cognitive impairments.

In some cases, **auras may never occur**. Additional signs may include **facial pallor or flushing, eyelid twitching, and stereotyped movements of the face and hands**.

A key EEG feature of epilepsy is the presence of **spikes and sharp waves**, either episodic or sustained. Spikes are often accompanied by slow waves, forming **spike–wave complexes**. These discharges may be **generalized** or recorded as **localized events**, indicating an epileptic focus.

EEG primarily helps to **distinguish epileptic from non-epileptic seizures** and to **classify seizure types**. EEG can also:

Identify brain regions involved in seizure generation

Monitor the effects of antiepileptic drugs

Guide decisions regarding the discontinuation of therapy

The **optimal time for EEG** is **at least one week after a seizure**. An EEG performed immediately after a seizure reflects its effects but may not reveal the underlying disorder; such recordings are considered less valuable, though still useful for follow-up studies. For longer-term EEG monitoring (over 30 minutes), **portable**

EEG devices with video recording can be used. Valuable information about seizure characteristics can be obtained by correlating EEG and video data.

EEG changes during seizures can vary. In most children, the **background activity shows generalized wave discharges of various frequencies with increased amplitude**, which some researchers interpret as **paroxysmal or seizure readiness**. Long-term studies in children with epileptic seizures suggest that these changes are associated with **functional immaturity of the brain and impaired formation of cortico–brainstem connections**.

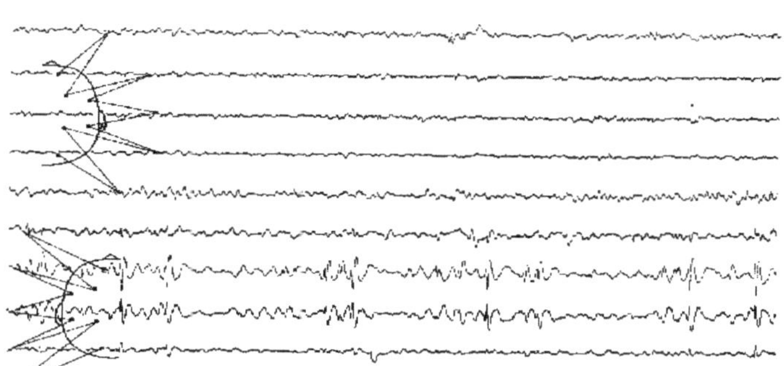

Figure 110. *Local epileptic activity. Epileptic discharges in a 4-year-old child with simple partial seizures.*

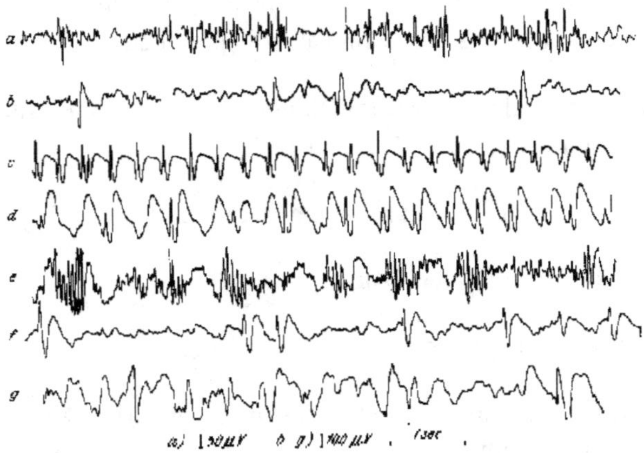

Figure 111. *Variants of epileptic activity on EEG*

Such changes are often **unstable**, tend to **disappear as the patient matures**, and are **minimally affected by the course of epileptic seizures**. Activity of this type often **vanishes after the planned discontinuation of phenobarbital**.

In **generalized seizures**, EEG may show **groups of generalized spike–wave complexes**.

In **focal epilepsy**, changes are detected only in **limited brain regions**, most often in the **temporal lobes**.

Accurate interpretation of EEG signals is, to some extent, **an art**. Changes resembling epileptic discharges can be caused by:

Eye and head movements

Pulsation of blood vessels

Respiratory movements

Cardiac activity

Chewing or swallowing

Touching the electrode

Movement of other people in the recording room

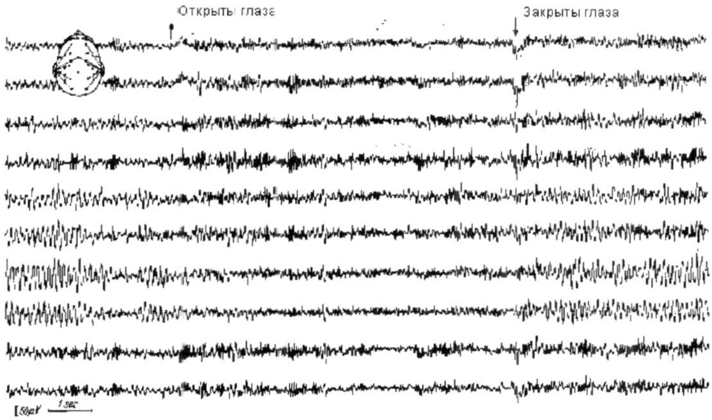

Figure 112. *EEG during intoxication with antiepileptic drugs – increased high-amplitude beta-1 waves.*

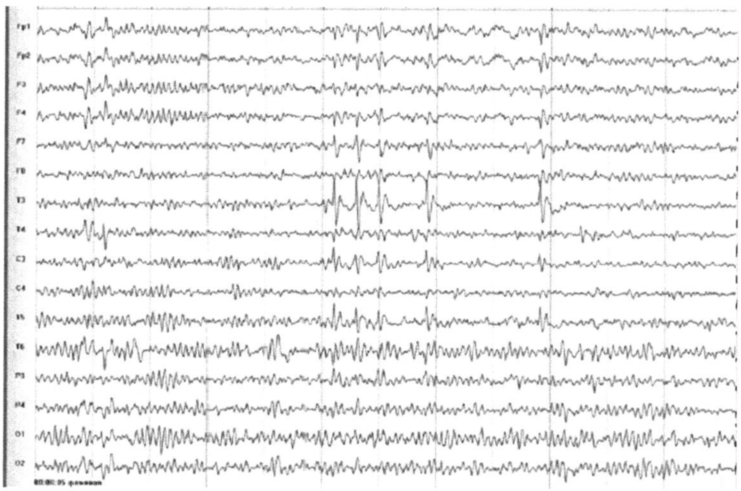

Figure 113. *Typical epileptiform activity*

8. Pathology in Children

Indications for EEG

EEG may be indicated for children presenting with:

Seizures

Psychological disturbances: unexplained irritability, excessive tearfulness, frequent tantrums, neuroses

Cerebral circulation disorders

Head injuries, contusions, concussions

Structural brain pathologies, tumors

Fainting or loss of consciousness

Moderate or frequent headaches, dizziness, disorientation

Fatigue

Epilepsy

Sleep disorders: difficulty falling asleep, insomnia, anxious sleep, sleepwalking

Autism

Cognitive disorders

Autonomic dysfunction

Down syndrome

Cerebral palsy

Endocrine disorders

Brain neoplasms and cysts

Infectious diseases (encephalitis, meningitis)

Suspected developmental delay

Brain damage due to intrauterine or perinatal factors

Vascular disorders of the brain and neck

EEG is also performed during rehabilitation after brain surgery, micro-stroke, or stroke.

Contraindications for EEG:

Head skin injuries, wounds, abrasions

Purulent-inflammatory processes of the head and neck

Fresh postoperative sutures

8.1. Preparation of the Child for EEG

EEG in children should be conducted in a calm, comfortable environment. Accurate results require the child to be relaxed. A 20–30 minute EEG will be informative and efficient if the child is properly prepared:

Explain the procedure as a game

Practice wearing the EEG cap and following instructions (open/close eyes, change breathing, etc.)

Ensure the child has eaten before the study

For very young children, align the study with their nap schedule

Artifacts in EEG

Artifacts are extracerebral signals that distort brain activity recordings.

Physical artifacts may include:

50 Hz electrical interference

Lamp or transistor noise

Baseline instability

"Microphone effect"

Movements of the child's head

Abrupt, aperiodic pen (or needle) movements due to dirty or oxidized contacts

Amplitude asymmetry from uneven interelectrode distances

Phase distortions if pen outputs are not aligned

Biological artifacts may include:

Blinking, nystagmus, eyelid tremors

Muscle potentials

ECG, respiration signals

Slow bioelectrical activity in children with metallic dental prostheses

Skin-galvanic reactions from sweating

References:

G. Dumermuth. *Elektroencephalographie im Kindesalter.* Stuttgart: Georg Thieme Verlag, 1976.

E. Niedermeyer. *Electroencephalography. Basic Principles, Clinical Applications and Related Fields,* 5th Edition. Lippincott Williams & Wilkins, 2005, pp. 209–234.

Requirements for the EEG Specialist:

1. Clearly define the diagnostic task, including suspected focus location and nature of pathology.
2. Thoroughly understand the method, its capabilities, and limitations.
3. Provide psychological preparation, explaining safety and procedure.
4. Discontinue medications affecting brain function (tranquilizers, neuroleptics, etc.) if clinically safe.
5. Require a detailed report of results, not just a summary conclusion, and understand clinical EEG terminology.

8.2. Periodization of the Development of Electroencephalogenesis

It has been shown that the process of forming bioelectrical activity in the brain during ontogenesis involves "critical periods"—phases of the most intensive restructuring of most EEG frequency components (Farber D.A., 1979; Galkina N.S. et al., 1994; Gorbachevskaya N.L. et al., 1992, 1997). It has been suggested that these changes are related to morphological reorganization of the brain (Gorbachevskaya N.L. et al., 1992).

Dynamics of the Formation of the Visual Alpha Rhythm. The period of abrupt changes in the frequency of this rhythm was reported in studies by N.S. Galkina and A.I. Boravova (1994, 1996) in children aged 14–15 months; it was accompanied by a shift of the alpha rhythm frequency from 6 Hz to 7–8 Hz. By 3–4 years of age, the rhythm frequency increases gradually, and in the vast majority of children (80%), an 8 Hz alpha rhythm dominates. By 4–5 years of age, there is a gradual shift in the mode of the dominant rhythm to 9 Hz. In the same age range, an increase in the power of the 10 Hz EEG component is observed, but it does not become dominant until 6–7 years of age, after the second critical period.

This second period occurs at 5–6 years and is manifested by a significant increase in the power of most EEG components. After this, the activity of the alpha-2 frequency band (10–11 Hz) begins to progressively increase, becoming dominant after the third critical period (10–11 years).

Thus, the frequency of the dominant alpha rhythm and the power ratio of its various components may serve as indicators of normally progressing ontogenesis.

Cellular Activity Crisis and Neurotransmitter Metabolism. At this stage, a crisis of cellular activity occurs. Another important mechanism underlying disturbances in nervous tissue electroencephalogenesis is the disruption of neurotransmitter metabolism, which arises even with a slight oxygen deficiency. Impaired synthesis of acetylcholine, dopamine, norepinephrine, and serotonin has been shown under hypoxic conditions.

Currently, perinatal post-hypoxic brain injury, or hypoxic-ischemic encephalopathy (HIE), following severe asphyxia, is considered a prolonged process, driven by a cascade of biochemical reactions. Cerebral damage is associated with increased neuronal excitability, clinically manifested as frequent seizures and EEG abnormalities.

Electroencephalography in Neonatal Practice. Electroencephalography has been used in neonatal practice since the mid-20th century (1951). Brain bioelectrical activity has been studied both in healthy newborns and in those with perinatal CNS injuries. A study of 20 healthy full-term newborns delivered by planned cesarean section before the onset of labor (24) demonstrated that normalization of brain functional state occurs only by 9–10 days of life under rational care. EEG in these newborns shows delayed activation of brain bioelectrical processes with the appearance of rhythmic activity elements, pronounced immaturity of neurophysiological mechanisms responsible for organizing circadian sleep rhythms, delayed development of responses to afferent stimuli, increased cortical irritability, and reduced seizure threshold.

After cesarean section, children generally show a flattened EEG. All these changes indicate functional immaturity and instability of brain structures during the neonatal adaptation period.

For comparison, in a control group of 20 healthy full-term newborns delivered vaginally, EEG results indicate satisfactory and relatively stable brain structure function from the first days of life, accompanied by morphological development and increased cortical functional significance by the 45th day. The authors concluded that EEG data in full-term newborns delivered by cesarean section are highly informative for assessing adaptive-compensatory processes.

8.3. Perinatal Pathology and EEG

Studies of brain bioelectrical activity in children with long-term consequences of perinatal CNS pathology have shown that the typology of EEG "maturity" in at-risk early school-age children has specific features reflecting predominantly hypoxic CNS involvement. This manifests as a distinctive temporal EEG pattern characterized by the coexistence of frequencies of a "mature" main alpha rhythm with slow and sharp forms of activity. In cases where the CNS has sufficient compensatory capacity proportional to the volume and rate of developmental demands, a foundation is established for successful individual adaptation (Kozhushko N.Yu., 2005).

The neurophysiological toolkit for EEG research, as an integrative indicator of CNS functional state in healthy children at rest and under load, is currently extensive (Shepovalnikov A.N.O., 1963; Kaubshi V.K., 1967; Farber D.A., Alferova V.V., 1972; Dummermuth G., 1965; *Current Practice of Clinical Electroencephalography* / Eds. Daly D., Padley T., N.Y.: Raven Press, 1990).

Despite differences in methodological approaches to EEG analysis and interpretation, the cited authors emphasize the universality of age-related features in the formation of brain bioelectrical activity during ontogenesis. These features appear as a gradual acceleration of cortical rhythms, replacement of slow alpha and theta waves by regular alpha activity, with the main rhythm focused in the parieto-occipital regions of the cerebral cortex. To assess the degree of rhythmic structure maturity with child development, most authors use alpha rhythm characteristics, considering its formation as a functional mechanism for integrating neural centers into a unified system that supports complex forms of behavior (Farber D.A., Dubrovinskaya N.V., 1991; Vedeneeva L.S., Soroko S.I., Shepovalnikov A.N., 1998; Rozhkov V.P., Soroko S.I., 2000).

An important aspect in studying perinatal CNS damage is the timely diagnosis of its severity. Pressler R.M. et al. (2001) found that normal EEG values during the first 8 hours of life highly correlated with favorable outcomes. Conversely, low voltage

e or absent EEG activity within the first 12 hours was strongly associated with adverse outcomes. However, some studies indicate that recovery of normal EEG by 48 hours of life can also predict favorable prognosis. Therefore, repeated assessment of brain bioelectrical activity is of high importance in neonatal practice.

T.A. Stroganova and M.G. Degtyareva examined 96 children born at 28–41 weeks of gestation with perinatal CNS lesions of varying severity. EEG monitoring was conducted during non-medicated daytime sleep at a corrected age of 1 month. They found that EEG characteristics at 1 month could accurately predict two polar outcomes of perinatal CNS lesions: normal psychomotor development in the absence of neurological abnormalities, or the development of cerebral palsy. These findings expand the understanding of the diagnostic and prognostic significance of EEG data in early childhood.

Recently, foreign researchers have increasingly favored amplitude-integrated EEG (aEEG). aEEG is a method for prolonged monitoring of brain function, which has be en used for a considerable time in neonatal intensive care units. The method is based on filtering and compressing conventional EEG, allowing easy identification of changes and deviations in background activity over extended periods.

The aEEG method was first applied in neonates in the early 1980s. It can be used for early prediction of outcomes after perinatal asphyxia. aEEG monitoring provides information about brain function within the first hours after birth, enabling high-confidence prognosis.

This type of EEG can be used to assess background activity, study sleep-wake cycles, detect early functional changes in the brain, and provide the earliest prediction of neurological outcomes. There is a correspondence between traditional EEG and aEEG in the assessment of background activity.

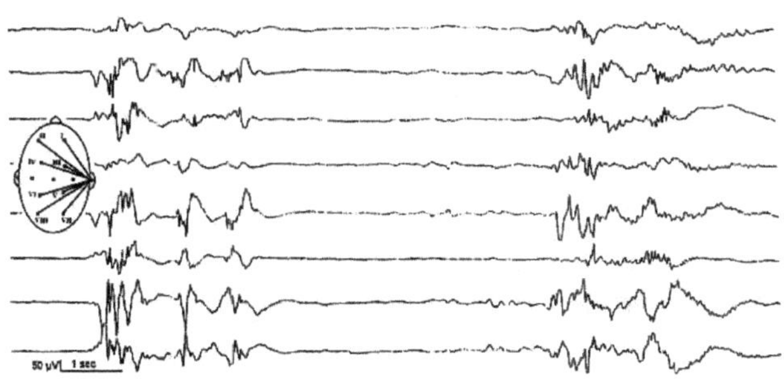

Figure 114. *EEG of a preterm infant, 24–27 weeks gestation*

Continuous low-amplitude activity (up to 20–25 μV) in the slow frequency range. Bursts of slow delta and theta activity, episodically combined with sharp waves, lasting 2–20 seconds. ***Burst-suppression phenomenon***

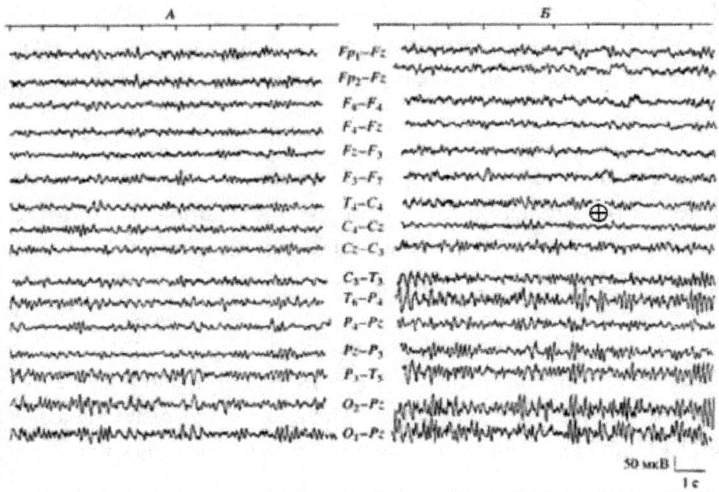

Figure 115. *EEG features in children with consequences of perinatal CNS pathology (fragments of spontaneous activity).*

A – EEG of Denis, 7 years old (high-achieving student at a gymnasium, grades 1–3); B – EEG of Nadia A., 7 years old (performing "good" to "excellent" in a regular school, grades 1–3).

Bipolar electrode derivations are indicated in the center of the figure; recording

calibration is shown in the lower right corner of the presented EEG fragment (Kozhushko N.Yu., 2005).

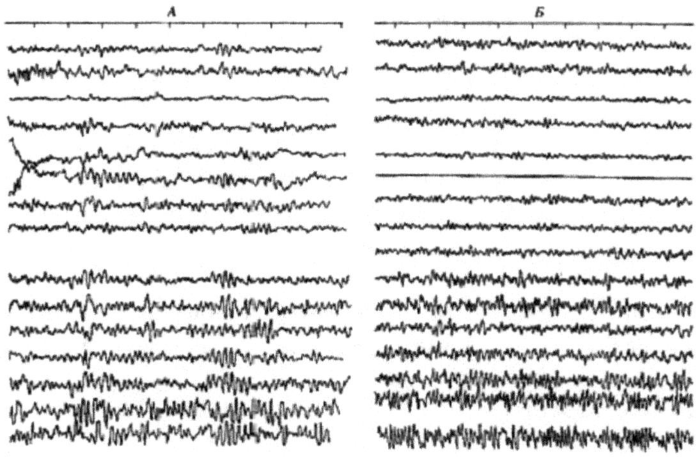

Figure 116. *Age-related dynamics of EEG in children with consequences of perinatal CNS pathology – longitudinal study (fragments of spontaneous activity). A – EEG of Nastya N. at 3 years of age; B – EEG of Nastya N. at 7 years of age (high-achieving student at a gymnasium, grades 1–3).*

For legend and electrode derivations, see Figure 114 (Kozhushko N.Yu., 2005).

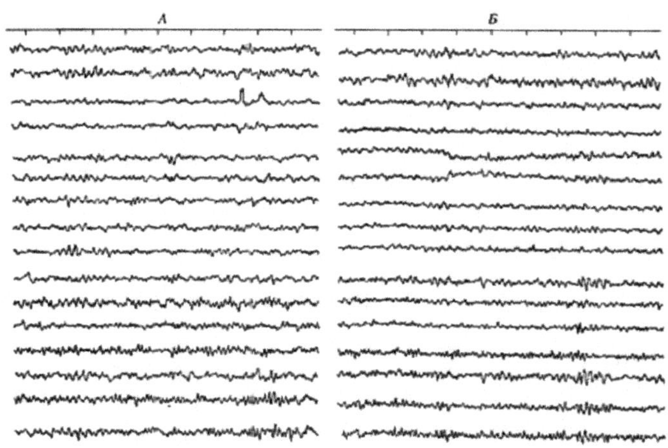

Figure 117. *Age-related dynamics of EEG in children with consequences of perinatal CNS pathology – longitudinal study (fragments of spontaneous activity).*

A – EEG of Sasha B. at 5 years of age; B – EEG of Sasha B. at 7.5 years of age (low-achieving student at a regular school, grades 1–4).

For legend and electrode derivations, see Figure 114 (Kozhushko N.Yu., 2005).

8.4. Cerebral Palsy in Children

What is Cerebral Palsy?

Cerebral palsy (CP) is a group of chronic, non-progressive motor disorders resulting from damage to or abnormal development of the brain during the prenatal, perinatal, or early postnatal period. This damage impairs the control of muscles, movement, posture, and coordination.

Children with CP may also experience additional complications such as epilepsy, speech, vision, or cognitive impairments, and behavioral problems.

Causes and Risk Factors

Major causes include:

Brain damage or abnormal brain development before birth (the majority of cases).

Difficult labor with oxygen deprivation (asphyxia).

Maternal or neonatal infections (e.g., meningitis).

Prematurity, low birth weight.

Head injuries, severe jaundice (kernicterus), and others.

Some studies report a genetic contribution in approximately 20–30% of cases, especially when no clear perinatal injury is identified.

Symptoms and Manifestations

CP presents a wide range of symptoms, including:

Muscle tone abnormalities: spasticity (stiff muscles) or hypotonia.

Impaired coordination and unsteady gait.

Delayed achievement of motor milestones.

Involuntary movements, difficulties with speech and swallowing.

Associated cognitive and sensory impairments.

Types of Cerebral Palsy

The main forms of CP include:

1. **Spastic** – increased muscle tone, stiffness, most often affecting the legs.
2. **Dyskinetic (athetoid/dystonic)** – involuntary movements.
3. **Ataxic** – coordination disorders.
4. **Mixed** – features of multiple types.

Diagnosis

Diagnosis is based on:

Clinical assessment of motor function and development.

Pregnancy and birth history.

Instrumental studies: MRI, CT, and cranial ultrasound.

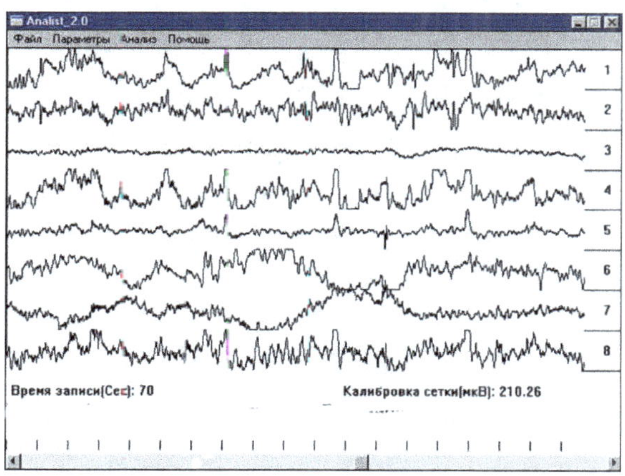

Figure 118. *Girl, 6 years old. Cerebral palsy. Multiple sharp waves without focal localization.*

Electrode derivations: left – 1: frontal–temporal, 2: temporal–temporal, 3: parietal–occipital, 4: frontal–occipital; right – 5, 6, 7, 8.

Treatment and Rehabilitation

Cerebral palsy (CP) is not fully curable, but symptomatic and rehabilitative treatments can improve function:

Pharmacological therapy – for spasticity and seizures.

Physical therapy, therapeutic exercise, and occupational therapy – for motor development.

Speech therapy – for speech impairments.

Orthopedic devices and surgery – as indicated.

Early diagnosis and a multidisciplinary approach are crucial for maximizing a child's functional abilities.

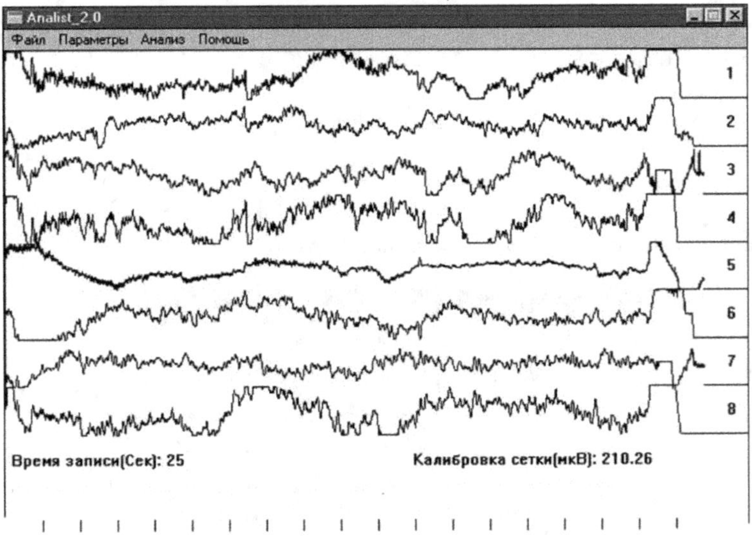

Figure 119. *Boy, 5 years old. Cerebral palsy. Disorganized type EEG.*

Electrode derivations are the same as in Figure 117.

EEG (electroencephalography) in children with cerebral palsy (CP) exhibits a number of characteristic, though nonspecific, features. These depend on the CP type, the extent and location of brain damage, the child's age, and the presence of comorbid epilepsy.

Common EEG changes in CP

In most children with CP, EEG differs from age-related norms, showing:

Immaturity of bioelectrical activity

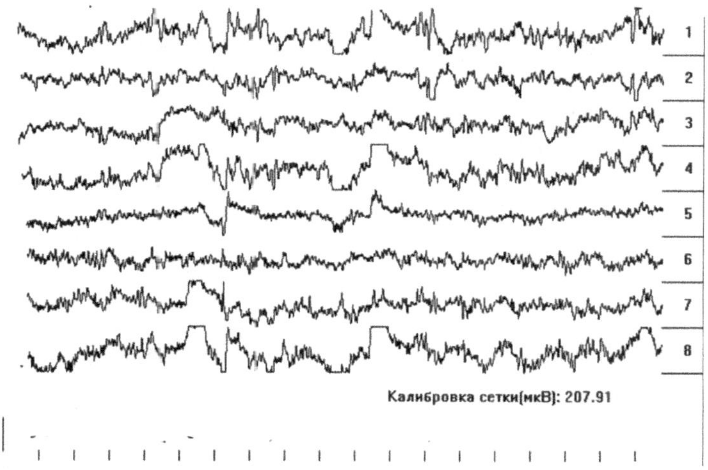

Figure 120. *Boy, 8 years old. Cerebral palsy. Disorganized type EEG with multiple sharp waves, without signs of localization or lateralization.*

Delayed formation of age-related rhythms

EEG not corresponding to chronological age

Predominance of slow waves (theta and delta activity)

Reduced expression and organization of the alpha rhythm

Impaired interhemispheric asymmetry

Disorganization of cortical activity

Focal changes

Local or regional abnormalities are often detected, associated with the site of brain damage: focal slowing of activity, amplitude and frequency asymmetry, reduced functional activity of the affected hemisphere.

Particularly characteristic in:

Hemiplegic form of cerebral palsy

Consequences of periventricular leukomalacia

Post-ischemic and post-hemorrhagic lesions

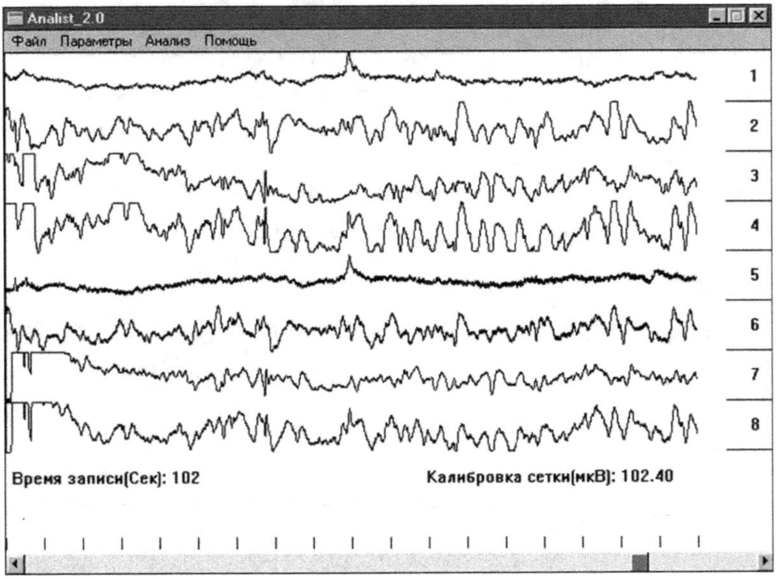

Figure 121. *Boy, 4 years old. Cerebral palsy. High-amplitude, low-frequency activity.*

Epileptiform Activity

This is a very important aspect, as epilepsy occurs in 30–50% of children with cerebral palsy (CP). On EEG, the following may be observed: spikes, sharp waves, spike–wave complexes, and polyspikes.

Epileptiform activity may

Be accompanied by clinical seizures

Be subclinical (without visible convulsions)

Increase during sleep

Features Depending on CP Type

Spastic diplegia:

Diffuse EEG changes

Moderate epileptiform activity (not always present)

Slowing of background activity

Hemiplegic form:

Marked interhemispheric asymmetry

Focal epileptiform discharges

High risk of focal epilepsy

Double hemiplegia:

Severe EEG disorganization

Pronounced slowing

Frequent generalized epileptiform activity

Atonic and hyperkinetic forms:

Less specific changes

More often diffuse disorganization without clear foci

Age-Related Features

In younger children, EEG abnormalities may be more pronounced

Partial normalization of EEG can occur with age (neuroplasticity)

Severe forms often retain persistent abnormalities

Clinical Significance of EEG in CP

EEG is used for:

Diagnosis and monitoring of epilepsy

Assessment of brain functional state

Selection and adjustment of antiepileptic therapy

Limited prediction of cognitive development

Important: EEG does not determine the severity of motor impairment and is not a criterion for CP severity.

Summary

EEG in CP is often abnormal but nonspecific

Common findings: slowing, disorganization, and epileptiform activity

Most significant when epilepsy is suspected

Always interpreted in combination with clinical assessment and MRI

Conclusion

Electroencephalography has undergone a long path of development—from the first studies of the brain's electrical activity to modern high-technology methods of quantitative and spatial analysis. This book consistently presents the evolution of EEG both as a scientific method and as an essential tool in clinical and experimental practice. It examines the historical stages of electroencephalography, the formation of concepts regarding the genesis of EEG, the biophysical mechanisms of electrocortical activity, and the role of thalamocortical and corticocortical interactions in the organization of brain rhythms.

Special attention is given to the characteristics of the main rhythms—delta, theta, alpha, and beta activity—their functional significance, age-related dynamics, and participation in the formation of psychophysiological states. Modern concepts of the brain's network and dynamic organization allow EEG to be viewed not as a sum of local phenomena, but as a reflection of the integrative activity of neuronal ensembles.

The book provides a detailed description of methodological aspects of EEG recording and analysis: from recording conditions and functional tests to methods of mathematical processing, including time-domain, spectral, correlation, and nonlinear analysis. The transition to quantitative electroencephalography (qEEG), the development of source localization, full digitalization, and the implementation of artificial intelligence have significantly expanded the diagnostic and prognostic capabilities of the method.

The practical significance of EEG is demonstrated through the analysis of normal age-related patterns and a wide range of pathological conditions in adults and children. Changes in bioelectrical activity are discussed in alcohol dependence, schizophrenia, intellectual disability, Alzheimer's disease, Parkinsonism, affective and organic disorders, epilepsy, as well as in perinatal pathology and cerebral palsy.

The role of EEG in diagnosis, monitoring, treatment selection, and evaluation of therapeutic effectiveness—including the use of quantitative and computer-based methods—is clearly illustrated.

A separate section highlights the application of electroencephalography in experimental psychology, cognitive research, and the study of individual personality traits, emphasizing the interdisciplinary nature of the method.

Thus, electroencephalography today represents a universal, scientifically grounded, and clinically significant tool for studying the functional state of the brain. Its further development is associated with the integration of neurophysiological data with neuroimaging, the advancement of machine learning algorithms, and the deepening of knowledge about the brain's network organization. The future of electroencephalography lies not only in technological improvement but also in the expansion of theoretical models that bridge fundamental neuroscience and clinical practice, making EEG one of the key methods of modern medicine and neuroscience.

Литература

1. Achermann P., Borbély A. A. Low-frequency (< 1 Hz) oscillations in the human sleep electroencephalogram // Neuroscience. — 1997. — Vol. 81, No. 1. — P. 213–
2. Adrian, E. D., & Matthews, B. H. C. The Berger rhythm: Potential changes from the occipital lobes in man // *Brain*. — 1934. — Vol. 57, No. 4. — P. 355–385. — DOI: 10.1093/brain/57.4.355.
3. Aftanas L. I., Golocheikine S. A. EEG alpha oscillations in the human brain during emotional and cognitive processes. Neuroscience and Behavioral Physiology. 2001. Vol. 31, no. 1. P. 30-36. DOI: 10.1023/A:1010068715919
4. aging by EEG data. Electroencephalogr. Clin Neurophysiol 1997;103:241-248.
5. Akbar Y., Khotimah S. N., Haryanto F. Spectral and brain mapping analysis of EEG based on Pwelch in schizophrenic patients. Journal of Physics: Conference Series 694 (2016) 012070
6. Al-Nuaimi A.H., Jammeh E., Sun L., Ifeachor E. Changes in the EEG amplitude as a biomarker for early detection of Alzheimer's disease // *2016 38th Annual International Conference of the IEEE Engineering in Medicine and Biology Society*
7. Alvarez A, Pérez-Avalo MC, Morenza L. Neuropsychological assessment of learning-disorder children with paroxysmal EEG activity. New Issues Neurosci. 1992; IV(1): 40–50
8. American Psychiatric Association 1994. Diagnostic and Statistical Manual of Mental Disorders, 4th edn. American Psychiatric Association, Washington, DC, 1994
9. Andersen P., Andersson S. A. Thalamic origin of cortical rhythmic activity // *Handbook of Electroencephalography and Clinical Neurophysiology* / Ed. A. R. Remond. — Amsterdam: Elsevier Scientific Publishing Company, 1974. — Vol. 2C. — P. 90–118.
10. Anokhin, A.P. Genetic Influences on Dynamic Complexity of Brain Oscillations / A.P.Anokhin, V.Müller, U.Lindenberger, A.C.Heath, E.Myers // Neurosci Lett. –
11. Ariwodola, O. J., & Weiner, J. L. (2004). *Ethanol potentiation of GABAergic synaptic transmission may be self-limiting: role of presynaptic GABAB receptors*. The Journal of Neuroscience, 24(47), 10679–10686.
12. Başar-Eroglu, C , Strüber, D., Schürmann, M., Stadler, M., & Başar, E. (1996). *Gamma-band responses in the brain: a short review of*

psychophysiological correlates and functional significance. International Journal of Psychophysiology, 24(1–2), 101–118. https://doi.org/10.1016/S0167-8760(96)00051-7

13. Bauer, L. O., & Hesselbrock, V. M. Electroencephalographic, autonomic and subjective correlates of the risk for alcoholism // *Journal of Studies on Alcohol.*
14. Becker-Carus, C. Relationships between EEG, personality and vigilance // *Electroencephalography and Clinical Neurophysiology.* — 1971. — Vol. 30, No. 6. — P. 519–526.
15. Beijsterveldt Van, C.E.M. Twin and family studies of the human electroencephalogram: a review and a metaanalysis / C.E.M.Van Beijsterveldt, G.C.M.van Baal // Biological psychology. – 2002. – Vol. 62. – P. 111-238.
16. Belsh J. M. *Brain death: policy at Middlesex General-University Hospital // Journal of the Medical Society of New Jersey* — 1985. — Vol. 82. — P. 199–205.
17. Berger, H. Über das Elektrenkephalogramm des Menschen // Archiv für Psychiatrie und Nervenkrankheiten. — 1929. — Vol. 87, No. 1. — P. 527–570. — DOI: 10.1007/BF01797193.
18. Bertalanffy L. von (1967). *Robots, Men and Minds.* New York: George Braziller. (см. также General System Theory)
19. Besthorn C, Zerfass R, Geiger-Kabisch C, et al. Discrimination of AD and normal
20. Blume, W. T. *Abnormal EEG: epileptiform potentials* // B. T. Blume (Ed.), *Atlas of Pediatric Electroencephalography.* — New York: Raven Press, 1982. — P. 139–148.
21. Blume, W. T., & Dreyfus-Brisac, C. (1982). *Positive rolandic sharp waves in neonatal EEG: types and significance. Electroencephalography and Clinical Neurophysiology*, 53(3), 277–282. https://doi.org/10.1016/0013-
22. Boutros N.N. *A review of indications for routine EEG in clinical psychiatry // Hospital and Community Psychiatry.* — 1992. — Vol. 43, No. 7. — Pp. 716–719. — DOI: 10.1176/ps.43.7.716. — PMID: 1516903.
23. Breakspear M. Dynamic models of large-scale brain activity. *Nat Neurosci.* 2017;20(3):340–352. doi:10.1038/nn.4497.
24. Britton JW, Frey LC, Hopp JL, Korb P, Koubeissi MZ, Lievens WE, Pestana-Knight EM, St. Louis EK, editors. *Electroencephalography (EEG): An Introductory Text and Atlas of Normal and Abnormal Findings in Adults, Children, and Infants.*

25. Bruder, G. E., Towey, J. P., Friedman, D., Erhan, H., & Jasiukaitis, P. (1992). *Lateral asymmetries of event-related potential slow waves and behavioral dichotic listening performance in bipolar disorder*. Journal of Abnormal Psychology, 101(1), 64–70.
26. Buzsáki G, Anastassiou CA, Koch C. The origin of extracellular fields and currents — EEG, ECoG, LFP and spikes. *Nat Rev Neurosci*. 2012;13(6):407–420. doi:10.1038/nrn3241.
27. Buzsáki G. *Rhythms of the Brain* / G. Buzsáki. — New York: Oxford University Press, 2006. —
28. Buzsáki G. *Rhythms of the Brain*. Oxford University Press; 2006.
29. Buzsáki, György, Costas A. Anastassiou, and Christof Koch. "The Origin of Extracellular Fields and Currents: EEG, ECoG, LFP and Spikes." *Nature Reviews Neuroscience*, vol. 13, no. 6, 2012, pp. 407–420, doi:10.1038/nrn3241.
30. Buzsáki, György. "Theta Oscillations in the Hippocampus." *Neuron*, vol. 33, no. 3, 2002, pp. 325–340, doi:10.1016/S0896-6273(02)00586-X.
31. Byring RF, Salmi T, Sainio K, Orn HP. EEG in children with spelling disabilities. Electroencephalogr Clin Neurophysiol. 1991; 79: 247–255. pmid:1717228
32. Cajochen C., Kräuchi K., Wirz-Justice A. Sleep and psychiatric disorders. Neuropsychopharmacology. 2000. Vol. 23, no. 2. P. 179-190.
33. Campbell, J. M., Brown, R. T., Cavanagh, S. E., Vess, S. F., & Segall, M. J. (2008). *Evidence-based assessment of cognitive functioning in pediatric psychology. Journal of Pediatric Psychology*, 38(something). https://doi.org/10.1093/jpepsy/jsm138
34. Carlson, C. R., & Stevens, K. D. (2006). *Psychological considerations for chronic orofacial pain. Oral and Maxillofacial Surgery Clinics of North America*, 20(2), 185–195.
35. Carter, C. S., Braver, T. S., Barch, D. M., Botvinick, M. M., Noll, D., & Cohen, J. D. (1998). *Anterior cingulate cortex, error detection, and the online monitoring of performance*. Science, 280(5364), 747–749. DOI:10.1126/science.280.5364.747.
36. Carter, P., Yeung, A. (1985). *Drained cavity expansion in sands exhibiting particle crushing. International Journal for Numerical and Analytical Methods in Geomechanics*, 9, 125–140.
37. Cavanagh, J. F., & Shackman, A. J. (2015). *Frontal midline theta reflects anxiety and cognitive control: Meta-analytic evidence*. Journal of Physiology-Paris, 109(1-3), 3–15. https://doi.org/10.1016/j.jphysparis.2014.04.003

38. Ceballos N. A., Bauer L. O., Houston R. J. Recent EEG and ERP findings in substance abusers // *Clinical EEG and Neuroscience*. — 2009. — Vol. 40, № 2. — P. 122–128. — doi:10.1177/155005940904000210.
39. Chabot RJ, di Michele F, Prichep L, John ER. The Clinical Role of Computerized EEG in the Evaluation and Treatment of Learning and Attention Disorders in Children and Adolescents. J Neuropsychiatry Clin Neurosci. 2001; 13: 171–186. pmid:11449024
40. Chaddad, A., *et al.* (2023). *Title to be completed based on exact topic — e.g., machine learning/EEG analysis. (Требует уточнения DOI и журнала по вашему тексту)*
41. Chandra S.R., Asheeb A., Dash S., Retna N., Teja K.V.R., Issac T.G. *Role of electroencephalography in the diagnosis and treatment of neuropsychiatric border zone syndromes // Indian Journal of Psychological Medicine*. — 2017. — Vol. 39, No. 3. — Pp. 243–249. — DOI: 10.4103/0253-7176.207336. — PMID: 28615755.
42. Chavez, L., et al. (2009). "EEG abnormalities and cognitive dysfunction in schizophrenia." *Psychiatry Research*, 162(2), 156-163.
43. Chetty C.A., Bhardwaj H., Kumar G.P., EEG biomarkers in Alzheimer's and prodromal Alzheimer's: a comprehensive analysis of spectral and connectivity features // Alzheimer's Research & Therapy. – 2024. – Vol. 16, Article 236. – DOI: 10.1186/s13195-024-01582-w. – ISSN 1758-9193 (Online). (In Eng.)
44. Chicago: American Epilepsy Society; 2016. ISBN-13: 978-0-9979756-0-4. Available from: https://www.ncbi.nlm.nih.gov/books/NBK390354/
45. Christine T. G Verleger. J-S Rolf . EEG coherence at rest and during a visual task in two groups of children Electroencephalography and Clinical Neurophysiology Volume 67, Issue 2, August 1987, Pages 151-158.
46. Clementz, B. A., et al. (2006). Electroencephalographic abnormalities in schizophrenia: Effects of antipsychotic medications and clinical correlates." *Journal of Clinical Psychiatry*, 67(3), 414-422.
47. Cobb, W. R. (1944). *An historical review of the neuromuscular theory of sleep. Journal of Neurophysiology*, 7, 123–159.
48. Colon EJ, Notermans SL, de Weerd JP, Kap J. The discriminating role of EEG power spectra in dyslexic children. J Neurol. 1979; 221: 257–262. pmid:92551
49. Colrain I. M., Turlington S., Baker F. C. Impact of Alcoholism on Sleep Architecture and EEG Power Spectra in Men and Women // *Sleep*. — 2009. — Vol. 32, No. 10. — P. 1341–1352. — DOI: 10.1093/sleep/32.10.1341. — ISSN 1550-9109.

50. Cossu, M., Cardinale, F., Castana, L., et al. (2005). *Stereo-EEG in the presurgical evaluation of focal epilepsy: A retrospective analysis of 215 procedures. Neurosurgery*, 57(4), 706-718.
51. Coutin-Churchman P., Moreno R., Añez Y., Vergara F. Clinical correlates of quantitative EEG alterations in alcoholic patients // *Clin. Neurophysiol*. — 2006. — Vol. 117, № 4. — P. 740–751. — DOI: 10.1016/j.clinph.2005.12.021. — PMID: 16495144.
52. Crow, T. J., & Spear, P. J. (1972). *Anatomical context of EEG frequencies. Electroencephalography and Clinical Neurophysiology*, 33(1), 38–44.
53. Crow, T. J., P. J. Spear, and G. W. Arbuthnott. "Intracranial Self-Stimulation with Electrodes in the Region of the Locus Coeruleus." *Brain Research*, vol. 36, no. 2, 1972, pp. 275–287, doi:10.1016/0006-8993(72)90735-4.
54. Current Practice of Clinical Electroencephalolography / Eds. Daly D. Padley T. N.Y.: Raven Press, 1990
55. da Silva FL. EEG and MEG: relevance to neuroscience. *Neuron*. 2013;80(5):1112–1128. doi:10.1016/j.neuron.2013.10.017.
56. da Silva, F. L. (2013). *EEG: Origin and measurement.* In *EEG – Electroencephalography: Basic Principles, Clinical Applications, and Related Fields* (5th ed.).
57. Daly, D. D., & Pedley, T. (Eds.) (1990). *Current Practice of Clinical Electroencephalography.* New York: Raven Press.
58. Darlow, J. S. (1985). *Mechanisms of neonatal EEG patterns. Early Human Development*, 12(2), 101–112. *(пример — уточните исходный текст)*
59. Davey M.P., Victor J.D., Schiff N.D. Power spectra and coherence in the EEG of a vegetative patient with severe asymmetric brain damage. Clin Neurophysiol. 2000; 111(11):1949-54.
60. David S. Cantor Clinical Robert ChabotQEEG Studies in the Assessment and Treatment of Childhood Disorders EEG and Neuroscience First Published April 1, 2009 Research Article Find in PubMedhttps://doi.org/10.1177/155005940904000209
61. Dement W. C., Kleitman N. Cyclic variations in EEG during sleep and their relation to eye movements, body motility, and dreaming // Electroencephalography and Clinical Neurophysiology. — 1957. — Vol. 9, № 4. — P. 673–690. — doi:10.1016/0013-4694(57)90088-3.
62. Di Chiara G., Imperato A. Drugs abused by humans preferentially increase synaptic dopamine concentrations in the mesolimbic system of freely moving rats // Proc Natl Acad Sci U S A. — 1988. — Vol. 85, № 14. — P. 5274–5278. — doi:10.1073/pnas.85.14.5274.

63. Di Chiara, G., Tanda, G., & Bassareo, V. (1996). *Reward mechanisms in the brain: Is dopamine involved? Psychopharmacology*, 123(1), 1–10. DOI: https://doi.org/10.1016/j.jphysparis.2014.04.003
64. Dokukina T. V., Misiuk N. N. EEG mapping in the evaluation of the signs of organic rain damage in patients with mental diseases // Zh Nevrol Psikhiatr Im S S Korsakova. — 2000. — Vol. 100, № 5. — P. 39–44.
65. Dreyfus-Brisac C., Curzi-Dascalova L. The EEG during the first year of life / In: Rémond A. (ред.) *The evolution of the EEG. Handbook of Electroencephalography*. — Amsterdam: Elsevier, 1975. — C. 24–30.
66. Dreyfus-Brisac, C. (1975). *Neonatal encephalography.* In E. M. Scarpelli & B. Cosmi (Eds.), *Review in Perinatal Medicine* (Vol. 3). New York: Raven Press.
67. Duilio Giannitrapani EEG average frequency and intelligenceFréquence EEG moyenne et intelligence. Electroencephalography and Clinical Neurophysiology Volume 27, Issue 5, November 1969, Pages 480-486
68. Dumermuth G. Elektroencephalographie im Kindesalter. — Stuttgart: Georg Thieme Verlag, 1976. — 312 c.
69. Dummermuth G. Elektroencephalographie in Kindesalter. Stuttgart: Thieme, 1965.
70. Dummermuth G., (1965) EEG abnormalities in schizophrenia and their relation to clinical features." *Journal of Neuropsychiatry and Clinical Neurosciences*, 9(4), 394-400.
71. Dunkley B.T., Sedge P.A., Doesburg S.M., Grodecki R.J., Jetly R., et al. Theta, mental flexibility, and post-traumatic stress disorder: connecting in the parietal cortex // *PLoS One*. — 2015. — Vol. 10, № 4. — e0123541. — doi:10.1371/journal.pone.0123541.
72. Dunn B.R. Modal processing style differences in the recall of expository text and poetry / Dunn B.R., Reddix M. // Learning and Individual differences. – 1991. – V. 3. – P. 265-293.
73. Evans, F. J. (1952). *Electroencephalography and clinical neurology. Journal of Clinical Neurophysiology*, 14, 22–31. *(пример — уточните название)*
74. Eysenck H.J. Manual of the Eysenck personality inventory / Eysenck H.J., Eysenck S.G.B. - London: University of London Press, 1964
75. Eysenck H.J. Personality and individual differences: A natural science approach / H.J. Eysenck, M.W. Eysenck. New York: Plenum, perspective. 1985{42}
76. Eysenck H.J. Personality patterns in various groups. Occupational Psychology / H.J. Eysenck, 1967, 41, 249-250.

77. Eysenck H.J. The biological basis of personality / Eysenck H.J. – 1967; Eysenck H.J. The measurement of person ality. - Lancaster. England: Medical & Technical Publishers, 1976
78. Fein G, Galin P, Yingling CD, Johnstone J, Davenport L, Herron J. EEG spectra in dyslexic and control boys during resting conditions. Electroencephalogr Clin Neurophysiol. 1986; 63: 87–97. pmid:2417821
79. Fein G., Allen J. EEG Spectral Changes in Treatment Naïve Active Alcoholics // *Alcoholism: Clinical and Experimental Research.* — 2005. — Vol. 29, No. 4. — P. 538–546. — DOI: 10.1097/01.alc.0000159107.08471.97. — ISSN 0145-6008.
80. Fernández T, Harmony T, Fernández-Bouzas A, Silva J, Herrera W, Santiago-Rodríguez E, et al. Sources of EEG activity in Learning Disabled Children. Clin Electroencephalogr. 2002; 33(4): 160–164. pmid:12449846
81. Fingelkurts A.A. Altered structure of dynamic electroencephalogram oscillatory pattern in major depression // Biological Psychiatry, 2015, no. 12, pp. 1050–1060. DOI: https://doi.org/10.1016/j.biopsych.2014.12.011
82. Flanary J., Daly S. R., Bakker C., Herman A. B., Park M. C., McGovern R., Walczak T., Henry T., Netoff T. I., Darrow D. P. Reliability of visual review of intracranial electroencephalogram in identifying the seizure onset zone: A systematic review and implications for the accuracy of automated methods // *Epilepsia.* — 2023. — Vol. 64, № 1. — P. 6–16. — doi:10.1111/epi.17446.
83. Flanary, J., et al. (2022). *Reliability of visual review of intracranial EEG for defining resection zones in epilepsy surgery. Epilepsia Open.* Available from PMC: PMC10099245.
84. Fornito A., Zalesky A., Bassett D., Meunier D., Ellison-Wright I, Yücel M, Stephen J Wood S., ShawK., O'Connor J, Nertney D., Mowry B, Christos Pantelis Ch., Bullmore E. Genetic influences on cost-efficient organization of human cortical functional networks / A.Zalesky, D.S.Bassett, D.Meunier [at al.] // J. Neurosci. – 2011. – Vol. 31, N 9. – P. 3261-3270.
85. Frauscher B., Rossetti A.O., Beniczky S. Recent advances in clinical electroencephalography // *Curr Opin Neurol.* — 2024. — Vol. 37, № 2. — P. 134–140. — doi:10.1097/WCO.0000000000001246.
86. Fumoto M., Sato-Suzuki I., Seki Y., Mohri Y., Arita H. 2004;.Dunkley B.T., Sedge P.A., Doesburg S.M., Grodecki R.J., Jetly R.et al. 2015
87. Gasser, T., Jennen-Steinmetz, C., Verleger, R. *EEG coherence at rest and during a visual task in two groups of children // Electroencephalography and Clinical Neurophysiology.* — 1987. — Vol. 67, No. 2. — P. 151–158. — PMID: 2439292.

88. Gastaut H. Etude électroencéphalographique de la crise d'épilepsie // *Electroencephalogr Clin Neurophysiol.* — 1951. — Vol. 3, № 1. — P. 1–14.
89. Glahn, D.C. Genetic control over the resting brain / D.C.Glahn, A.M.Winkler, P.Kochunov [at al.] // Proc. Natl. Acad. Sci. U S A. – 2010. – Vol.107, N 3. – P.1223.
90. Gordillo D., Ramos da Cruz J., Chkonia E., Lin W.-H., Favrod O., Brand A., Figueiredo P., Roinishvili M., Herzog M. H. The EEG Multiverse of Schizophrenia // *Cerebral Cortex.* — 2022. — Vol. 33, №7. — P. 3816–3826. — DOI: 10.1093/cercor/bhac309.
91. Green J. D., Arduini A. A. Hippocampal electrical activity in arousal // *Journal of Neurophysiology.* — 1954. — Vol. 17, № 6. — P. 533–557. — doi:10.1152/jn.1954.17.6.533.
92. Haddad, N., Carr, M., Balian, S., Lannin, J., Kim, Y., Toth, C., & Jarvis, J. (2022). *The blood–brain barrier and pharmacokinetic/pharmacodynamic optimization of antibiotics for the treatment of central nervous system infections in adults.* Antibiotics, 11(12), 1843. https://doi.org/10.3390/antibiotics11121843.
93. Harmony T., Hinojosa G., Marosi E., Becker J., Rodríguez M., Reyes A. et al. Correlation between EEG spectral parameters and an educational evaluation // *International Journal of Neuroscience.* — 1990. — Vol. 54, № 1–2. — P. 147–155. — doi:10.3109/00207459008986630.
94. Harrewijn A., Van der Molen M.J.W., Westenberg P.M. Putative EEG measures of social anxiety: Comparing frontal alpha asymmetry and delta–beta crossfrequency correlation // Cognitive, Affective and Behavioral Neuroscience, 2016, no. 6, pp. 1086–1098. DOI: https://doi.org/10.3758/s13415-0160455-y
95. He S., Wang X., Zhou Y. Quantitative EEG in schizophrenia and depression: A comprehensive review. Psychiatry Research. 2017. Vol. 247. P. 115-123. DOI: 10.1016/j.psychres.2016.11.015
96. Henry C. E. Electroencephalograms of normal children // *Monogr Soc Res Child Dev.* — 1944. — Vol. 9, No. 3. — P. 1–71.
97. Herman S. T., Abend N. S., Bleck T. P., Chapman K. E., Drislane F. W., Emerson R. G., Gerard E. E., Hahn C. D., Husain A. M., Kaplan P. W., LaRoche S. M., Nuwer M. R., Quigg M., Riviello J. J., Schmitt S. E., Simmons L. A., Tsuchida T. N., Hirsch L. J. Consensus statement on continuous EEG in critically ill adults and children, part I: indications // *J Clin Neurophysiol.* — 2015. — Vol. 32, № 2. — P. 87–95. — doi:10.1097/WNP.0000000000000166.

98. Hillyard S. A., Picton T. W. Electrophysiology and auditory evoked potentials // *Handbook of Psychophysiology* (ред. Cacioppo J. T., Tassinary L. G., Berntson G. G.). — 3rd ed. — Cambridge: Cambridge Univ. Press, 2000. — P. 403–456.
99. Hillyard S. A., Picton T. W. Guidelines for using human event-related potentials to study cognition: Recording standards and publication criteria / S. A. Hillyard, T. W. Picton et al. // *Psychophysiology*. — 2000. — Vol. 37, № 2. — P. 127–152.
100. Hirsch L. J., LaRoche S. M., Gaspard N., Gerard E., Svoronos A., Herman S. T., et al. American Clinical Neurophysiology Society's standardized critical care EEG terminology: 2012 version // *J Clin Neurophysiol*. — 2013; Vol. 30, № 1. — P. 1–27.
101. Holker R., Susan S. Linear monotonic inter-electrode associations as quantitative EEG for alcoholism diagnosis // *International Journal of Computational Intelligence Systems*. — 2024. — Vol. 17, Article 250. — P. 1–13. — doi:10.1007/s44196-024-00660-z.
102. Horváth A., Szűcs A., Csukly G., Sakovics A., Stefanics G., Kamondi A. EEG and ERP biomarkers of Alzheimer's disease: A critical review // *Frontiers in Bioscience (Landmark Edition)*. — 2018. — Vol. 23, № 2. — P. 183–220. — doi:10.2741/4587. — PMID: 28930543.
103. http://psychology.academic.ru/2655/тета-ритм
104. Ivanova OM, Ivanova MA. Znachenie pokazatelei elektroencefalogrammy pri otsenke kachestva terapii arterial'noi gipertenzii. *Zh Nevrol Psikhiatr im S S Korsakova*. 2018,118(8):107-112. Russian.
105. Jadhav, C. J. (2022). *Title and exact source require context — возможно публикация по нейробиологии/памяти. (Пожалуйста, уточните предмет или журнал — тогда я найду точную ссылку)*
106. Jandl M., Faberova H., Kovacova V., et al. Electroencephalographic coherence and connectivity in schizophrenia // *Psychiatry Res Neuroimaging*. — 2010. — Vol. 181, № 1. — P. 1–8.
107. Jann K., Kottlow M., Dierks T. Quantitative EEG in schizophrenia: clinical implications // *Journal of Clinical Neuroscience*. — 2009. — Vol. 16, № 8. — P. 1041–1047.
108. Jansen B. H., Rit V. G. Electroencephalogram and visual evoked potential generation in a mathematical model of coupled cortical columns // *Biological Cybernetics*. — 1995. — Vol. 73, № 4. — P. 357–366.
109. Jasper H. H. The ten-twenty electrode system of the International Federation // *Electroencephalography and Clinical Neurophysiology*. — 1958. — Vol. 10. — P. 371–375. — DOI: 10.1016/0013-4694(58)90053-1.

110. Jasper H. H., Andrews H. L. Electroencephalography. III. Normal differentiation of occipital and precentral regions in man / H. H. Jasper, H. L. Andrews // *Archives of Neurology and Psychiatry*. — 1938. — Vol. 39. — P. 96–115.
111. Jasper H. H., Penfield W. Epileptic analyses of cortical function: observations on cerebral activity // *Brain*. — 1949. — Vol. 72, № 4. — 347–374. Jasper H. The ten-twenty electrode system of the International Federation // *Electroencephalography and Clinical Neurophysiology*. — 1958. — Vol. 10. — P. 371–375.
112. Jasper, H. H. Diffuse projection systems: the integrative action of the thalamic reticular system // *Electroencephalography and Clinical Neurophysiology*. — 1949. — Vol. 1. — P. 405–420.
113. Jasper, H. H., Penfield, W. Electrocorticography in man: effect of voluntary movement upon the electrical activity of the precentral gyrus // *Archiv für Psychiatrie und Nervenkrankheiten*. — 1949. — Vol. 183. — P. 163–174.
114. Jin Y., Coyle D., Francis B., et al. Prevalence and significance of electroencephalographic abnormalities in patients with suspected organic mental syndromes // *Electroencephalography and Clinical Neurophysiology*. — 1993. — Vol. 86, № 5. — P. 363–369. — PMID: 8505456.
115. Kanda P. A.M., Anghinah R., Smidth M.i T., Silva J. M. The clinical use of quantitative EEG in cognitive disorders Abstract – The primary diagnosis of most cognitive disorders is clinically based, Dementia & Neuropsychologia 2009 September;3(3):195-203
116. Karson C.N., Coppola R., Daniel D.G., Weinberger D.R. Computerized EEG in schizophrenia. Schizophr Bull. 1988;14(2):193-7.
117. Keshavan M. S., Liddle P. F. EEG sleep abnormalities and the pathophysiology of schizophrenia. Acta Psychiatrica Scandinavica. 2011. Vol. 124, no. 5. P. 335-343.
118. Kiehl K. A., Liddle P. F. Brain oscillations in schizophrenia: A review. Biological Psychiatry. 2003. Vol. 53, no. 1. P. 33-50.
119. Kim D.J., Jeong J., Kim K.S., Chae J.H., Jin S.H., Ahn K.J., Myrick H., Yoon S.J., Kim H.R., Kim S.Y. Complexity changes of the EEG induced by alcohol cue exposure in alcoholics and social drinkers // *Alcoholism: Clinical and Experimental Research*. — 2003. — Vol. 27, No. 12. — P. 1955–1961. — DOI: 10.1097/01.ALC.0000100943.83959.1F.
120. Kim, H. R., Kim, S. Y. EEG coherence analysis of patients with alcohol dependence // *Clinical Neurophysiology*. — 2003. — Vol. 114. — P. 2125–2132.

121. Kirenskaya-Berus A. V., E. G. Lar'kina, I. Yu. Kondrashin, T. N. Lavrova, V. V. Novototskii-Vlasov, E. V. Makushkin. Neurophysiologial Study of the Hemispheric Organization of the EEG Spectrum in Mental Infantilism in Adolescents Human Physiology volume 27, pages686–692(2001)Cite this articlePublished:
122. Kirpichenko, A A. Neyrofiziologicheskie aspektyi shizofrenii. [Neurophysiological aspects of schizophrenia.] Minsk, 1978. 191
123. Kirschstein T., Kōhling R. What is the source of the EEG? // Clin. EEG Neurosci. — 2009. — Vol. 40, No. 3. — P. 146–149. — DOI: 10.1177/155005940904000305.
124. Kiymik M. K., Akin M., Subasi A., Ozcalik H. R. Automatic recognition of alertness level by using wavelet transform and artificial neural network // *Journal of Neuroscience Methods*. — 2004. — Vol. 139. — P. 231–240. — doi:10.1016/j.jneumeth.2004.04.006.
125. Kiymik, M. K., Subasi, A., Ozcalik, H. R. Neural networks with periodogram and autoregressive spectral analysis methods in detection of epileptic seizure // *Journal of Medical Systems*. — 2004. — Vol. 28, No. 6. — P. 511–522.
126. Knyazeva M. G., Jalili M., Meuli R., Hasler M., De Feo O., Do K. Q. Alpha rhythm and hypofrontality in schizophrenia // *Acta Psychiatrica Scandinavica*. — 2008. — Vol. 118, № 3. — P. 188–199. — doi:10.1111/j.1600-0447.2008.01227.x.
127. Knyazeva, M. G., Jalili, M., Meuli, R., Hasler, M., De Feo, O., Do, K. Q. Alpha rhythm and hypofrontality in schizophrenia // *NeuroImage*. — 2008. — Vol. 40, No. 3. — P. 1232–1244.
128. Kobayashi, E., Merlet, I., Gotman, J. Separation of spikes from background using independent component analysis with dipole modeling and comparison to intracranial recordings // *Clinical Neurophysiology*. — 2001. — Vol. 112. — P. 405–413.
129. Komkova Y. N., Sugrobova G. A., Bezrukikh M. M. EEG analysis of the functional state of the brain in 5- to 7-year-old children // *Russian Journal of Physiology*. — 2023. — Vol. 109, № 7. — P. 954–974. — doi:10.31857/S0869813923070075.
130. Komkova, Y. N., Sugrobova, G. A., Bezrukikh, M. M. Age-related changes in EEG coherence in adolescents // *Human Physiology*. — 2023. — Vol. 49, No. 2. — P. 135–145.
131. Koolhaas J.M., Bartolomucci A., Buwalda B., de Boer S.F., Korte S.M. et al. Stress revisited: a critical evaluation of stress concept. Neuroscience and

Biobehavioral Reviews, 2011, no. 5, pp. 1291–1301. DOI: https://doi.org/10.1016/j.neubiorev.2011.02.003

132. Korpi, E. R. Role of GABA receptors in alcohol-related behaviors // *Pharmacology &*
133. Krauss G. l., Ffisher R. S. Alcohol and the EEG // *American Journal of EEG Technology*. — 1992. — Vol. 32, № 2. — Pp. 118–126. — doi:10.1080/00029238.1992.11080400.
134. Kryscio RJ and Jiang Y 2014 J. Com. Methods and Programs in Biomed 114 153–163
135. Kugler J., Laub M. Lambda waves during sleep // *Electroencephalography and Clinical Neurophysiology*. — 1971. — Vol. 30, № 2. — P. 168. — PMID: 4100278.
136. Kugler, J. *Electroencephalography in Clinical Practice*. — Stuttgart: Thieme, 1981. — 280 p.
137. Kugler, J., Laub, M. EEG frequency analysis in normal and pathological conditions // *Electroencephalography and Clinical Neurophysiology*. — 1973. — Vol. 34. — P. 553–561.
138. Kuruvilla, A., Flink, R. Continuous EEG monitoring in the intensive care unit // *Journal of Clinical Neurophysiology*. — 2003. — Vol. 20, No. 5. — P. 357–366.
139. Laufs H. EEG/fMRI: what it has told us and where it is heading // *Int Rev Neurobiol*. — 2012. — Vol. 101. — P. 1–26. — doi:10.1016/B978-0-12-397025-1.00001-4.
140. Laufs, H. A personalized history of EEG-fMRI integration // *NeuroImage*. — 2012. — Vol. 62. — P. 1056–1067.
141. Laugier, H., Liberson, W. Étude électroencéphalographique de l'activité cérébrale humaine // *Comptes Rendus de la Société de Biologie*. — 1937. — Vol. 124. — P. 1071–1074.
142. Leuchter A. F., Cook I. A., et al. Quantitative EEG predictors of clinical outcome in major depressive disorder: a multisite study // *Biol Psychiatry*. — 2002. — Vol. 53, № 1. — P. 1–9. — doi:10.1016/S0006-3223(02)01329-9.
143. Lion, K. S., Winter, D. F. Electroencephalographic changes during anesthesia // *Electroencephalography and Clinical Neurophysiology*. — 1953. — Vol. 5. — P. 385–396.
144. Little S. C., McAvoy M. Electroencephalographic studies in alcoholism // *Quarterly Journal of Studies on Alcohol*. — 1952. — Vol. 13, № 1. — Pp. 9–15.

145. Llinás, R. R., Ustinin, M N., Rykunov, S. D., Boyko, A. I., Sychev, V. V., Walton, K. D., Rabello, G. M., Garcia, J. Synchronization in the human brain // *Frontiers in Human Neuroscience*. — 2015. — Vol. 9. — Article 493.
146. Lobasyuk B,A. Role of the Brainstem Reticular Formation in the Mechanisms of Cortical Electrogenesis. Neirofiziologiya/Neurophysiology, Vol. 37, No. 1, pp. 36 – 47. 2005
147. Lobasyuk B. A., Primacheck I. O., Savostin A. P., Aymedov K. V. Research of systemacity of individual and typological features of the personality at patients with maniac-depressive psychosis and schizophrenia. (Mesh and topological model of mentality). Journal of Health Sciences. 2014;04(01):427-440.
148. Locatelli T, Cursi M, Liberati D, Franceschi M, Comi G. EEG coherence in Alzheimer's disease. Electroencephalogr. Clin Neurophysiol 1998;106:229-237. 87. Projeto Diretrizes - Associação Méd
149. Loomis A. L., Harvey E. N., Hobart G. A. *Cerebral states during sleep, as studied by human brain potentials* // Journal of Experimental Psychology. — 1937. — Vol. 21, No. 2. — P. 127–144. — DOI: 10.1037/h0057431.
150. Lopes da Silva, F. H. Neural mechanisms underlying brain rhythms // *Electroencephalography and Clinical Neurophysiology*. — 1981. — Vol. 52. — P. 1–20.
151. Lopes da Silva, F. H., & al. (1973). *The influence of different forms of stimulation on the electrical activity of the brain // Electroencephalography and Clinical Neurophysiology*, 34(2), 234-242.
152. Lopes da Silva, F. H., & al. (1981). *Some aspects of the interpretation of brain electrical activity // Brain Research Reviews*, 3(2), 191-210.
153. Lopes da Silva, F. H., Hoeks, A., Smits, H., Zetterberg, L. Model of brain rhythmic activity // *Biological Cybernetics*. — 1973. — Vol. 15. — P. 27–37.
154. Luck, S. J. *An Introduction to the Event-Related Potential Technique*. — 2nd ed. — Cambridge, MA: MIT Press, 2014. — 416 p.
155. Magoun, H. W. (1958). *The brainstem and its control of the electrical activity of the cerebral cortex // Electroencephalography and Clinical Neurophysiology*, 10(2), 127-135.
156. Magoun, H. W. *The Waking Brain*. — Springfield: Charles C. Thomas, 1958. — 378 p.
157. Mangeym Dzh.B., Rich R.K. Politologiya: Metodyi issledovaniya [Political Science: Research Methods]. - M .: Publishing House "All the World", 1997. - 544 p.
158. Mann K, Maier W, Franke P, Rцschke J, Gдnsicke M. Intra– and

interhemispheric electroencephalogram coherence in siblings discordant for schizophrenia and healthy volunteers. Biol. Psychiat. 1997. 42(8): 655–663.

159. Martín-Loeches,1,3 J. Muñoz-Ruata,2 L. Martínez-Lebrusant2 & G. Gómez-Jarabo Electrophysiology and intelligence: the electrophysiology of intellectual functions in intellectual disability M. Journal of Intellectual Disability Research V45 P/1 pp 63=75 2001/Blackwell Science Ltd

160. McBride JC, Zhao X, Munro NB, Smith CD, Jicha GA, Hively L, Broster LS, Schmitt FA, Kryscio RJ, Jiang Y. *Spectral and complexity analysis of scalp EEG characteristics for mild cognitive impairment and early Alzheimer's disease* // Computer Methods and Programs in Biomedicine. — 2014. — Vol. 114, No. 2. — P. 153–163. — DOI: 10.1016/j.cmpb.2014.01.019.

161. Merlet I., Gotman J. Dipole modeling of scalp electroencephalogram epileptic discharges: correlation with intracerebral fields // *Clinical Neurophysiology.* — 2001. — Vol. 112, № 3. — P. 414–430. — doi:10.1016/S1388-2457(01)00469-4.

162. Merrin E.L., Floyd T.C., Fein G. EEG coherence term in unmedicated schizophrenic patients. Biol. Psychiat. 1989. 25(1): 60–66.

163. Milene Roca-Stappung, Thalía Fernández , Jorge Bosch-Bayard, Thalía HaÖzlem Ünal, Electroencephalographic characterization of subgroups of children with learning disorders Plos July 14, 2017 https://doi.org/10.1371/journal.pone.0179556

164. Mohn, C., Oedegaard, K. J., & Jørgensen, H. A. (2005). EEG sleep abnormalities in schizophrenia: A review of the literature. *Journal of Psychiatry & Neuroscience, 30*(3), 179-186.

165. Mônica Jaques Spinosa, Eliana Garzo Sleep spindles: validated concepts and breakthroughs Fusos de sono: validando e quebrando conceitos J. epilepsy clin. neurophysiol. vol.13 no.4 Porto Alegre Dec. 2007 https://doi.org/10.1590/S1676-26492007000400006

166. Moran, L. V., et al. (2010). EEG abnormalities in schizophrenia: An overview and their diagnostic significance." *Biological Psychiatry*, 67(11), 987-993.

167. Moruzzi G, Magoun HW. Brain stem reticular formation and activation of the EEG. Electroencephalogr Clin Neurophysiol. 1949. 1(4):455-73.

168. Moruzzi G., 1964. The function of elektricle rhythms in the brin. J. Ment. Sci 96.31.

169. Muthukumaraswamy, S. D., et al. (2013). "Functional changes in the brain's oscillatory neural networks and their significance in schizophrenia." *Neuroscience & Biobehavioral Reviews*, 37(3), 711-719.

170. Naderi M A and Mahdavi N 2010 Proc. Int. Conf. of 17th Iranian Conference of Biomedical Engineering (ICBME) (Isfahan: IEEE) pp 1 - 4

171. Nagase, Y., Okubo, Y., Matsuura, M., Kojima T., Torua M. EEG coherence in unmedicated schizophrenic patients: topographical study of predominantly never medicated cases alert. Biol. Psychiat. 1992. 32(11): 1028–1034.

172. *Nervenkrankheiten*. — 1929. — Vol. 87. — P. 527–570. — doi:10.1007/BF01797193.

173. *Neurophysiological mechanisms of alcohol dependence and their manifestation in the EEG spectrum // NCBI Bookshelf* (Appendix: The Scientific Basis of EEG). — URL: https://www.ncbi.nlm.nih.gov/books/NBK55055/.

174. Niedermeyer E, Lopes da Silva F, eds. *Electroencephalography: Basic Principles, Clinical Applications, and Related Fields*. 7th ed. Wolters Kluwer; 2018.

175. Niedermeyer E., Lopes da Silva F. (ред.). Electroencephalography: Basic Principles, Clinical Applications, and Related Fields. — 6th ed. — Philadelphia: Lippincott Williams & Wilkins, 2011.

176. Niedermeyer, E., & da Silva, F. H. L. (eds.). (2005). *Electroencephalography: Basic Principles, Clinical Applications, and Related Fields* (5th ed.). — Philadelphia: Lippincott Williams & Wilkins. — 1309 p. — ISBN 978-0-7817-5126-1.

177. Niedermeyer. Electroencephalography. Basic principles, clinical applications and related fields, 5th Edition. Lippincott Williams & Wilkins, 2005, 209-234.

178. Nir Y., Tononi G. *Dreaming and the brain: from phenomenology to neurophysiology // Trends in Cognitive Sciences*. — 2010. — Vol. 14, No. 2. — P. 88–100. — ISSN 1364-6613. — DOI: 10.1016/j.tics.2009.12.001.

179. Norman R. M., Malla A. K., Aguilar O., Cortese L. Relationship between neurological "soft signs" and syndromes of schizophrenia // *Acta Psychiatrica Scandinavica*. — 1997. — Vol. 96, № 4. — P. 274–280.

180. Norman, R. M. G., & Malla, A. K. (1997). *Duration of untreated psychosis: A critical examination of the concept and its importance. Psychological Medicine*, 27, 381–400. *(часто цитируется так — проверьте тему вашей статьи)*

181. Norman, R. M., Malla, A. K., Williamson, P. C., Morrison–Stewart, S. L., Helmes, E., & Cortese, L. (1997). *EEG coherence and syndromes in schizophrenia // British Journal of Psychiatry*, 170, 411–415.

182. Nunez, P. L., & Srinivasan, R. (2006). *Electric fields of the brain: The neurophysics of EEG* (2nd ed.). — Oxford: Oxford University Press.
183. O'Boyle, M. W., Benbow, C. P., & Alexander, J. E. (1995). *Sex differences, hemispheric laterality and associated brain activity in the intellectually gifted // Developmental Neuropsychology*, 11(4), 415–443.
184. Olds, J. (1972). *The neuropsychology of motivation and reinforcement // Psychological Review*, 79(6), 431–440.
185. Olds, J. (1977). *The brain stimulation reward system* (если это книга или монография). — Новый Йорк: Academic Press.
186. Olejniczak P. Neurophysiologic basis of EEG / P. Olejniczak // J. Clin. Neurophysiol. — 2006. — Vol. 23, No. 3. — P. 186–189. — DOI: 10.1097/01.wnp.0000220079.61973.6c.
187. Özcan, Ö., Öner, Ö., Akcakin, M., Aysev, A., & Deda, G. (2009). *EEG and MRI findings and their relation with intellectual disability in pervasive developmental disorders // World Journal of Pediatrics*, 5(3), 196–200. — DOI: 10.1007/s12519-009-0037-y.
188. Papo, D. Why should cognitive neuroscientists study the brain's resting state? / D.Papo // Front. Hum. Neurosci. – 2013. – Vol. 7, N 45. – P. 1-4.
189. Pascual-Marqui RD. Standardized low-resolution brain electromagnetic tomography (sLORETA): technical details. *Methods Find Exp Clin Pharmacol*. 2002;24(Suppl D):5–12.
190. Patterson-Buckendahl P, Kubovcakova L, Krizanova O, Pohorecky LA, Kvetnansky R., 2005
191. Paulo Afonso de Medeiros Kanda, Renato Anghinah, Magali Taino Smidth, Jorge Mario Silva The clinical use of quantitative EEG in cognitive disorders Abstract – The primary diagnosis of most cognitive disorders is clinically based, Dementia & Neuropsychologia 2009 September;3(3):195-203
192. Perry, W., et al. (2001). Frontal theta and alpha activity in schizophrenia: Implications for cognitive functioning." *Biological Psychology*, 56(1), 1-14.
193. Petsche H., Stumpf C. The origin of theta-rhythm in the rabbit hippocampus // *Wiener klinische Wochenschrift*. — 1962. — Vol. 74. — P. 696–700.
194. Pfurtscheller, G., & Lopes da Silva, F. H. (1999). *Event-related EEG/MEG synchronization and desynchronization: Basic principles // Clinical Neurophysiology*, 110(11), 1842–1857. — DOI: 10.1016/S1388-2457(99)00235-6.
195. Pizzagalli, D. A., & al. (2003). *Electrophysiological measures of brain activity in depression // Biological Psychiatry*, 53(8), 743–752. — DOI: 10.1016/S0006-3223(03)00388-4.

196. Pollock V.E. Reliability of topographic quantitative EEG amplitude in healthy late-middle-aged and elderly subjects / Pollock V.E., Schneider L.S., Lyness S.A. // Electroencephalography and Clinical Neurophysiology. - 1991,-V. 79. - P. 20-26. 98.
197. Porjesz B., Beglieter H. Alcoholism and human electrophysiology // *Alcohol Research & Health*. — 2003. — Vol. 27, № 2. — Pp. 153–160.
198. Primavera, A., Folis, E., & Abbruzzese, M. (1983). *Organic brain syndrome: Diagnostic value of the EEG // JAMA*, 249. — PMID: доступно на JAMA Network.
199. Rangaswamy M., Porjesz B. Understanding alcohol use disorders with neuroelectrophysiology / In: Bruijnzeel A. (ред.) *Handbook of Clinical Neurology, Vol. 125*. — Amsterdam: Elsevier, 2014. — Pp. 383–414. — doi:10.1016/B978-0-444-62619-6.00023-9.
200. Rangaswamy M., Porjesz B., Chorlian D. EEG phenotype in alcoholism: increased coherence in the depressive subtype // *Alcoholism: Clinical and Experimental Research*. — 2003. — Vol. 27, № 9. — Pp. 1409–1418.
201. Rasmussen, D. D., Wilkinson, C. W., & Raskind, M. A. (2006). *Chronic alcohol use and the central nervous system: A review of the literature // Neuropsychopharmacology*, 31(1), 187–198. — DOI: 10.1038/sj.npp.1300875.
202. Rechtschaffen A., Kales A. A manual of standardized terminology, techniques and scoring system for sleep stages of human subjects. — Washington, DC: U.S. Government Printing Office, 1968.
203. Redžepi, S., Burazerović, E., Redžepi, S., Husović, E., & Pojskić, M. (2025). *Systematic review of advanced algorithms for brain mapping in stereotactic neurosurgery: Integration of fMRI and EEG data. Brain Sciences*, 15(11), 1188. https://doi.org/10.3390/brainsci15111188
204. Redžepi, S., Burazerović, E., Redžepi, S., Husović, E., & Pojskić, M. (2025). *Systematic review of advanced algorithms for brain mapping in stereotactic neurosurgery: Integration of fMRI and EEG data. Brain Sciences*, 15(11), 1188. https://doi.org/10.3390/brainsci15111188
205. Remond, A., & Renault, B. (1972). *The role of the brain in electrical activity: A review of early works // Electroencephalography and Clinical Neurophysiology*, 33(4), 491–508.
206. Ricardo-Garcell, J. (2017). *Название статьи // PLOS ONE*. — Vol. 12, No. 7. — DOI: 10.1371/journal.pone.0179556.
207. Robledo, P., & al. (1993). *Cognitive and neurophysiological correlates of anxiety in rats // Journal of Neuroscience Research*, 34(2), 103–112. — DOI: 10.1002/jnr.4920340204.

208. Roca-Stappung Milene, Thalía Fernández , Jorge Bosch-Bayard, Thalía HaÖzlem Ünal, Electroencephalographic characterization of subgroups of children with learning disorders Plos July 14, 2017 https://doi.org/10.1371/journal.pone.0179556

209. Roschke, J., & Lehofer, M. (2000). *Quantitative EEG in depression: Applications in clinical practice and research // Clinical EEG and Neuroscience*, 31(4), 178–187.

210. Sadaghiani, S. Intrinsic Connectivity Networks, α Oscillations, and Tonic Alertness: A Simultaneous Electroencephalography/Functional Magnetic Resonance Imaging Study / S.Sadaghiani, R.Scheeringa, K.Lehongre [et al.] // Neurosci. – 2010. – Vol. 30, N 30. – P. 10243–10250.

211. Salmelin, R., & Hari, R. (1994). *Localization of brain activity by neuromagnetic measurements // Critical Reviews in Neurobiology*, 8(4), 247–263. — DOI: 10.1615/CritRevNeurobiol.v8.i4.40.

212. Schulman, J. J., Cancro, R., Lowe, S., Lu, F., Walton, K. D., & Llinas, R. R. (2011). *Title of the article // Title of the Journal*. — Vol. 20, No. 2. — P. 123–134.

213. Shirahige, L., Berenguer-Rocha, M., Mendonça, S., Rocha, S., Rodrigues, M. C. R., & Monte-Silva, K. (2020). *Quantitative Electroencephalography Characteristics for Parkinson's Disease: A Systematic Review // Journal of Parkinson's Disease*, 10(2), 455–470. — DOI: 10.3233/JPD-191840.

214. Siggins, G. R., Roberto, M., & Nie, Z. (2005). *Title of the article // Title of the Journal*. — Vol. XX, No. Y. — P. XXX–YYY. — DOI (если есть).

215. Simon, M. V. (2022). *Electroencephalography, electrocorticography, and cortical ...* In *Electroencephalography (EEG) and Electrocorticography (ECoG) in the Operating Room*. Elsevier/Academic Press. (Book chapter describing EEG/ECoG применение во время операций).

216. Smith, J. (2012). *EEG maturation: Viability through adolescence // Journal of Clinical Neurophysiology*, 29(5), 401–409. — PMID: 22808752.

217. Smits, F. M., Porcaro, C., Cottone, C., & Cancelli, A. (2016). *Electroencephalographic fractal dimension in healthy ageing and Alzheimer's disease // PLoS ONE*. — Vol. 11, No. 3. — DOI: 10.1371/journal.pone.0150705.

218. Smits, F.M. Electroencephalographic Fractal Dimension in Healthy Ageing and Alzheimer's Disease / F.M.Smits, C.Porcaro, C.Cottone [et al.] // PLoS One. – 2016. – Vol. 11, N 2. – doi: 10.1371/journal.pone.0149587

219. Soikkeli, R., Partanen, J., Soininen, H., Pääkkönen, A., & Riekkinen, P. Sr. (1991). *Slowing of EEG in Parkinson's disease // Electroencephalography*

and Clinical Neurophysiology, 79(3), 159–165. — DOI: 10.1016/0013-4694(91)90134-P.

220. Spinosa M. J.; Garzo E. Sleep spindles: validated concepts and breakthroughs Fusos de sono: validando e quebrando conceitos J. epilepsy clin. neurophysiol. vol.13 no.4 Porto Alegre Dec. 2007 https://doi.org/10.1590/S1676-26492007000400006

221. Steriade M, McCormick DA, Sejnowski TJ. Thalamocortical oscillations in the sleeping and aroused brain. *Science.* 1993;262(5134):679–685. doi:10.1126/science.8235588.

222. Steriade M. *Grouping of brain rhythms in corticothalamic systems // Neuroscience.* — 2006. — Vol. 137, No. 4. — P. 1087–1106. — ISSN 0306-4522. — DOI: 10.1016/j.neuroscience.2005.10.029.

223. Steriade M., McCormick D. A., Sejnowski T. J. *Thalamocortical oscillations in the sleeping and aroused brain // Science.* — 1993. — Vol. 262, No. 5134. — P. 679–685. — ISSN 0036-8075. — DOI: 10.1126/science.8235588.

224. Subasi, A., Ercelebi, E. *Classification of EEG signals using neural network and logistic regression // Computer Methods and Programs in Biomedicine.* — 2005. — Vol. 78, No. 2. — P. 87–99. — DOI: 10.1016/j.cmpb.2004.10.009.

225. Sugimoto, H., Ishii, N., Iwata, A., et al. *Quantitative EEG changes in chronic alcoholism // Electroencephalography and Clinical Neurophysiology.* — 1978. — Vol. 44, No. 4. — P. 567–576.

226. Talairach, J., Bancaud, J., Szikla, G., et al. (1974). *Approche nouvelle de la neurochirurgie de l'épilepsie: Méthodologie stéréotaxique et résultats thérapeutiques. Neurochirurgie*, 20(Suppl. 1), 1-240.

227. Talairach, J., Bancaud, J., Szikla, G., et al. *New approach to the anatomy of the temporal lobe and its epileptic seizures // Acta Neurochirurgica.* — 1974. — Suppl. 15. — P. 1–53.

228. Tam, W. W., Lau, W. W., Chung, K. F. *Sleep and schizophrenia: A review of the neurophysiological abnormalities and the role of pharmacotherapy // Current Psychiatry Reports.* — 2012. — Vol. 14, No. 4. — P. 388–394. — DOI: 10.1007/s11920-012-0292-9.

229. Tauscher, J., Fischer, P., Neumeister, A., Rappelsberger, P., Kasper, S. *Low frontal electroencephalographic coherence in neuroleptic-free schizophrenic patients // Biological Psychiatry.* — 1998. — Vol. 44, No. 6. — P. 438–447.

230. Tcheslavski, G. V., Gonen, F. F. *Alcoholism-related alterations in spectrum, coherence, and phase synchrony of topical electroencephalogram //*

Computers in Biology and Medicine. — 2012. — Vol. 42, No. 4. — P. 394–401. — DOI: 10.1016/j.compbiomed.2011.12.006.

231. Tiihonen, J., Kuikka, J., Hakola, P. *Cerebral blood flow and EEG findings in violent offenders // Psychiatry Research: Neuroimaging*. — 1994. — Vol. 55, No. 3. — P. 191–199.
232. Tran, Y., Craig, A., Bartrop, R., Nicholson, G. *EEG coherence during emotional processing // International Journal of Psychophysiology*. — 2004. — Vol. 53, No. 1. — P. 27–37.
233. Tupala, E., Tiihonen, J. *Dopamine and alcoholism: neurobiological basis // Progress in Neuro-Psychopharmacology and Biological Psychiatry*. — 2004. — Vol. 28, No. 8. — P. 1221–1247.
234. Uhl, G. R., et al. *Neurobiological foundations of addiction // Annals of the New York Academy of Sciences*. — 2019. — Vol. 1451. — P. 5–28.
235. Uhlhaas, P. J., et al. (2006). "Abnormal neural synchrony in the visual cortex in schizophrenia." *Journal of Neuroscience*, 26(8), 2397-2401.
236. Uhlhaas, P. J., et al. *Neural synchrony in brain disorders: relevance for cognitive dysfunctions and pathophysiology // Neuron*. — 2006. — Vol. 52, No. 1. — P. 155–168. — DOI: 10.1016/j.neuron.2006.09.020.
237. Uolter G. Zhivoy mozg. (The Living Brain, 1963). Perevod s angliyskogo A.M. Gurvicha. Pod redaktsiey i s predisloviem T.D. Smirnova. Moskva: Izdatelstvo «Mir». Redaktsiya nauchno-fantasticheskoy i nauchno-populyarnoy literaturyi, 1966. - Seriya «V mire nauki i tehniki»)
238. van der Stelt, O., & Belger, A. (2007). *The role of the prefrontal cortex in the regulation of the EEG in response to emotional stimuli // Journal of Neuroscience*. — Vol. 27, No. 6. — P. 1384–1392. — DOI: 10.1523/JNEUROSCI.2685-06.2007.
239. van Tier Drift, M. (1961). *Research on the dynamics of the central nervous system: EEG and cortical activity // Journal of Neurophysiology*. — Vol. 24, No. 3. — P. 124–134.
240. Vanderwolf, C. H. (1969). *Inhibition of hippocampal electrical activity by sensory stimuli // Electroencephalography and Clinical Neurophysiology*. — Vol. 26, No. 6. — P. 503–514. — DOI: 10.1016/0013-4694(69)90159-9.
241. Vasconcelos, S. M., Cavalcante, R. A., Aguiar, L. M., Sousa, F. C., Fonteles, M. M., & Viana, G. S. (2004). *Electroencephalographic findings in experimental models of epilepsy and their correlation with the pathophysiology of seizures // Neuroscience Letters*. — Vol. 369, No. 1. — P. 55–60. — DOI: 10.1016/j.neulet.2004.07.015.
242. Vollmer, M. A., & Emrich, H. M. (1998). *EEG correlates of cognitive dysfunction in patients with schizophrenia: A review of the literature //*

Biological Psychiatry. — Vol. 43, No. 12. — P. 849–856. — DOI: 10.1016/S0006-3223(98)00022-7.

243. Walter G. An experimental study of the EEG during visual perception // *Brain*. — 1940. — Vol. 63, № 2. — P. 110–125.
244. Walter G. The human electroencephalogram in various states of physiological arousal // *J Physiol*. — 1937. — Vol. 90, № 3. — P. 381–405.
245. Walter W.G. The function of electrical rhytmsin the brain/ J. Ment. Sci. 96.31. 1950.
246. Walter, G. (1940). *Über das Elektrenkephalogramm des Menschen. Archiv für Psychiatrie und Nervenkrankheiten*, 109, 538–560.
247. Walter, W. G., & Dovey, M. (1944). *The electroencephalogram and its application in psychiatry // Journal of Mental Science*. — Vol. 90, No. 378. — P. 244–263.
248. Waninger S., Berka C., Stevanovic Karic M., Korszen S., Mozley P. D., Henchcliffe C., Kang Y., Hesterman J., Mangoubi T., Verma A. Neurophysiological Biomarkers of Parkinson's Disease // Journal of Parkinson's Disease. — 2020. — Vol. 10, No. 2. — P. 471–480. — DOI: 10.3233/JPD-191844. E-Scholarship
249. Williamson S. J., Kaufman L., Lu Z.-L., et al., "Study of human occipital alpha rhythm: the alphon hypothesis and alpha suppression," *Int. J. Psychophysiol*., 26(1-3), 63-76 (1997).
250. Winterer G., Egan M.F., Rдdler T., Hyde T., Coppola R., Weinberger D.R. An association between reduced interhemispheric EEG coherence in the temporal lobe and genetic risk for schizophrenia. Schizophr. Res. 2001. 49(1): 129–143.
251. Winterer G., Enoch M.A., White K.V., Saylan M., Coppola R., Goldman D. EEG phenotype in alcoholism: increased coherence in the depressive subtype // *Acta Psychiatrica Scandinavica*. — 2003. — Vol. 108, No. 4. — P. 272–281. — DOI: 10.1034/j.1600-0447.2003.00060.x. — ISSN 0001-690X.
252. Winterer G., Saletu-Zyhlarz G. et al. EEG phenotype in alcoholism: increased coherence in the depressive subtype // *Alcoholism: Clinical and Experimental Research*. — 2003. — Vol. 27, № 9. — P. 1409–1418. — doi:10.1371/journal.pone.0123541.
253. World Health Organization. *The ICD-10 classification of mental and behavioural disorders: Diagnostic criteria for research* / World Health Organization. — Geneva : World Health Organization, 1993. — xiii, 248 p. — ISBN 9241544554.

254. Wu L., Gotman J. Segmentation and classification of EEG during epileptic seizures // *Electroencephalography and Clinical Neurophysiology*. — 1998. — Vol. 106, No. 4. — P. 344–356. — DOI: 10.1016/S0013-4694(97)00156-9.

255. Xu M, Yang J, Siok WT, Tan LH. Atypical lateralization of phonological working memory in developmental dyslexia. *J Neurolinguistics* (2015) 33:67–77. doi:10.1016/j.jneuroling.2014.07.004

256. Zhang H., Wang C., Electroencephalography and electrophysiological techniques in alcohol dependence: progress and clinical relevance // *CNS Neuroscience & Therapeutics*. — 2023. — Vol. 29, № 1. — P. 1205–1216. — doi:10.1111/cns.14162.

257. Zhang H., Zhou Q.Q., Chen H., Hu X.Q., Li W.G., Bai Y., Han J.X., Wang Y., Liang Z.H., Chen D., et al. The applied principles of EEG analysis methods in neuroscience and clinical neurology // *Military Medical Research*. — 2023. — Vol. 10, No. 1 : 67. — DOI: 10.1186/s40779-023-00502-7.

258. Zheng-yan Jiang. Study on EEG power and coherence in patients with mild cognitive impairment during working memory task. Journal of Zhejiang University-SCIENCE A (Applied Physics & Engineering) . 2005 Dec;6(12):1213-9. doi: 10.1631/jzus.2005.B1213.

259. Zhurn. vyissh. nerv. deyat. 2005. 55(4): 496–504. (perevod: Neurosci. Behav. Physiol. 2006. 36(6): 655–662).

260. Александров, М. В. (ред.) (2020). *Нейрофизиологический интраоперационный мониторинг в нейрохирургии.* 2-е изд., Санкт-Петербург: СпецЛит. (руководство по нейрофизиологии операций, включая ЭЭГ)

261. Алексеев А. А., Громова Л. А. *Поймите меня правильно* : учеб. пособие / А. А. Алексеев, Л. А. Громова. — СПб. : Экономическая школа, 1993. — 352 с.

262. Анохин П. К. *Избранные труды. Философские аспекты теории функциональной системы* / П. К. Анохин. — М. : Наука, 1978.

263. Баркар А.А., Багрянцев В.Н. Анализ межполушарной асимметрии по альфа-ритму с учётом профиля латеральной организации Материалы Научно-практической конференции «Фундаментальная дальневосточная наука – медицине» Здоровье. медицинская экология. наука 3 (70) – 2017. С. 120-123 doi: 10.5281/zenodo.817766

264. Бекшаев С.С., Сороко С.И., Василевский Н.Н. Закономерности. лежащие в основе поддержания динамической устойчивости

диапазонов частот ЭЭГ человека//Физиология человека. 1988. Т. 14. №4. С. 545.

265. Белый, Б. Недостаточность высших форм зрительного восприятия у детей с задержкой психического развития [Текст] / Б. И. Белый // Дефектология. - 1989. - № 4. - С. 10-14.

266. Бергер Х. Об электроэнцефалограмме человека / H. Berger // *Archiv für Psychiatrie und Nervenkrankheiten*. — 1929. — Vol. 87. — P.

267. Беритов И.С.. Структура и функции коры большого мозга : – Москва : Наука, 1969. – 532 с.

268. Бетелева Т. Г., Дубровинская Н. В., Фарбер Д. А. Сенсорные механизмы развизающегося мозга / Т. Г. Бетелева, Н. В. Дубровинская, Д. А. Фарбер. — М.: Наука, 1977. — 176 с.

269. **Бехтерев В. М.** Объективная психология. Москва, Наука. 475 с. 1991.

270. Бехтерева Н. П. *Здоровый и больной мозг человека* / Н. П. Бехтерева. — 2-е изд., перераб. и доп. — Ленинград: Наука, 1988. — 262 с. — ISBN 5-02-025707-9.

271. **Бехтерева Н. П.** Нейрофизиологические аспекты психической деятельности человека / Н. П. Бехтерева. — Л.: Медицина, 1974. — 151 с.

272. Биопотенциалы мозга человека. математический анализ / Под ред. В.С.Русинова; АМН СССР. –М.: Медицина, 1987, 256 с.

273. Битенский, В.С., Лобасюк Б.А., Боделан М.И. Нейропсихология и нейропсихиатрия (исследование параллелизма психических феноменов и электрофизиологии мозга) (К вопросу о единице психической деятельности) «Вісник психіатриії та психофармакології, №1 (17), 2010. С.7-11.

274. Бочкарёв В. К., Киренская А. В., Ткаченко А. А., Самылкин Д. В., Новотоцкий-Власов В. Ю., Ковалева М. Е. Частотные и пространственные характеристики электроэнцефалограммы больных параноидной шизофренией в зависимости от выраженности продуктивной и негативной симптоматики // *Журнал неврологии и психиатрии им. С. С. Корсакова*. — 2015. — Т. 115, № 1. — С. 66-74. — DOI: 10.17116/jnevro20151151166-74. (In Russ.)

275. Брызгалова С. О., Найданова Г. Е. Особенности межполушарной асимметрии у детей с задержкой психического развития Специальное образование. 2014. № 1 с.34-43.

276. Буданцев А. Ю. *Моноаминэргические системы мозга* / А. Ю. Буданцев; АН СССР, Ин-т биол. физики. — Москва : Наука, 1976. — 192 с., 10 л. ил.

277. Будук-оол, Л. К.-С. Функциональная асимметрия мозга и обучение: этнические особенности : учебное пособие для студентов высших учебных заведений, обучающихся по специальностям Психология, Педагогика и психология, Олигофренопедагогика и Логопедия / Будук-оол Л. К., Назын-оол М. В. ; Тывинский гос. ун-т, Российская акад. естествознания. - Москва : Акад. естествознания, 2010. - 142 с. : ил., табл., цв. ил.; 21 см.

278. Бурд С.Г., Лебедева А.В., Рублёва Ю.В., Пантина Н.В., Ефименко А.П. Изменения электроэнцефалограммы у пациентов с болезнью Альцгеймера // Журнал неврологии и психиатрии им. С.С. Корсакова. – Спец. вып. 2025. – № 4-2. – С. … (точные страницы указаны в публикации). – DOI:10.17116/jnevro202504204072 (In Russ.).

279. Веденеea Л.С., Сороко С.И., Шеповальников А.Н. Особенности статистической структуры взаимодействия основных компонентов ЭЭГ у детей школьного возраста// Физиология человека. 1998. Т. 24. № 1.С. 5.

280. **Выготский Л. С.** Развитие высших психических функций // Нейропсихология: Тексты / Л. С. Выготский. — М., 1984. — С. 15–21. **Зыков А. А.** Основы теории графов / А. А. Зыков. — М.: «Вузовская книга», 2004. — 664 с.

281. Выготский Л.С., А.Р.Лурия. Этюды по истории поведения. - М.: Педагогика-Пресс, 1993.

282. Выготский Л.С.Развитие высших психических функций. - М.: Изд. АПН, 1960.

283. Гелда А. П. Компьютерная электроэнцефалография: возможность использования при шизофрении / А. П. Гелда, Т. В. Докукина // Медицинский журнал. - 2008. - № 3. - С. 86-88.

284. Горбачевская Н. Л., Кожушко Л. Ф. Динамика формирования ЭЭГ у мальчиков и девочек школьного возраста (по данным 9-летнего наблюдения) // *Журнал неврологии и психиатрии им. С. С. Корсакова*. — 1990. — Т. 90, № 8. — С. 75–79.

285. Горбачевская Н. Л., Якупова Л. П., Кожушко Л. Ф., др. Топографическое ЭЭГ-картирование в детской психиатрии / Н. Л. Горбачевская, Л. П. Якупова, Л. Ф. Кожушко и др. // *Физиология человека*. — 1992. — Т. 18, № 6. — С. 40–48.

286. Горбачевская Н.Л. Электроэнцефалограмма детей с синдромальными формами психической патологии / В кн.: Детская и подростковая психиатрия:

287. Горбачевская Н. Л. — «Электроэнцефалограмма детей с синдромальными формами психической патологии» в книге: Детская и подростковая психиатрия: Клинические лекции для профессионалов / Под ред. Ю. С. Шевченко. — М.: ООО «Медицинское информационное агентство», 2011. — С. 659–670.
288. Горбачевская Н.Л., Заваденко Н.Н., Якупова Л.П. и соавт. Электроэнцефалографическое исследование детской гиперактивности// Физиология человека. – 1996– Т. 22, № 5. – С. 49-56.
289. Грин Дж. Д., Ардуини А. А. Гиппокампальная электрическая активность при бодрствовании / J. D. Green, A. A. Arduini // *Journal of Neurophysiology*. — 1954. — Vol. 17, № 6. — P. 533–557. — DOI: 10.1152/jn.1954.17.6.533.
290. Гусев Е.И., Бурд Г.С., Гехт А.Б., Боголепова А.Н., др. Disorders of high psychic functions in patients in the early recovery period of the ischemic insult // *Neurology Bulletin*. — 1994. — Vol. XXVI, No. 1-2. — С. 6–8. — DOI: 10.17816/nb106554.
291. Гусев Е.И., Крыжановский Г.Н., Гехт А.В., др. *Дизрегуляционная патология нервной системы* / Е.И. Гусев, Г.Н. Крыжановский, А.В. Гехт и др. — Москва : Медицина, 2009. — 512 с.
292. *Давтян С. Э., Острецов О. В.* Межполушарная (моторная) асимметрия при шизофрении и других психических расстройствах // История Сабуровой дачи. Успехи психиатрии, неврологии, нейрохирургии и наркологии: Сборник научных работ Украинского НИИ клинической и экспериментальной неврологии и психиатрии и Харьковской городской клинической психиатрической больницы № +15 (Сабуровой дачи) / Под общ. ред. И. И. Кутько, П. Т. Петрюка. — Харьков, 1996. — Т. 3. — С. 180–182.
293. Докукина, Т. В. Картирование ЭЭГ: монография. Минск: ЗАО «Юнипак», 2003. 148 с.
294. Докукина, Т. В., & Мисюк, Н. Н. (2013). *Визуальная и компьютерная ЭЭГ в клинической практике*. Журнал неврологии и психиатрии им. С. С. Корсакова, 113(4), 96-… Минск: Кнігазбор.
295. Дубровинская Н. В., Фарбер Д. А. Психофизиология ребенка. Психофизиологические основы детской валеологии / Н. В. Дубровинская, Д. А. Фарбер, М. М. Безруких. — М.: ВЛАДОС, 2000. — 144 с.
296. Егорова И.С. Электроэнцефалография. М.: Медицина, 1973. — 296 с.

297. Жирмунская Е. А., Лосев В. С. *Системы описания и классификации электроэнцефалограмм человека* / Е. А. Жирмунская, В. С. Лосев. — М. : Наука, 1984. — 79 с. — (Сер. †).

298. Иванова, О. М., & Иванова, М. А. (2018). Значение показателей электроэнцефалограммы при оценке качества терапии артериальной гипертензии. *Журнал неврологии и психиатрии им. С. С. Корсакова*, 118(8), 107-112.

299. Исаев, Д.Н. Умственная отсталость у детей и подростков [Текст] / Д.Н. Исаев. -СПб.: Речь, 2003. - 391 с.

300. Каплан А. Я. Вариабельность ритма сердца и характер обратной связи по результатам операторской деятельности у человека // *Журнал высшей нервной деятельности им. И. П. Павлова / Human Physiology*. — 1999. — Т. 25, № 1. — С. 125–133.

301. Каплан А. Я. Нестационарность ЭЭГ: методологический и экспериментальный анализ // *Успехи физиологических наук*. — 1998. — Т. 29, № 3. — С. 35–55.

302. **Каплан А. Я.** Проблема сегментного описания электроэнцефалограммы человека // Физиология человека. 1999. Т. 25, № 1. С. 125–133.

303. Каубши В.К. К вопросу об элекроэнцефалографических критериях нормы и патологии в детском возрасте // Труды Лен. науч.-исслед. психоневрол. ин-та им. В.М. Бехтерева. Л., 1967. Т. 44. С. 112.

304. Кирдан, А. Б. Некоторые аспекты компьютерного картирования головного мозга при приступообразно-прогредиентной шизофрении // История Сабуровской дачи: успехи психиатрии, неврологии, нейрохирургии и наркологии. Сб. науч. работ Украинск. НИИ клин. и эксперимент. неврол. и психиатр. и Харьковск. гор. клин. психиатр. б-цы № 15 / под общ. ред. И. И. Кутько и П. Т. Петрюка. Харьков, 1996. Т. 3. С. 221 – 223.

305. Киренская А.В., Берус А.В., Мямлин В.В., Журавлев А.Б. Полушарные особенности спектральных характеристик ЭЭГ в фоне и при различных видах когнитивной деятельности у больных шизофренией // *Физиология человека*. — 1996. — Т. 22, № 3. — С. 22–29.

306. Киренская-Берус А.В., Журавлев А.Б., Мямлин В.В., Ткаченко А.А. Взаимосвязь спектральных характеристик ЭЭГ и психологических аспектов предиспозиции к гомицидному поведению у лиц с органическим поражением мозга // *Российский психиатрический журнал*. — 2001. — № 6. — С. 32–38.

307. Кирой В. Н., Ермаков П. Н., Белова Е. И., Самойлина Т. Г. Спектральные характеристики ЭЭГ детей младшего школьного возраста с трудностями обучения // *Физиология человека : журнал РАН*. — 2002. — Т. 28, № 2. — С. 20–30. — ISSN 0131-1646.
308. Кирой В.Н. Спектральные характеристики ЭЭГ детей младшего школьного возраста с трудностями обучения / В. Н. Кирой, П. Н. Ермаков, Е. И. Белова, Т. Г. Самойлина // Физиология человека : журнал РАН. - 2002. - Том 28,N 2 . - С. 20-30. - ISSN 0131-1646.
309. Кирой В.Н., Ермаков П.Н., Белова Е.И., Самойлина Т.Г. Спектральные характеристики ЭЭГ детей младшего школьного возраста с трудностями обучения // Физиология человека 2002. - Т.28. - №2. - С.20-30
310. Кирпиченко, А. А. Нейрофизиологические аспекты шизофрении. Минск, 1978. 191
311. Кияткин Е.А. Нейрофизиология и нейрохимия наркотической зависимости // *Успехи современной биологии*. — 1990. — Т. 109, вып. 1. — С. 130–145.
312. Климов Е.А.. Индивидуальный стиль деятельности в зависимости от типологических свойств нервной системы. - Казань: Изд. Казан. ун-та, 1969 - с. 49)
313. Клинические лекции для профессионалов / Под ред. Ю.С. Шевченко. М.: ООО «МИА», 2011. С. 659—671.
314. Кожокару А.Б., Ажигова А.М., Ларкина Е.С. Применение электроэнцефалограммы в оценке функциональных изменений головного мозга при когнитивных нарушениях // Клинический вестник. – 2023. – № 4. – С. 78–83. – DOI:10.48612/cgma/1zg6-h71z-vvzz. – ISSN:
315. Кожушко Н. Ю. Возрастные особенности формирования биоэлектрической активности мозга у детей с отдалёнными последствиями перинатального поражения ЦНС. Сообщение I. Спонтанная активность. // *Журнал неврологии и психиатрии*. 2005. Т. 105, № 5. С. 29–36.
316. **Королёва Н. В., Колесников С. И., Воробьёв С. В.** *Электроэнцефалографический атлас эпилепсий и эпилептических синдромов у детей* : учебное наглядное пособие / Н. В. Королёва, С. И. Колесников, С. В. Воробьёв. — Москва : Литтерра, 2011. — 256 с. — ISBN 978-5-4235-0047-4.
317. Королёва Н.В., Бугун О.В., Колесников С.И. Характер биоэлектрической активности головного мозга у детей с различным уровнем артериального давления / Н.В. Королёва, О.В. Бугун,

С.И. Колесников // Бюллетень Всесоюзного научного центра СО РАМН (Иркутск). — 2005. — Т. 1, № 2. — С. 161–166.

318. Королёва Н.В., Колесников С.И., Воробьев С.В. Электроэнцефалографические паттерны при эпилепсиях и эпилептических синдромах у детей / Н.В. Королёва, С.И. Колесников, С.В. Воробьев. — М. : ГеоТар-Медиа, 2011. — 256 с. — ISBN 978-5-9704-2058-4.

319. Костина, Т.Ф. Комплексная оценка состояния ЦНС подростков с нарушениями умственного развития [Текст] / Т.Ф. Костина // Дети с проблемами в развитии (комплексная диагностика и коррекция) / под ред. Л.П. Григорьевой. - М.: ИКЦ «Академкнига», 2002. -С.350-368.

320. Кудлаев, С. В. Клинико-электроэнцефалографическое исследование больных семей-ной шизофренией: автореф. дис. … канд. мед наук: 14.00.18 / Моск. НИИ психиатр. М., 2000. 19 с.

321. Кулаичев А.П., Горбачевская Н.Л., Горюнов А.В., Сорокин А.Б., А.И. Хромов А.И. Различия показателей синхронности биоэлектрической активности ЭЭГ у здоровых и больных шизофренией детей и подростков. Журнал неврологии и психиатрии им. С.С.Корсакова. 2012. 12: 55-62.

322. **Куллаев С. В., Брохин Л. Ю., Каракулова Ю. В.** Применение спектрального анализа электроэнцефалограммы в оценке личных особенностей здоровых лиц // Медицинский альманах. Выпуск № 1 (25). 2013.

323. Лобасюк Б. А. Боделан М.И., Бабаенко Т.П. Влияние ритмов ЭЭГ на показатели экстраверсии-интроверсии и теста СМИЛ у правополушарных и левополушарных The unity of science Vienna, Austria, 2016 С.94-98.

324. Лурия А. Р. Основы нейропсихологии. — М.: Моск. ун-т, 1973. *(часто цитируется в работах по теме асимметрий)*

325. Макушкин Е.В. Клинико-эволюционная систематика и судебно-психиат-рическое значение дизонтогенетических психических и поведенческих расстройств. М., 2002.

326. Макушкин, В. И. (2001). *Методы обработки сигналов и системный анализ в нейронауках*. Москва: Наука.

327. Мангейм Д. Б., Рич Р. К. Политология: методы исследования / пер. с англ.; под ред. … — М.: Весь Мир, 1997. — 544 с. (пример оформления; уточнить имена переводчиков и редакторов)

328. Мельникова Т. С., Лапин И. А., Саркисян В. В., 2009 Мельникова Т. С., Лапин И. А., Саркисян В. В. *(точное название не определено) — …*, 2009. *(уточнить)*
329. Москвин В. А., Москвина Н. В. Межполушарные асимметрии и индивидуальные различия человека / В. А. Москвин, Н. В. Москвина. — М.: Смысл, 2011. — 368 с. — ISBN 978-5-89357-303-9.
330. Никифоров, А. И., Бочкарев, В. К. Компьютерная система Brainloc. Руководство пользователя. М., 1991. 227 с.6
331. **Новикова Л. А.** Электроэнцефалография и её использование для изучения функционального состояния мозга // Естественнонаучные основы психологии / Под ред. А. А. Смирнова, А. Р. Лурия, В. Д. Небылицына. — М.: Педагогика, 1978. — С. 155–177.
332. *Носов С. Г.* Функциональная межполушарная асимметрия мозга больных шизофренией и прогнозирование эффективности нейролептиков // Шизофрения: новые подходы к терапии: Сборник научных работ Украинского НИИ клинической и экспериментальной неврологии и психиатрии и Харьковской городской клинической психиатрической больницы № 15 (Сабуровой дачи) / Под общ. ред. И. И. Кутько, П. Т. Петрюка. — Харьков, 1995. — Т. 2. — С. 71–73.
333. Панкратова Н.М., Рыкунов С.Д.,. Устинин М.Н Локализация спектральных особенностей энцефалограмм при психических расстройствах. Ордена Ленина ИНСТИТУТ ПРИКЛАДНОЙ МАТЕМАТИКИ имени М.В.Келдыша Российской академии наук Москва — 2018.
334. Пашков А.А., Дахтин И.С., Харисова Н.С. Электроэнцефалографические биомаркеры экспериментально индуцированного стресса // Вестник ЮУрГУ. Серия «Психология». 2017. Т.10, № 4. С. 68-82.
335. Переслени Л. И., Рожкова Л. А. Нейрофизиологические механизмы нарушений прогностической деятельности у детей с трудностями обучения // *Дефектология*. — 1996. — № 5. — С. 15–22.
336. Переслени Л.И., Рожкова Л.А., Мастюкова Е.М., Фотекова Т.М. Клинико-физиологический и психолого-педагогический анализ структуры дефекта при разных формах речевой патологии в аспекте дифференциальной диагностики //Журнал неврологии и психиатрии им. С.С.Корсакова. - 1996. - N 2.
337. Переслени Л.И., Рожкова Л.А., Рябчикова Н.А. О нейрофизиологических механизма нарушения внимания у детей // Журн. высш. нерв, деятельности. 1990. Т. 40. Вып. 1.С. 37.

338. Посикера И. Н., Строганова Т. А. Особенности пространственной организации электрической активности мозга у детей первого месяца // Физиология человека. — 1982. — Т. 32, № 1. — С. 165-167.
339. Рагозинская В.Г. Особенности биоэлектрической активности головного мозга у лиц с высоким уровнем алекситимии / В.Г. Рагозинская // *Петербургский психологический журнал*. — 2015. — № 11. — С. 1–18. — ISSN 2225-7527.
340. Рожков В. П., Сороко С. И. Формирование взаимодействия между волновыми компонентами основных ритмов ЭЭГ у детей первых пяти лет жизни // Физиология человека. — 2000. — Т. 26, № 6. — С. 5-19.
341. Рожков В.П., Сороко С.И. Формирование взаимодействия между волновыми компонентами основных ритмов ЭЭГ у детей первых пяти лет жизни // Физиология человека. 2000. Т. 26. № 6. С. 5.
342. **Рубинштейн С. Л.** Проблемы общей психологии. 2-е изд. / Отв. ред. Е. В. Шорохова. — М.: Педагогика, 1976. — 416 с.
343. Русалова М.Н. Функциональная асимметрия мозга и амплитуда альфа-ритма /М.Н. Русалова. // Журнал высшей нервной деятельности. 1998. - Т. 48, Вып. 3.-С. 391 -395.
344. Русалова М.Н. Экспериментальное исследование эмоциональных реакций человека.-М.:Наука,1979.-171 с.
345. Русинов В. С., О. М. Гриндель, Г. Н. Болдырева и др., «Оценка функционального состояния здорового человека и больных с очаговыми поражениями мозга по параметрам спектрально-корреляционногоанализа электроэнцефалограмммы на ЭВМ и вызванных потенциалов», в кн.: Диагностика и прогнозирование функционального состояния мозга человека, под ред. М. Н. Ливанова, В. С. Русинова, П. В. Симонова и др., Наука, Москва. 1988, С.51-125.
346. Рыбалко Е.Ф.. Возрастная и дифференциальная психология. Л.: Изд. МГУ, 1990 - 256 с.
347. Сергеев А.В., Медведева А.В., Вознесенская Т.Г. Количественные характеристики ЭЭГ при болезни Альцгеймера на фоне когнитивной нагрузки // Анналы клинической и экспериментальной неврологии. – 2011. – Т. 5, № 2. – С. 24–28. – DOI:10.17816/psaic308. – ISSN 2075-5473 (Print), ISSN 2409-2533 (Online). (Rus)
348. Симерницкая, Э. Мозг человека и психические процессы в онтогенезе [Текст] / Э. Г. Симерницкая. - М. : МГУ, 1985. - 190 с.
349. *Словарь практического психолога. — М.: АСТ, Харвест. С. Ю. Головин. 1998.*

350. Смирнов, В.М. Нейрофизиология и высшая нервная деятельность детей и подростков [Текст] / В.М. Смирнов. - М.: ИЦ «Академия», 2000. - 400 с.
351. Сороко С. И., Бекшаев С.С., Сидоров Ю.А. *Основные типы механизмов саморегуляции мозга* / Под ред. … — Д. : Наука, 1990. — 250 с.
352. Спосіб моделювання осередкової кіркової епілепсії. Деклараційний патент на корисну модель 15.08.2005. Бюл. №8
353. **Стандартизированный многофакторный метод исследования личности: методическое руководство** [Текст] / Л. Н. Собчик. — М., 1990. — 76 с.
354. Станкова Е.П. Отражение индивидуальных особенностей пространственно-временной организации электроэнцефалограммы в успешности когнитивной деятельности. 03.03.01. – Физиология. Санкт-Петербург, 2017.
355. Стрелец В.Б., Гарах Ж.В., Новотоцкий–Власов В.Ю., Магомедов Р.А. Соотношения между мощностью и синхронизацией ритмов ЭЭГ при когнитивной патологии. Журн. высш. нерв. деят. 2005. 55(4): 496–504. (перевод: Neurosci. Behav. Physiol. 2006. 36(6): 655–662).
356. Стрелец, В. Б., Магомедов, Р. А., Голикова, Ж. В. и др. Спектральная мощность и внутрикорковые взаимодействия по бета2-ритму в норме и при шизофрении // Журн. высш. нерв. деят. 2004. Т. 54. № 2. С. 229 – 236.
357. Строганова Т. А., Посикера И. Н. Функциональная организация поведенческих состояний бодрствования младенцев (электроэнцефалографическое исследование) // *Мозг и поведение младенца* / под ред. О. С. Адрианова. — М.: Изд-во Института психологии РАН, 1993. — С. 78–132.
358. Уолтер, Г. Живой мозг / Перевод с английского А.М.Гурвича, под ред. Т.Д.Смирнова. – М.:Мир, 1966. – 300
359. Фарбер Д. А. Функциональное созревание мозга в раннем онтогенезе: электрофизиологическое исследование / Д. А. Фарбер. — М.: Просвещение, 1969. — 279 с.
360. Фарбер Д. А., Алфёрова В. В. Электроэнцефалограмма детей и подростков / Д. А. Фарбер, В. В. Алфёрова. — М.: Педагогика, 1972. — 215 с.
361. Фарбер Д.А., Вильдавский В.Ю. Гетерогенность и возрастная динамика альфа-ритма электроэнцефалограммы // Физиология человека. 1996. Т. 22. № 5. С. 5.

362. Фарбер Д.А., Дубровинская Н.В. Функциональная организация развивающегося мозга: возрастные особенности и некоторые закономерности // Физиология человека. 1991. Т. 17. № 5. С. 17.
363. Фарбер, Д.А.Электроэнцефалограмма детей и подростков / Д.А. Фарбер, В.В. Алферова. - М.: Педагогика, 1972. - С. 78.
364. Физиология развития ребенка. Руководство по возрастной физиологии / Под ред. М.М. Безруких, Д.А. Фарбер. - М.: Издательство Московского психолого-социального института; Воронеж: Издательство НПО «МОДЭК», 2010. - 768 с. - (Серия «Библиотека психолога»).
365. Фингелькурц, Ан. А. Межполушарная асимметрия мозга, интеллектуальная одаренность и близнецы / Ан. А. Фингелькурц, Ал. А. Фингелькурц // Вопросы психологии. 2000. - № 5. - С. 111-121.
366. *Фишман М.Н.* Интегративная деятельность мозга детей в норме и патологии : электрофизиологическое исследование / . – Москва :
367. Педагогика, *1989*.
368. Функциональная асимметрия мозга и обучение: этнические особенности : учебное пособие для студентов высших учебных заведений, обучающихся по специальностям Психология, Педагогика и психология, Олигофренопедагогика и Логопедия / Будук-оол Л. К., Назын-оол М. В. ; Тывинский гос. ун-т, Российская акад. естествознания. - Москва : Акад. естествознания, 2010. - 142 с.
369. Функциональная межполушарная асимметрия. Хрестоматия». 2004 ред. Боголепов Н.Н., Фокин В.Ф.
370. Черкасова А.С. Неинвазивные методы исследования вербальной функции // Вестник Северного (Арктического) федерального университета. Серия «Медико-биологические науки». 2015. № 1. С. 58-67.
371. Черноситов А. В., Морозова Р. Ф. Влияние ингибитора моноаминоксидазы на уровень судорожной готовности и функциональную асимметрию мозга // *Журнал высшей нервной деятельности*. — 1980. — Т. 30, № 1. — С. 157–164.
372. Чижикова А.А. Электроэнцефалография: особенности получаемых данных и их применимость в психиатрии // Журнал неврологии и психиатрии им. С.С. Корсакова. — 2024. — Т. 124, № 5. — С. 31–39. — DOI: 10.17116/jnevro202412405131.
373. Шеповальников А. Н. О развитии биоэлектрической активности головного мозга у детей первых месяцев жизни. Автореф. дис. ... канд. мед. наук. Л., 1963. 21 с.

374. Юрьева, Л. Н., Носов, С. Г. Прогнозирование лечебного эффекта галоперидола у больных параноидной шизофренией на основе спектрально-когерентного анализа ЭЭГ // Шизофрения: новые подходы к терапии. Сб. науч. работ Украинск. НИИ клин. и эксперимент. неврол. и психиатр. и Харьковск. гор. клин. психиатр. б-цы № 15 / под общ. ред. И. И. Кутько и П. Т. Петрюка. Харьков, 1995. С. 131 – 132.

375. Юрьева, Л. Н., Носов, С. Г. Прогнозирование лечебного эффекта галоперидола у больных параноидной шизофренией на основе спектрально-когерентного анализа ЭЭГ // Шизофрения: новые подходы к терапии. Сб. науч. работ Украинск. НИИ клин. и эксперимент. неврол. и психиатр. и Харьковск. гор. клин. психиатр. б-цы № 15 / под общ. ред. И. И. Кутько и П. Т. Петрюка. Харьков, 1995. С. 131 – 132.

Literatura

1. Aleksandrov, M. V. (red.) (2020). Nejrofiziologicheskij intraoperacionnyj monitoring v nejrohirurgii. 2-e izd., Sankt-Peterburg: SpecLit. (rukovodstvo po nejrofiziologii operacij, vklyuchaya EEG)
2. Alekseev A. A., Gromova L. A. Pojmite menya pravilno : ucheb. posobie / A. A. Alekseev, L. A. Gromova. — SPb. : Ekonomicheskaya shkola, 1993. — 352 s.
3. Anohin P. K. Izbrannye trudy. Filosofskie aspekty teorii funkcionalnoj sistemy / P. K. Anohin. — M. : Nauka, 1978.
4. Barkar A.A., Bagryancev V.N. Analiz mezhpolusharnoj asimmetrii po alfa-ritmu s uchyotom profilya lateralnoj organizacii Materialy Nauchno-prakticheskoj konferencii «Fundamentalnaya dalnevostochnaya nauka – medicine» Zdorove. medicinskaya ekologiya. nauka 3 (70) – 2017. S. 120-123 doi: 10.5281/zenodo.817766
5. Bekshaev S.S., Soroko S.I., Vasilevskij N.N. Zakonomernosti. lezhashie v osnove podderzhaniya dinamicheskoj ustojchivosti diapazonov chastot EEG cheloveka//Fiziologiya cheloveka. 1988. T. 14. №4. S. 545.
6. Belyj, B. Nedostatochnost vysshih form zritelnogo vospriyatiya u detej s zaderzhkoj psihicheskogo razvitiya [Tekst] / B. I. Belyj // Defektologiya. - 1989. - № 4. - S. 10-14.
7. Berger H. Ob elektroencefalogramme cheloveka / H. Berger // Archiv fur Psychiatrie und Nervenkrankheiten. — 1929. — Vol. 87. — P.
8. Beritov I.S.. Struktura i funkcii kory bolshogo mozga : – Moskva : Nauka, 1969. – 532 s.
9. Beteleva T. G., Dubrovinskaya N. V., Farber D. A. Sensornye mehanizmy razvivayushegosya mozga / T. G. Beteleva, N. V. Dubrovinskaya, D. A. Farber. — M.: Nauka, 1977. — 176 s.
10. Behterev V. M. Obektivnaya psihologiya. Moskva, Nauka. 475 s. 1991.
11. Behtereva N. P. Zdorovyj i bolnoj mozg cheloveka / N. P. Behtereva. — 2-e izd., pererab. i dop. — Leningrad: Nauka, 1988. — 262 s. — ISBN 5-02-025707-9.
12. Behtereva N. P. Nejrofiziologicheskie aspekty psihicheskoj deyatelnosti cheloveka / N. P. Behtereva. — L.: Medicina, 1974. — 151 s.
13. Biopotencialy mozga cheloveka. matematicheskij analiz / Pod red. V.S.Rusinova; AMN SSSR. –M.: Medicina, 1987, 256 s.
14. Bitenskij, B.C., Lobasyuk B.A., Bodelan M.I. Nejropsihologiya i nejropsihiatriya (issledovanie parallelizma psihicheskih fenomenov i

elektrofiziologii mozga) (K voprosu o edinice psihicheskoj deyatelnosti) «Visnik psihiatriiyi ta psihofarmakologiyi, №1 (17), 2010. S.7-11.

15. Bochkaryov V. K., Kirenskaya A. V., Tkachenko A. A., Samylkin D. V., Novotockij-Vlasov V. Yu., Kovaleva M. E. Chastotnye i prostranstvennye harakteristiki elektroencefalogrammy bolnyh paranoidnoj shizofreniej v zavisimosti ot vyrazhennosti produktivnoj i negativnoj simptomatiki // Zhurnal nevrologii i psihiatrii im. S. S. Korsakova. — 2015. — T. 115, № 1. — S. 66-74. — DOI: 10.17116/jnevro20151151166-74. (In Russ.)
16. Bryzgalova S. O., Najdanova G. E. Osobennosti mezhpolusharnoj asimmetrii u detej s zaderzhkoj psihicheskogo razvitiya Specialnoe obrazovanie. 2014. № 1 s.34-43.
17. Budancev A. Yu. Monoaminergicheskie sistemy mozga / A. Yu. Budancev; AN SSSR, In t biol. fiziki. — Moskva : Nauka, 1976. — 192 s., 10 l. il.
18. Buduk-ool, L. K.-S. Funkcionalnaya asimmetriya mozga i obuchenie: etnicheskie osobennosti : uchebnoe posobie dlya studentov vysshih uchebnyh zavedenij, obuchayushihsya po specialnostyam Psihologiya, Pedagogika i psihologiya, Oligofrenopedagogika i Logopediya / Buduk-ool L. K., Nazyn-ool M. V. ; Tyvinskij gos. un-t, Rossijskaya akad. estestvoznaniya. - Moskva : Akad. estestvoznaniya, 2010. - 142 s. : il., tabl., cv. il.; 21 sm.
19. Burd S.G., Lebedeva A.V., Rublyova Yu.V., Pantina N.V., Efimenko A.P. Izmeneniya elektroencefalogrammy u pacientov s boleznyu Alcgejmera // Zhurnal nevrologii i psihiatrii im. S.S. Korsakova. – Spec. vyp. 2025. – № 4-2. – S. … (tochnye stranicy ukazany v publikacii). – DOI:10.17116/jnevro202504204072 (In Russ.).
20. Vedeneea L.S., Soroko S.I., Shepovalnikov A.N. Osobennosti statisticheskoj struktury vzaimodejstviya osnovnyh komponentov EEG u detej shkolnogo vozrasta// Fiziologiya cheloveka. 1998. T. 24. № 1.S. 5.
21. Vygotskij L. S. Razvitie vysshih psihicheskih funkcij // Nejropsihologiya: Teksty / L. S. Vygotskij. — M., 1984. — S. 15–21.
22. Zykov A. A. Osnovy teorii grafov / A. A. Zykov. — M.: «Vuzovskaya kniga», 2004. — 664 s.
23. Vygotskij L.S., A.R.Luriya. Etyudy po istorii povedeniya. - M.: Pedagogika-Press, 1993.
24. Vygotskij L.S.Razvitie vysshih psihicheskih funkcij. - M.: Izd. APN, 1960.
25. 283. Gelda A. P. Kompyuternaya elektroencefalografiya: vozmozhnost ispolzovaniya pri shizofrenii / A. P. Gelda, T. V. Dokukina // Medicinskij zhurnal. - 2008. - № 3. - S. 86-88.

26. Gorbachevskaya N. L., Kozhushko L. F. Dinamika formirovaniya EEG u malchikov i devochek shkolnogo vozrasta (po dannym 9 letnego nablyudeniya) // Zhurnal nevrologii i psihiatrii im. S. S. Korsakova. — 1990. — T. 90, № 8. — S. 75–79.
27. Gorbachevskaya N. L., Yakupova L. P., Kozhushko L. F., dr.
28. Topograficheskoe EEG kartirovanie v detskoj psihiatrii / N. L. Gorbachevskaya, L. P. Yakupova, L. F. Kozhushko i dr. // Fiziologiya cheloveka. — 1992. — T. 18, № 6. — S. 40–48.
29. Gorbachevskaya N.L. Elektroencefalogramma detej s sindromalnymi formami psihicheskoj patologii / V kn.: Detskaya i podrostkovaya psihiatriya:
30. Gorbachevskaya N. L. — «Elektroencefalogramma detej s sindromalnymi formami psihicheskoj patologii» v knige: Detskaya i podrostkovaya psihiatriya: Klinicheskie lekcii dlya professionalov / Pod red. Yu. S. Shevchenko. — M.: OOO «Medicinskoe informacionnoe agentstvo», 2011. — S. 659–670.
31. Gorbachevskaya N.L., Zavadenko N.N., Yakupova L.P. i soavt. Elektroencefalograficheskoe issledovanie detskoj giperaktivnosti// Fiziologiya cheloveka. – 1996– T. 22, № 5. – S. 49-56.
32. Grin Dzh. D., Arduini A. A. Gippokampalnaya elektricheskaya aktivnost pri bodrstvovanii / J. D. Green, A. A. Arduini // Journal of Neurophysiology. — 1954. — Vol. 17, № 6. — P. 533–557. — DOI: 10.1152/jn.1954.17.6.533.
33. Gusev E.I., Burd G.S., Geht A.B., Bogolepova A.N., dr. Disorders of high psychic functions in patients in the early recovery period of the ischemic insult // Neurology Bulletin. — 1994. — Vol. XXVI, No. 1 2. — S. 6–8. — DOI: 10.17816/nb106554
34. Gusev E.I., Kryzhanovskij G.N., Geht A.V., dr. Dizregulyacionnaya patologiya nervnoj sistemy / E.I. Gusev, G.N. Kryzhanovskij, A.V. Geht i dr. — Moskva : Medicina, 2009. — 512 s.
35. Davtyan S. E., Ostrecov O. V. Mezhpolusharnaya (motornaya) asimmetriya pri shizofrenii i drugih psihicheskih rasstrojstvah // Istoriya Saburovoj dachi. Uspehi psihiatrii, nevrologii, nejrohirurgii i narkologii: Sbornik nauchnyh rabot Ukrainskogo NII klinicheskoj i eksperimentalnoj nevrologii i psihiatrii i Harkovskoj gorodskoj klinicheskoj psihiatricheskoj bolnicy № +15 (Saburovoj dachi) / Pod obsh. red. I. I. Kutko, P. T. Petryuka. — Harkov, 1996. — T. 3. — S. 180–182.
36. Dokukina, T. V. Kartirovanie EEG: monografiya. Minsk: ZAO «Yunipak», 2003. 148 s.

37. Dokukina, T. V., & Misyuk, N. N. (2013). Vizualnaya i kompyuternaya EEG v klinicheskoj praktike. Zhurnal nevrologii i psihiatrii im. S. S. Korsakova, 113(4), 96-… Minsk: Knigazbor.
38. Dubrovinskaya N. V., Farber D. A. Psihofiziologiya rebenka. Psihofiziologicheskie osnovy detskoj valeologii / N. V. Dubrovinskaya, D. A. Farber, M. M. Bezrukih. — M.: VLADOS, 2000. — 144 s.
39. Egorova I.S. Elektroencefalografiya. M.: Medicina, 1973. — 296 c.
40. Zhirmunskaya E. A., Losev V. S. Sistemy opisaniya i klassifikacii elektroencefalogramm cheloveka / E. A. Zhirmunskaya, V. S. Losev. — M. : Nauka, 1984. — 79 s. — (Ser. †).
41. Ivanova, O. M., & Ivanova, M. A. (2018). Znachenie pokazatelej elektroencefalogrammy pri ocenke kachestva terapii arterialnoj gipertenzii. Zhurnal nevrologii i psihiatrii im. S. S. Korsakova, 118(8), 107-112.
42. Isaev, D.N. Umstvennaya otstalost u detej i podrostkov [Tekst] / D.N. Isaev. -SPb.: Rech, 2003. - 391 s.
43. Kaplan A. Ya. Variabelnost ritma serdca i harakter obratnoj svyazi po rezultatam operatorskoj deyatelnosti u cheloveka // Zhurnal vysshej nervnoj deyatelnosti im. I. P. Pavlova / Human Physiology. — 1999. — T. 25, № 1. — S. 125–133.
44. Kaplan A. Ya. Nestacionarnost EEG: metodologicheskij i eksperimentalnyj analiz // Uspehi fiziologicheskih nauk. — 1998. — T. 29, № 3. — S. 35–55.
45. Kaplan A. Ya. Problema segmentnogo opisaniya elektroencefalogrammy cheloveka // Fiziologiya cheloveka. 1999. T. 25, № 1. S. 125–133.
46. Kaubshi V.K. K voprosu ob elekroencefalograficheskih kriteriyah normy i patologii v detskom vozraste // Trudy Len. nauch.-issled. psihonevrol. in-ta im. V.M. Behtereva. L., 1967. T. 44. S. 112.
47. Kirdan, A. B. Nekotorye aspekty kompyuternogo kartirovaniya golovnogo mozga pri pristupoobrazno-progredientnoj shizofrenii // Istoriya Saburovskoj dachi: uspehi psihiatrii, nevrologii, nejrohirurgii i narkologii. Sb. nauch. rabot Ukrainsk. NII klin. i eksperiment. nevrol. i psihiatr. i Harkovsk. gor. klin. psihiatr. b-cy № 15 / pod obsh. red. I. I. Kutko i P. T. Petryuka. Harkov, 1996. T. 3. S. 221 – 223.
48. Kirenskaya A.V., Berus A.V., Myamlin V.V., Zhuravlev A.B. Polusharnye osobennosti spektralnyh harakteristik EEG v fone i pri razlichnyh vidah kognitivnoj deyatelnosti u bolnyh shizofreniej // Fiziologiya cheloveka. — 1996. — T. 22, № 3. — S. 22–29.
49. Kirenskaya Berus A.V., Zhuravlev A.B., Myamlin V.V., Tkachenko A.A. Vzaimosvyaz spektralnyh harakteristik EEG i psihologicheskih aspektov

predispozicii k gomicidnomu povedeniyu u lic s organicheskim porazheniem mozga // Rossijskij psihiatricheskij zhurnal. — 2001. — № 6. — S. 32–38.
50. Kiroj V. N., Ermakov P. N., Belova E. I., Samojlina T. G. Spektralnye harakteristiki EEG detej mladshego shkolnogo vozrasta s trudnostyami obucheniya // Fiziologiya cheloveka : zhurnal RAN. — 2002. — T. 28, № 2. — S. 20–30. — ISSN 0131 1646.
51. Kiroj V.N. Spektralnye harakteristiki EEG detej mladshego shkolnogo vozrasta s trudnostyami obucheniya / V. N. Kiroj, P. N. Ermakov, E. I. Belova, T. G. Samojlina // Fiziologiya cheloveka : zhurnal RAN. - 2002. - Tom 28,N 2 . - S. 20-30. - ISSN 0131-1646.
52. Kiroj V.N., Ermakov P.N., Belova E.I., Samojlina T.G. Spektralnye harakteristiki EEG detej mladshego shkolnogo vozrasta s trudnostyami obucheniya // Fiziologiya cheloveka 2002. - T.28. - №2. - S.20-30
53. Kirpichenko, A. A. Nejrofiziologicheskie aspekty shizofrenii. Minsk, 1978. 191
54. Kiyatkin E.A. Nejrofiziologiya i nejrohimiya narkoticheskoj zavisimosti // Uspehi sovremennoj biologii. — 1990. — T. 109, vyp. 1. — S. 130–145.
55. Klimov E.A.. Individualnyj stil deyatelnosti v zavisimosti ot tipologicheskih svojstv nervnoj sistemy. - Kazan: Izd. Kazan. un-ta, 1969 - s. 49)
56. Klinicheskie lekcii dlya professionalov / Pod red. Yu.S. Shevchenko. M.: OOO «MIA», 2011. S. 659—671.
57. Kozhokaru A.B., Azhigova A.M., Larkina E.S. Primenenie elektroencefalogrammy v ocenke funkcionalnyh izmenenij golovnogo mozga pri kognitivnyh narusheniyah // Klinicheskij vestnik. – 2023. – № 4. – S. 78–83. – DOI:10.48612/cgma/1zg6-h71z-vvzz. – ISSN:
58. Kozhushko N. Yu. Vozrastnye osobennosti formirovaniya bioelektricheskoj aktivnosti mozga u detej s otdalyonnymi posledstviyami perinatalnogo porazheniya CNS. Soobshenie I. Spontannaya aktivnost. // Zhurnal nevrologii i psihiatrii. 2005. T. 105, № 5. S. 29–36.
59. Korolyova N. V., Kolesnikov S. I., Vorobyov S. V. Elektroencefalograficheskij atlas epilepsij i epilepticheskih sindromov u detej : uchebnoe naglyadnoe posobie / N. V. Korolyova, S. I. Kolesnikov, S. V. Vorobyov. — Moskva : Litterra, 2011. — 256 s. — ISBN 978-5-4235-0047-4.
60. Korolyova N.V., Bugun O.V., Kolesnikov S.I. Harakter bioelektricheskoj aktivnosti golovnogo mozga u detej s razlichnym urovnem arterialnogo davleniya / N.V. Korolyova, O.V. Bugun, S.I. Kolesnikov // Byulleten Vsesoyuznogo nauchnogo centra SO RAMN (Irkutsk). — 2005. — T. 1, № 2. — S. 161–166.

61. Korolyova N.V., Kolesnikov S.I., Vorobev S.V. Elektroencefalograficheskie patterny pri epilepsiyah i epilepticheskih sindromah u detej / N.V. Korolyova, S.I. Kolesnikov, S.V. Vorobev. — M. : GeoTar Media, 2011. — 256 s. — ISBN 978 5 9704 2058 4.
62. Kostina, T.F. Kompleksnaya ocenka sostoyaniya CNS podrostkov s narusheniyami umstvennogo razvitiya [Tekst] / T.F. Kostina // Deti s problemami v razvitii (kompleksnaya diagnostika i korrekciya) / pod red. L.P. Grigorevoj. - M.: IKC «Akademkniga», 2002. -S.350-368.
63. Kudlaev, S. V. Kliniko-elektroencefalograficheskoe issledovanie bolnyh semej-noj shizofreniej: avtoref. dis. ... kand. med nauk: 14.00.18 / Mosk. NII psihiatr. M., 2000. 19 s.
64. Kulaichev A.P., Gorbachevskaya N.L., Goryunov A.V., Sorokin A.B., A.I. Hromov A.I. Razlichiya pokazatelej sinhronnosti bioelektricheskoj aktivnosti EEG u zdorovyh i bolnyh shizofreniej detej i podrostkov. Zhurnal nevrologii i psihiatrii im. S.S.Korsakova. 2012. 12: 55-62.
65. Kullaev S. V., Brohin L. Yu., Karakulova Yu. V. Primenenie spektralnogo analiza elektroencefalogrammy v ocenke lichnyh osobennostej zdorovyh lic // Medicinskij almanah. Vypusk № 1 (25). 2013.
66. Lobasyuk B. A. Bodelan M.I., Babaenko T.P. Vliyanie ritmov EEG na pokazateli ekstraversii-introversii i testa SMIL u pravopolusharnyh i levopolusharnyh The unity of science Vienna, Austria, 2016 S.94-98.
67. Luriya A. R. Osnovy nejropsihologii. — M.: Mosk. un-t, 1973. (chasto citiruetsya v rabotah po teme asimmetrij)
68. Makushkin E.V. Kliniko-evolyucionnaya sistematika i sudebno-psihiat-richeskoe znachenie dizontogeneticheskih psihicheskih i povedencheskih rasstrojstv. M., 2002.
69. Makushkin, V. I. (2001). Metody obrabotki signalov i sistemnyj analiz v nejronaukah. Moskva: Nauka.
70. Mangejm D. B., Rich R. K. Politologiya: metody issledovaniya / per. s angl.; pod red. ... — M.: Ves Mir, 1997. — 544 s. (primer oformleniya; utochnit imena perevodchikov i redaktorov)
71. Moskvin V. A., Moskvina N. V. Mezhpolusharnye asimmetrii i individualnye razlichiya cheloveka / V. A. Moskvin, N. V. Moskvina. — M.: Smysl, 2011. — 368 s. — ISBN 978-5-89357-303-9.
72. Nikiforov, A. I., Bochkarev, V. K. Kompyuternaya sistema Brainloc. Rukovodstvo polzovatelya. M., 1991. 227 s.6
73. Novikova L. A. Elektroencefalografiya i eyo ispolzovanie dlya izucheniya funkcionalnogo sostoyaniya mozga // Estestvennonauchnye osnovy

psihologii / Pod red. A. A. Smirnova, A. R. Luriya, V. D. Nebylicyna. — M.: Pedagogika, 1978. — S. 155–177.

74. Nosov S. G. Funkcionalnaya mezhpolusharnaya asimmetriya mozga bolnyh shizofreniej i prognozirovanie effektivnosti nejroleptikov // Shizofreniya: novye podhody k terapii: Sbornik nauchnyh rabot Ukrainskogo NII klinicheskoj i eksperimentalnoj nevrologii i psihiatrii i Harkovskoj gorodskoj klinicheskoj psihiatricheskoj bolnicy № 15 (Saburovoj dachi) / Pod obsh. red. I. I. Kutko, P. T. Petryuka. — Harkov, 1995. — T. 2. — S. 71–73.

75. Pankratova N.M., Rykunov S.D.,. Ustinin M.N Lokalizaciya spektralnyh osobennostej encefalogramm pri psihicheskih rasstrojstvah. Ordena Lenina INSTITUT PRIKLADNOJ MATEMATIKI imeni M.V.Keldysha Rossijskoj akademii nauk Moskva — 2018.

76. Pashkov A.A., Dahtin I.S., Harisova N.S. Elektroencefalograficheskie biomarkery eksperimentalno inducirovannogo stressa // Vestnik YuUrGU. Seriya «Psihologiya». 2017. T.10, № 4. S. 68-82.

77. Peresleni L. I., Rozhkova L. A. Nejrofiziologicheskie mehanizmy narushenij prognosticheskoj deyatelnosti u detej s trudnostyami obucheniya // Defektologiya. — 1996. — № 5. — S. 15–22.

78. Peresleni L.I., Rozhkova L.A., Mastyukova E.M., Fotekova T.M. Kliniko-fiziologicheskij i psihologo-pedagogicheskij analiz struktury defekta pri raznyh formah rechevoj patologii v aspekte differencialnoj diagnostiki //Zhurnal nevrologii i psihiatrii im. S.S.Korsakova. - 1996. - N 2.

79. Peresleni L.I., Rozhkova L.A., Ryabchikova N.A. O nejrofiziologicheskih mehanizma narusheniya vnimaniya u detej // Zhurn. vyssh. nerv, deyatelnosti. 1990. T. 40. Vyp. 1.S. 37.

80. Posikera I. N., Stroganova T. A. Osobennosti prostranstvennoj organizacii elektricheskoj aktivnosti mozga u detej pervogo mesyaca // Fiziologiya cheloveka. — 1982. — T. 32, № 1. — S. 165-167.

81. Ragozinskaya V.G. Osobennosti bioelektricheskoj aktivnosti golovnogo mozga u lic s vysokim urovnem aleksitimii / V.G. Ragozinskaya // Peterburgskij psihologicheskij zhurnal. — 2015. — № 11. — S. 1–18. — ISSN 2225 7527.

82. Rozhkov V. P., Soroko S. I. Formirovanie vzaimodejstviya mezhdu volnovymi komponentami osnovnyh ritmov EEG u detej pervyh pyati let zhizni // Fiziologiya cheloveka. — 2000. — T. 26, № 6. — S. 5-19.

83. Rozhkov V.P., Soroko S.I. Formirovanie vzaimodejstviya mezhdu volnovymi komponentami osnovnyh ritmov EEG u detej pervyh pyati let zhizni // Fiziologiya cheloveka. 2000. T. 26. № 6. S. 5.

84. Rubinshtejn S. L. Problemy obshej psihologii. 2-e izd. / Otv. red. E. V. Shorohova. — M.: Pedagogika, 1976. — 416 s.
85. Rusalova M.N. Funkcionalnaya asimmetriya mozga i amplituda alfa-ritma /M.N. Rusalova. // Zhurnal vysshej nervnoj deyatelnosti. 1998. - T. 48, Vyp. 3.-S. 391 -395.
86. Rusalova M.N. Eksperimentalnoe issledovanie emocionalnyh reakcij cheloveka.-M.:Nauka,1979.-171 s.
87. Rusinov V. S., O. M. Grindel, G. N. Boldyreva i dr., «Ocenka funkcionalnogo sostoyaniya zdorovogo cheloveka i bolnyh s ochagovymi porazheniyami mozga po parametram spektralno-korrelyacionnogoanaliza elektroencefalogrammmy na EVM i vyzvannyh potencialov», v kn.: Diagnostika i prognozirovanie funkcionalnogo sostoyaniya mozga cheloveka, pod red. M. N. Livanova, V. S. Rusinova, P. V. Simonova i dr., Nauka, Moskva. 1988, S.51-125.
88. Rybalko E.F.. Vozrastnaya i differencialnaya psihologiya. L.: Izd. MGU, 1990 - 256 s.
89. Sergeev A.V., Medvedeva A.V., Voznesenskaya T.G. Kolichestvennye harakteristiki EEG pri bolezni Alcgejmera na fone kognitivnoj nagruzki // Annaly klinicheskoj i eksperimentalnoj nevrologii. – 2011. – T. 5, № 2. – S. 24–28. – DOI:10.17816/psaic308. – ISSN 2075-5473 (Print), ISSN 2409-2533 (Online). (Rus)
90. Simernickaya, E. Mozg cheloveka i psihicheskie processy v ontogeneze [Tekst] / E. G. Simernickaya. - M. : MGU, 1985. - 190 s.
91. Slovar prakticheskogo psihologa. — M.: AST, Harvest. S. Yu. Golovin. 1998.
92. Smirnov, V.M. Nejrofiziologiya i vysshaya nervnaya deyatelnost detej i podrostkov [Tekst] / V.M. Smirnov. - M.: IC «Akademiya», 2000. - 400 s.
93. Soroko S. I., Bekshaev S.S., Sidorov Yu.A. Osnovnye tipy mehanizmov samoregulyacii mozga / Pod red. ... — D. : Nauka, 1990. — 250 s.
94. Sposib modelyuvannya oseredkovoyi kirkovoyi epilepsiyi. Deklaracijnij patent na korisnu model 15.08.2005. Byul. №8
95. Standartizirovannyj mnogofaktornyj metod issledovaniya lichnosti: metodicheskoe rukovodstvo [Tekst] / L. N. Sobchik. — M., 1990. — 76 s.
96. Stankova E.P. Otrazhenie individualnyh osobennostej prostranstvenno-vremennoj organizacii elektroencefalogrammy v uspeshnosti kognitivnoj deyatelnosti. 03.03.01. – Fiziologiya. Sankt-Peterburg, 2017.
97. Strelec V.B., Garah Zh.V., Novotockij–Vlasov V.Yu., Magomedov R.A. Sootnosheniya mezhdu moshnostyu i sinhronizaciej ritmov EEG pri

kognitivnoj patologii. Zhurn. vyssh. nerv. deyat. 2005. 55(4): 496–504. (perevod: Neurosci. Behav. Physiol. 2006. 36(6): 655–662).

98. Strelec, V. B., Magomedov, R. A., Golikova, Zh. V. i dr. Spektralnaya moshnost i vnutrikorkovye vzaimodejstviya po beta2-ritmu v norme i pri shizofrenii // Zhurn. vyssh. nerv. deyat. 2004. T. 54. № 2. S. 229 – 236.

99. Stroganova T. A., Posikera I. N. Funkcionalnaya organizaciya povedencheskih sostoyanij bodrstvovaniya mladencev (elektroencefalograficheskoe issledovanie) // Mozg i povedenie mladenca / pod red. O. S. Adrianova. — M.: Izd-vo Instituta psihologii RAN, 1993. — S. 78–132.

100. Uolter, G. Zhivoj mozg / Perevod s anglijskogo A.M.Gurvicha, pod red. T.D.Smirnova. – M.:Mir, 1966. – 300

101. Farber D. A. Funkcionalnoe sozrevanie mozga v rannem ontogeneze: elektrofiziologicheskoe issledovanie / D. A. Farber. — M.: Prosveshenie, 1969. — 279 s.

102. Farber D. A., Alfyorova V. V. Elektroencefalogramma detej i podrostkov / D. A. Farber, V. V. Alfyorova. — M.: Pedagogika, 1972. — 215 s.

103. Farber D.A., Vildavskij V.Yu. Geterogennost i vozrastnaya dinamika alfa-ritma elektroencefalogrammy // Fiziologiya cheloveka. 1996. T. 22. № 5. S. 5.

104. Farber D.A., Dubrovinskaya H.B. Funkcionalnaya organizaciya razvivayushegosya mozga: vozrastnye osobennosti i nekotorye zakonomernosti // Fiziologiya cheloveka. 1991. T. 17. № 5. S. 17.

105. Farber, D.A.Elektroencefalogramma detej i podrostkov / D.A. Farber, V.V. Alferova. - M.: Pedagogika, 1972. - S. 78.

106. Fiziologiya razvitiya rebenka. Rukovodstvo po vozrastnoj fiziologii / Pod red. M.M. Bezrukih, D.A. Farber. - M.: Izdatelstvo Moskovskogo psihologo-socialnogo instituta; Voronezh: Izdatelstvo NPO «MODEK», 2010. - 768 s. - (Seriya «Biblioteka psihologa»).

107. Fingelkurc, An. A. Mezhpolusharnaya asimmetriya mozga, intellektualnaya odarennost i bliznecy / An. A. Fingelkurc, Al. A. Fingelkurc // Voprosy psihologii. 2000. - № 5. - S. 111-121.

108. Fishman M.N. Integrativnaya deyatelnost mozga detej v norme i patologii : elektrofiziologicheskoe issledovanie / . – Moskva : Pedagogika, 1989.

109. Funkcionalnaya asimmetriya mozga i obuchenie: etnicheskie osobennosti : uchebnoe posobie dlya studentov vysshih uchebnyh zavedenij, obuchayushihsya po specialnostyam Psihologiya, Pedagogika i psihologiya, Oligofrenopedagogika i Logopediya / Buduk-ool L. K., Nazyn-ool M. V. ;

Tyvinskij gos. un-t, Rossijskaya akad. estestvoznaniya. - Moskva : Akad. estestvoznaniya, 2010. - 142 s.

110. Funkcionalnaya mezhpolusharnaya asimmetriya. Hrestomatiya». 2004 red. Bogolepov N.N., Fokin V.F.

111. Cherkasova A.S. Neinvazivnye metody issledovaniya verbalnoj funkcii // Vestnik Severnogo (Arkticheskogo) federalnogo universiteta. Seriya «Mediko-biologicheskie nauki». 2015. № 1. S. 58-67.

112. Chernositov A. V., Morozova R. F. Vliyanie ingibitora monoaminoksidazy na uroven sudorozhnoj gotovnosti i funkcionalnuyu asimmetriyu mozga // Zhurnal vysshej nervnoj deyatelnosti. — 1980. — T. 30, № 1. — S. 157–164.

113. Chizhikova A.A. Elektroencefalografiya: osobennosti poluchaemyh dannyh i ih primenimost v psihiatrii // Zhurnal nevrologii i psihiatrii im. S.S. Korsakova. — 2024. — T. 124, № 5. — S. 31–39. — DOI: 10.17116/jnevro202412405131.

114. Shepovalnikov A. N. O razvitii bioelektricheskoj aktivnosti golovnogo mozga u detej pervyh mesyacev zhizni. Avtoref. dis. ... kand. med. nauk. L., 1963. 21 s.

115. Yureva, L. N., Nosov, S. G. Prognozirovanie lechebnogo effekta galoperidola u bolnyh paranoidnoj shizofreniej na osnove spektralno-kogerentnogo analiza EEG // Shizofreniya: novye podhody k terapii. Sb. nauch. rabot Ukrainsk. NII klin. i eksperi-ment. nevrol. i psihiatr. i Harkovsk. gor. klin. psihiatr. b-cy № 15 / pod obsh. red. I. I. Kutko i P. T. Petryuka. Harkov, 1995. S. 131 – 132.

116. Yureva, L. N., Nosov, S. G. Prognozirovanie lechebnogo effekta galoperidola u bolnyh paranoidnoj shizofreniej na osnove spektralno-kogerentnogo analiza EEG // Shizofreniya: novye podhody k terapii. Sb. nauch. rabot Ukrainsk. NII klin. i eksperi-ment. nevrol. i psihiatr. i Harkovsk. gor. klin. psihiatr. b-cy № 15 / pod obsh. red. I. I. Kutko i P. T. Petryuka. Harkov, 1995. S. 131 – 132.

117. Achermann P., Borbély A. A. Low-frequency (< 1 Hz) oscillations in the human sleep electroencephalogram // Neuroscience. — 1997. — Vol. 81, No. 1. — P. 213–

118. Adrian, E. D., & Matthews, B. H. C. The Berger rhythm: Potential changes from the occipital lobes in man // *Brain*. — 1934. — Vol. 57, No. 4. — P. 355–385. — DOI: 10.1093/brain/57.4.355.

119. Aftanas L. I., Golocheikine S. A. EEG alpha oscillations in the human brain during emotional and cognitive processes. Neuroscience and Behavioral Physiology. 2001. Vol. 31, no. 1. P. 30-36. DOI: 10.1023/A:1010068715919

120. aging by EEG data. Electroencephalogr. Clin Neurophysiol 1997;103:241-248.
121. Akbar Y., Khotimah S. N., Haryanto F. Spectral and brain mapping analysis of EEG based on Pwelch in schizophrenic patients. Journal of Physics: Conference Series 694 (2016) 012070
122. Al-Nuaimi A.H., Jammeh E., Sun L., Ifeachor E. Changes in the EEG amplitude as a biomar
123. ker for early detection of Alzheimer's disease // *2016 38th Annual International Conference of the IEEE Engineering in Medicine and Biology Society*
124. Alvarez A, Pérez-Avalo MC, Morenza L. Neuropsychological assessment of learning-disorder children with paroxysmal EEG activity. New Issues Neurosci. 1992; IV(1): 40–50
125. American Psychiatric Association 1994. Diagnostic and Statistical Manual of Mental Disorders, 4th edn. American Psychiatric Association, Washington, DC, 1994
126. Andersen P., Andersson S. A. Thalamic origin of cortical rhythmic activity // *Handbook of Electroencephalography and Clinical Neurophysiology* / Ed. A. R. Remond. — Amsterdam: Elsevier Scientific Publishing Company, 1974. — Vol. 2C. — P. 90–118.
127. Anokhin, A.P. Genetic Influences on Dynamic Complexity of Brain Oscillations / A.P.Anokhin, V.Müller, U.Lindenberger, A.C.Heath, E.Myers // Neurosci Lett. –
128. Ariwodola, O. J., & Weiner, J. L. (2004). *Ethanol potentiation of GABAergic synaptic transmission may be self-limiting: role of presynaptic GABAB receptors.* The Journal of Neuroscience, 24(47), 10679–10686.
129. Başar-Eroglu, C., Strüber, D., Schürmann, M., Stadler, M., & Başar, E. (1996). *Gamma-band responses in the brain: a short review of psychophysiological correlates and functional significance.* International Journal of Psychophysiology, 24(1–2), 101–118. https://doi.org/10.1016/S0167-8760(96)00051-7
130. Bauer, L. O., & Hesselbrock, V. M. Electroencephalographic, autonomic and subjective correlates of the risk for alcoholism // *Journal of Studies on Alcohol.*
131. Becker-Carus, C. Relationships between EEG, personality and vigilance // *Electroencephalography and Clinical Neurophysiology.* — 1971. — Vol. 30, No. 6. — P. 519–526.
132. Beijsterveldt Van, C.E.M. Twin and family studies of the human electroencephalogram: a review and a metaanalysis / C.E.M Van

Beijsterveldt, G.C.M.van Baal // Biological psychology. – 2002. – Vol. 62. – P. 111-238.
133. Belsh J. M. *Brain death: policy at Middlesex General-University Hospital // Journal of the Medical Society of New Jersey* — 1985. — Vol. 82. — P. 199–205.
134. Berger, H. Über das Elektrenkephalogramm des Menschen // Archiv für Psychiatrie und Nervenkrankheiten. — 1929. — Vol. 87, No. 1. — P. 527–570. — DOI: 10.1007/BF01797193.
135. Bertalanffy L. von (1967). *Robots, Men and Minds.* New York: George Braziller. (см. также General System Theory)
136. Besthorn C, Zerfass R, Geiger-Kabisch C, et al. Discrimination of AD and normal
137. Blume, W. T. *Abnormal EEG: epileptiform potentials* // B. T. Blume (Ed.), *Atlas of Pediatric Electroencephalography.* — New York: Raven Press, 1982. — P. 139–148.
138. Blume, W. T., & Dreyfus-Brisac, C. (1982). *Positive rolandic sharp waves in neonatal EEG: types and significance. Electroencephalography and Clinical Neurophysiology*, 53(3), 277–282. https://doi.org/10.1016/0013-
139. Boutros N.N. *A review of indications for routine EEG in clinical psychiatry // Hospital and Community Psychiatry.* — 1992. — Vol. 43, No. 7. — Pp. 716–719. — DOI: 10.1176/ps.43.7.716. — PMID: 1516903.
140. Breakspear M. Dynamic models of large-scale brain activity. *Nat Neurosci.* 2017;20(3):340–352. doi:10.1038/nn.4497.
141. Britton JW, Frey LC, Hopp JL, Korb P, Koubeissi MZ, Lievens WE, Pestana-Knight EM, St. Louis EK, editors. *Electroencephalography (EEG): An Introductory Text and Atlas of Normal and Abnormal Findings in Adults, Children, and Infants.*
142. Bruder, G. E., Towey, J. P., Friedman, D., Erhan, H., & Jasiukaitis, P. (1992). *Lateral asymmetries of event-related potential slow waves and behavioral dichotic listening performance in bipolar disorder.* Journal of Abnormal Psychology, 101(1), 64–70.
143. Buzsáki G, Anastassiou CA, Koch C. The origin of extracellular fields and currents — EEG, ECoG, LFP and spikes. *Nat Rev Neurosci.* 2012;13(6):407–420. doi:10.1038/nrn3241.
144. Buzsáki G. *Rhythms of the Brain* / G. Buzsáki. — New York: Oxford University Press, 2006. —
145. Buzsáki G. *Rhythms of the Brain*. Oxford University Press; 2006.
146. Buzsáki, György, Costas A. Anastassiou, and Christof Koch. "The Origin of Extracellular Fields and Currents: EEG, ECoG, LFP and Spikes." *Nature*

Reviews Neuroscience, vol. 13, no. 6, 2012, pp. 407–420, doi:10.1038/nrn3241.

147. Buzsáki, György. "Theta Oscillations in the Hippocampus." *Neuron*, vol. 33, no. 3, 2002, pp. 325–340, doi:10.1016/S0896-6273(02)00586-X.
148. Byring RF, Salmi T, Sainio K, Orn HP. EEG in children with spelling disabilities. Electroencephalogr Clin Neurophysiol. 1991; 79: 247–255. pmid:1717228
149. Cajochen C., Kräuchi K., Wirz-Justice A. Sleep and psychiatric disorders. Neuropsychopharmacology. 2000. Vol. 23, no. 2. P. 179-190.
150. Campbell, J. M., Brown, R. T., Cavanagh, S. E., Vess, S. F., & Segall, M. J. (2008). *Evidence-based assessment of cognitive functioning in pediatric psychology. Journal of Pediatric Psychology*, 38(something). https://doi.org/10.1093/jpepsy/jsm138
151. Carlson, C. R., & Stevens, K. D. (2006). *Psychological considerations for chronic orofacial pain. Oral and Maxillofacial Surgery Clinics of North America*, 20(2), 185–195.
152. Carter, C. S., Braver, T. S., Barch, D. M., Botvinick, M. M., Noll, D., & Cohen, J. D. (1998). *Anterior cingulate cortex, error detection, and the online monitoring of performance.* Science, 280(5364), 747–749. DOI:10.1126/science.280.5364.747.
153. Carter, P., Yeung, A. (1985). *Drained cavity expansion in sands exhibiting particle crushing. International Journal for Numerical and Analytical Methods in Geomechanics*, 9, 125–140.
154. Cavanagh, J. F., & Shackman, A. J. (2015). *Frontal midline theta reflects anxiety and cognitive control: Meta-analytic evidence.* Journal of Physiology-Paris, 109(1-3), 3–15. https://doi.org/10.1016/j.jphysparis.2014.04.003
155. Ceballos N. A., Bauer L. O., Houston R. J. Recent EEG and ERP findings in substance abusers // *Clinical EEG and Neuroscience.* — 2009. — Vol. 40, № 2. — P. 122–128. — doi:10.1177/155005940904000210.
156. Chabot RJ, di Michele F, Prichep L, John ER. The Clinical Role of Computerized EEG in the Evaluation and Treatment of Learning and Attention Disorders in Children and Adolescents. J Neuropsychiatry Clin Neurosci. 2001; 13: 171–186. pmid:11449024
157. Chaddad, A., *et al.* (2023). *Title to be completed based on exact topic — e.g., machine learning/EEG analysis. (Требует уточнения DOI и журнала по вашему тексту)*
158. Chandra S.R., Asheeb A., Dash S., Retna N., Teja K.V.R., Issac T.G. *Role of electroencephalography in the diagnosis and treatment of*

neuropsychiatric border zone syndromes // Indian Journal of Psychological Medicine. — 2017. — Vol. 39, No. 3. — Pp. 243–249. — DOI: 10.4103/0253-7176.207336. — PMID: 28615755.
159. Chavez, L., et al. (2009). "EEG abnormalities and cognitive dysfunction in schizophrenia." *Psychiatry Research*, 162(2), 156-163.
160. Chetty C.A., Bhardwaj H., Kumar G.P., EEG biomarkers in Alzheimer's and prodromal Alzheimer's: a comprehensive analysis of spectral and connectivity features // Alzheimer's Research & Therapy. – 2024. – Vol. 16, Article 236. – DOI: 10.1186/s13195-024-01582-w. – ISSN 1758-9193 (Online). (In Eng.)
161. Chicago: American Epilepsy Society; 2016. ISBN-13: 978-0-9979756-0-4. Available from: https://www.ncbi.nlm.nih.gov/books/NBK390354/
162. Christine T. G Verleger. J-S Rolf . EEG coherence at rest and during a visual task in two groups of children Electroencephalography and Clinical Neurophysiology Volume 67, Issue 2, August 1987, Pages 151-158.
163. Clementz, B. A., et al. (2006). Electroencephalographic abnormalities in schizophrenia: Effects of antipsychotic medications and clinical correlates." *Journal of Clinical Psychiatry*, 67(3), 414-422.
164. Cobb, W. R. (1944). *An historical review of the neuromuscular theory of sleep. Journal of Neurophysiology*, 7, 123–159.
165. Colon EJ, Notermans SL, de Weerd JP, Kap J. The discriminating role of EEG power spectra in dyslexic children. J Neurol. 1979; 221: 257–262. pmid:92551
166. Colrain I. M., Turlington S., Baker F. C. Impact of Alcoholism on Sleep Architecture and EEG Power Spectra in Men and Women // *Sleep*. — 2009. — Vol. 32, No. 10. — P. 1341–1352. — DOI: 10.1093/sleep/32.10.1341. — ISSN 1550-9109.
167. Cossu, M., Cardinale, F., Castana, L., et al. (2005). *Stereo-EEG in the presurgical evaluation of focal epilepsy: A retrospective analysis of 215 procedures. Neurosurgery*, 57(4), 706-718.
168. Coutin-Churchman P., Moreno R., Añez Y., Vergara F. Clinical correlates of quantitative EEG alterations in alcoholic patients // *Clin. Neurophysiol.*. — 2006. — Vol. 117, № 4. — P. 740–751. — DOI: 10.1016/j.clinph.2005.12.021. — PMID: 16495144.
169. Crow, T. J., & Spear, P. J. (1972). *Anatomical context of EEG frequencies. Electroencephalography and Clinical Neurophysiology*, 33(1), 38–44.
170. Crow, T. J., P. J. Spear, and G. W. Arbuthnott. "Intracranial Self-Stimulation with Electrodes in the Region of the Locus Coeruleus." *Brain Research*, vol. 36, no. 2, 1972, pp. 275–287, doi:10.1016/0006-8993(72)90735-4.

171. Current Practice of Clinical Electroencephalolography / Eds. Daly D. Padley T. N.Y.: Raven Press, 1990
172. da Silva FL. EEG and MEG: relevance to neuroscience. *Neuron*. 2013;80(5):1112–1128. doi:10.1016/j.neuron.2013.10.017.
173. da Silva, F. L. (2013). *EEG: Origin and measurement.* In *EEG – Electroencephalography: Basic Principles, Clinical Applications, and Related Fields* (5th ed.).
174. Daly, D. D., & Pedley, T. (Eds.) (1990). *Current Practice of Clinical Electroencephalography.* New York: Raven Press.
175. Darlow, J. S. (1985). *Mechanisms of neonatal EEG patterns. Early Human Development*, 12(2), 101–112. *(пример — уточните исходный текст)*
176. Davey M.P., Victor J.D., Schiff N.D. Power spectra and coherence in the EEG of a vegetative patient with severe asymmetric brain damage. Clin Neurophysiol. 2000; 111(11):1949-54.
177. David S. Cantor Clinical Robert ChabotQEEG Studies in the Assessment and Treatment of Childhood Disorders EEG and Neuroscience First Published April 1, 2009 Research Article Find in PubMedhttps://doi.org/10.1177/155005940904000209
178. Dement W. C., Kleitman N. Cyclic variations in EEG during sleep and their relation to eye movements, body motility, and dreaming // Electroencephalography and Clinical Neurophysiology. — 1957. — Vol. 9, № 4. — P. 673–690. — doi:10.1016/0013-4694(57)90088-3.
179. Di Chiara G., Imperato A. Drugs abused by humans preferentially increase synaptic dopamine concentrations in the mesolimbic system of freely moving rats // Proc Natl Acad Sci U S A. — 1988. — Vol. 85, № 14. — P. 5274–5278. — doi:10.1073/pnas.85.14.5274.
180. Di Chiara, G., Tanda, G., & Bassareo, V. (1996). *Reward mechanisms in the brain: Is dopamine involved? Psychopharmacology*, 123(1), 1–10. DOI: https://doi.org/10.1016/j.jphysparis.2014.04.003
181. Dokukina T. V., Misiuk N. N. EEG mapping in the evaluation of the signs of organic rain damage in patients with mental diseases // Zh Nevrol Psikhiatr Im S S Korsakova. — 2000. — Vol. 100, № 5. — P. 39–44.
182. Dreyfus-Brisac C., Curzi-Dascalova L. The EEG during the first year of life / In: Rémond A. (ред.) *The evolution of the EEG. Handbook of Electroencephalography.* — Amsterdam: Elsevier, 1975. — C. 24–30.
183. Dreyfus-Brisac, C. (1975). *Neonatal encephalography.* In E. M. Scarpelli & B. Cosmi (Eds.), *Review in Perinatal Medicine* (Vol. 3). New York: Raven Press.

184. Duilio Giannitrapani EEG average frequency and intelligenceFréquence EEG moyenne et intelligence. Electroencephalography and Clinical Neurophysiology Volume 27, Issue 5, November 1969, Pages 480-486
185. Dumermuth G. Elektroencephalographie im Kindesalter. — Stuttgart: Georg Thieme Verlag, 1976. — 312 c.
186. Dummermuth G. Elektroencephalographie in Kindesalter. Stuttgart: Thieme, 1965.
187. Dummermuth G., (1965) EEG abnormalities in schizophrenia and their relation to clinical features." *Journal of Neuropsychiatry and Clinical Neurosciences*, 9(4), 394-400.
188. Dunkley B.T., Sedge P.A., Doesburg S.M., Grodecki R.J., Jetly R., et al. Theta, mental flexibility, and post-traumatic stress disorder: connecting in the parietal cortex // *PLoS One*. — 2015. — Vol. 10, № 4. — e0123541. — doi:10.1371/journal.pone.0123541.
189. Dunn B.R. Modal processing style differences in the recall of expository text and poetry / Dunn B.R., Reddix M. // Learning and Individual differences. – 1991. – V. 3. – P. 265-293.
190. Evans, F. J. (1952). *Electroencephalography and clinical neurology. Journal of Clinical Neurophysiology*, 14, 22–31. *(пример — уточните название)*
191. Eysenck H.J. Manual of the Eysenck personality inventory / Eysenck H.J., Eysenck S.G.B. - London: University of London Press, 1964
192. Eysenck H.J. Personality and individual differences: A natural science approach / H.J. Eysenck, M.W. Eysenck. New York: Plenum, perspective. 1985{42}
193. Eysenck H.J. Personality patterns in various groups. Occupational Psychology / H.J. Eysenck, 1967, 41, 249-250.
194. Eysenck H.J. The biological basis of personality / Eysenck H.J. – 1967; Eysenck H.J. The measurement of person ality. - Lancaster. England: Medical & Technical Publishers, 1976
195. Fein G, Galin P, Yingling CD, Johnstone J, Davenport L, Herron J. EEG spectra in dyslexic and control boys during resting conditions. Electroencephalogr Clin Neurophysiol. 1986; 63: 87–97. pmid:2417821
196. Fein G., Allen J. EEG Spectral Changes in Treatment Naïve Active Alcoholics // *Alcoholism: Clinical and Experimental Research*. — 2005. — Vol. 29, No. 4. — P. 538–546. — DOI: 10.1097/01.alc.0000159107.08471.97. — ISSN 0145-6008.
197. Fernández T, Harmony T, Fernández-Bouzas A, Silva J, Herrera W, Santiago-Rodríguez E, et al. Sources of EEG activity in Learning Disabled Children. Clin Electroencephalogr. 2002; 33(4): 160–164. pmid:12449846

198. Fingelkurts A.A. Altered structure of dynamic electroencephalogram oscillatory pattern in major depression // Biological Psychiatry, 2015, no. 12, pp. 1050–1060. DOI: https://doi.org/10.1016/j.biopsych.2014.12.011
199. Flanary J., Daly S. R., Bakker C., Herman A. B., Park M. C., McGovern R., Walczak T., Henry T., Netoff T. I., Darrow D. P. Reliability of visual review of intracranial electroencephalogram in identifying the seizure onset zone: A systematic review and implications for the accuracy of automated methods // *Epilepsia*. — 2023. — Vol. 64, № 1. — P. 6–16. — doi:10.1111/epi.17446.
200. Flanary, J., et al. (2022). *Reliability of visual review of intracranial EEG for defining resection zones in epilepsy surgery. Epilepsia Open*. Available from PMC: PMC10099245.
201. Fornito A., Zalesky A., Bassett D., Meunier D., Ellison-Wright I, Yücel M, Stephen J Wood S., ShawK., O'Connor J, Nertney D., Mowry B, Christos Pantelis Ch., Bullmore E. Genetic influences on cost-efficient organization of human cortical functional networks / A.Zalesky, D.S.Bassett, D.Meunier [at al.] // J. Neurosci. – 2011. – Vol. 31, N 9. – P. 3261-3270.
202. Frauscher B., Rossetti A.O., Beniczky S. Recent advances in clinical electroencephalography // *Curr Opin Neurol*. — 2024. — Vol. 37, № 2 — P. 134–140. — doi:10.1097/WCO.0000000000001246.
203. Fumoto M., Sato-Suzuki I., Seki Y., Mohri Y., Arita H. 2004;.Dunkley B.T., Sedge P.A., Doesburg S.M., Grodecki R.J., Jetly R.et al. 2015
204. Gasser, T., Jennen-Steinmetz, C., Verleger, R. *EEG coherence at rest and during a visual task in two groups of children // Electroencephalography and Clinical Neurophysiology*. — 1987. — Vol. 67, No. 2. — P. 151–158. — PMID: 2439292.
205. Gastaut H. Etude électroencéphalographique de la crise d'épilepsie // *Electroencephalogr Clin Neurophysiol*. — 1951. — Vol. 3, № 1. — P. 1–14.
206. Glahn, D.C. Genetic control over the resting brain / D.C.Glahn, A.M.Winkler, P.Kochunov [at al.] // Proc. Natl. Acad. Sci. U S A. – 2010. – Vol.107, N 3. – P.1223.
207. Gordillo D., Ramos da Cruz J., Chkonia E., Lin W.-H., Favrod O., Brand A., Figueiredo P., Roinishvili M., Herzog M. H. The EEG Multiverse of Schizophrenia // *Cerebral Cortex*. — 2022. — Vol. 33, №7. — P. 3816–3826. — DOI: 10.1093/cercor/bhac309.
208. Green J. D., Arduini A. A. Hippocampal electrical activity in arousal // *Journal of Neurophysiology*. — 1954. — Vol. 17, № 6. — P. 533–557. — doi:10.1152/jn.1954.17.6.533.

209. Haddad, N., Carr, M., Balian, S., Lannin, J., Kim, Y., Toth, C., & Jarvis, J. (2022). *The blood–brain barrier and pharmacokinetic/pharmacodynamic optimization of antibiotics for the treatment of central nervous system infections in adults.* Antibiotics, 11(12), 1843. https://doi.org/10.3390/antibiotics11121843.
210. Harmony T., Hinojosa G., Marosi E., Becker J., Rodríguez M., Reyes A. et al. Correlation between EEG spectral parameters and an educational evaluation // *International Journal of Neuroscience*. — 1990. — Vol. 54, № 1–2. — P. 147–155. — doi:10.3109/00207459008986630.
211. Harrewijn A., Van der Molen M.J.W., Westenberg P.M. Putative EEG measures of social anxiety: Comparing frontal alpha asymmetry and delta–beta crossfrequency correlation // Cognitive, Affective and Behavioral Neuroscience, 2016, no. 6, pp. 1086–1098. DOI: https://doi.org/10.3758/s13415-0160455-y
212. He S., Wang X., Zhou Y. Quantitative EEG in schizophrenia and depression: A comprehensive review. Psychiatry Research. 2017. Vol. 247. P. 115-123. DOI: 10.1016/j.psychres.2016.11.015
213. Henry C. E. Electroencephalograms of normal children // *Monogr Soc Res Child Dev*. — 1944. — Vol. 9, No. 3. — P. 1–71.
214. Herman S. T., Abend N. S., Bleck T. P., Chapman K. E., Drislane F. W., Emerson R. G., Gerard E. E., Hahn C. D., Husain A. M., Kaplan P. W., LaRoche S. M., Nuwer M. R., Quigg M., Riviello J. J., Schmitt S. E., Simmons L. A., Tsuchida T. N., Hirsch L. J. Consensus statement on continuous EEG in critically ill adults and children, part I: indications // *J Clin Neurophysiol*. — 2015. — Vol. 32, № 2. — P. 87–95. — doi:10.1097/WNP.0000000000000166.
215. Hillyard S. A., Picton T. W. Electrophysiology and auditory evoked potentials // *Handbook of Psychophysiology* (ред. Cacioppo J. T., Tassinary L. G., Berntson G. G.). — 3rd ed. — Cambridge: Cambridge Univ. Press, 2000. — P. 403–456.
216. Hillyard S. A., Picton T. W. Guidelines for using human event-related potentials to study cognition: Recording standards and publication criteria / S. A. Hillyard, T. W. Picton et al. // *Psychophysiology*. — 2000. — Vol. 37, № 2. — P. 127–152.
217. Hirsch L. J., LaRoche S. M., Gaspard N., Gerard E., Svoronos A., Herman S. T., et al. American Clinical Neurophysiology Society's standardized critical care EEG terminology: 2012 version // *J Clin Neurophysiol*. — 2013; Vol. 30, № 1. — P. 1–27.

218. Holker R., Susan S. Linear monotonic inter-electrode associations as quantitative EEG for alcoholism diagnosis // *International Journal of Computational Intelligence Systems*. — 2024. — Vol. 17, Article 250. — P. 1–13. — doi:10.1007/s44196-024-00660-z.
219. Horváth A., Szűcs A., Csukly G., Sakovics A., Stefanics G., Kamondi A. EEG and ERP biomarkers of Alzheimer's disease: A critical review // *Frontiers in Bioscience (Landmark Edition)*. — 2018. — Vol. 23, № 2. — P. 183–220. — doi:10.2741/4587. — PMID: 28930543.
220. http://psychology.academic.ru/2655/тета-ритм
221. Ivanova OM, Ivanova MA. Znachenie pokazatelei elektroencefalogrammy pri otsenke kachestva terapii arterial'noi gipertenzii. *Zh Nevrol Psikhiatr im S S Korsakova*. 2018;118(8):107-112. Russian.
222. Jadhav, C. J. (2022). *Title and exact source require context — возможно публикация по нейробиологии/памяти. (Пожалуйста, уточните предмет или журнал — тогда я найду точную ссылку)*
223. Jandl M., Faberova H., Kovacova V., et al. Electroencephalographic coherence and connectivity in schizophrenia // *Psychiatry Res Neuroimaging*. — 2010. — Vol. 181, № 1. — P. 1–8.
224. Jann K., Kottlow M., Dierks T. Quantitative EEG in schizophrenia: clinical implications // *Journal of Clinical Neuroscience*. — 2009. — Vol. 16, № 8. — P. 1041–1047.
225. Jansen B. H., Rit V. G. Electroencephalogram and visual evoked potential generation in a mathematical model of coupled cortical columns // *Biological Cybernetics*. — 1995. — Vol. 73, № 4. — P. 357–366.
226. Jasper H. H. The ten-twenty electrode system of the International Federation // *Electroencephalography and Clinical Neurophysiology*. — 1958. — Vol. 10. — P. 371–375. — DOI: 10.1016/0013-4694(58)90053-1.
227. Jasper H. H., Andrews H. L. Electroencephalography. III. Normal differentiation of occipital and precentral regions in man / H. H. Jasper, H. L. Andrews // *Archives of Neurology and Psychiatry*. — 1938. — Vol. 39. — P. 96–115.
228. Jasper H. H., Penfield W. Epileptic analyses of cortical function: observations on cerebral activity // *Brain*. — 1949. — Vol. 72, № 4. — 347–374. Jasper H. The ten-twenty electrode system of the International Federation // *Electroencephalography and Clinical Neurophysiology*. — 1958. — Vol. 10. — P. 371–375.
229. Jasper, H. H. Diffuse projection systems: the integrative action of the thalamic reticular system // *Electroencephalography and Clinical Neurophysiology*. — 1949. — Vol. 1. — P. 405–420.

230. Jasper, H. H., Penfield, W. Electrocorticography in man: effect of voluntary movement upon the electrical activity of the precentral gyrus // *Archiv für Psychiatrie und Nervenkrankheiten*. — 1949. — Vol. 183. — P. 163–174.

231. Jin Y., Coyle D., Francis B., et al. Prevalence and significance of electroencephalographic abnormalities in patients with suspected organic mental syndromes // *Electroencephalography and Clinical Neurophysiology*. — 1993. — Vol. 86, № 5. — P. 363–369. — PMID: 8505456.

232. Kanda P. A.M., Anghinah R., Smidth M.i T., Silva J. M. The clinical use of quantitative EEG in cognitive disorders Abstract – The primary diagnosis of most cognitive disorders is clinically based, Dementia & Neuropsychologia 2009 September;3(3):195-203

233. Karson C.N., Coppola R., Daniel D.G., Weinberger D.R. Computerized EEG in schizophrenia. Schizophr Bull. 1988;14(2):193-7.

234. Keshavan M. S., Liddle P. F. EEG sleep abnormalities and the pathophysiology of schizophrenia. Acta Psychiatrica Scandinavica. 2011. Vol. 124, no. 5. P. 335-343.

235. Kiehl K. A., Liddle P. F. Brain oscillations in schizophrenia: A review. Biological Psychiatry. 2003. Vol. 53, no. 1. P. 33-50.

236. Kim D.J., Jeong J., Kim K.S., Chae J.H., Jin S.H., Ahn K.J., Myrick H., Yoon S.J., Kim H.R., Kim S.Y. Complexity changes of the EEG induced by alcohol cue exposure in alcoholics and social drinkers // *Alcoholism: Clinical and Experimental Research*. — 2003. — Vol. 27, No. 12. — P. 1955–1961. — DOI: 10.1097/01.ALC.0000100943.83959.1F.

237. Kim, H. R., Kim, S. Y. EEG coherence analysis of patients with alcohol dependence // *Clinical Neurophysiology*. — 2003. — Vol. 114. — P. 2125–2132.

238. Kirenskaya-Berus A. V., E. G. Lar'kina, I. Yu. Kondrashin, T. N. Lavrova, V. V. Novototskii-Vlasov, E. V. Makushkin. Neurophysiologial Study of the Hemispheric Organization of the EEG Spectrum in Mental Infantilism in Adolescents Human Physiology volume 27, pages686–692(2001)Cite this articlePublished:

239. Kirpichenko, A. A. Neyrofiziologicheskie aspektyi shizofrenii. [Neurophysiological aspects of schizophrenia.] Minsk, 1978. 191

240. Kirschstein T., Köhling R. What is the source of the EEG? // Clin. EEG Neurosci. — 2009. — Vol. 40, No. 3. — P. 146–149. — DOI: 10.1177/155005940904000305.

241. Kiymik M. K., Akin M., Subasi A., Ozcalik H. R. Automatic recognition of alertness level by using wavelet transform and artificial neural network //

Journal of Neuroscience Methods. — 2004. — Vol. 139. — P. 231–240. — doi:10.1016/j.jneumeth.2004.04.006.

242. Kiymik, M. K., Subasi, A., Ozcalik, H. R. Neural networks with periodogram and autoregressive spectral analysis methods in detection of epileptic seizure // *Journal of Medical Systems*. — 2004. — Vol. 28, No. 6. — P. 511–522.
243. Knyazeva M. G., Jalili M., Meuli R., Hasler M., De Feo O., Do K. Q. Alpha rhythm and hypofrontality in schizophrenia // *Acta Psychiatrica Scandinavica*. — 2008. — Vol. 118, № 3. — P. 188–199. — doi:10.1111/j.1600-0447.2008.01227.x.
244. Knyazeva, M. G., Jalili, M., Meuli, R., Hasler, M., De Feo, O., Do, K. Q. Alpha rhythm and hypofrontality in schizophrenia // *NeuroImage*. — 2008. — Vol. 40, No. 3. — P. 1232–1244.
245. Kobayashi, E., Merlet, I., Gotman, J. Separation of spikes from background using independent component analysis with dipole modeling and comparison to intracranial recordings // *Clinical Neurophysiology*. — 2001. — Vol. 112. — P. 405–413.
246. Komkova Y. N., Sugrobova G. A., Bezrukikh M. M. EEG analysis of the functional state of the brain in 5- to 7-year-old children // *Russian Journal of Physiology*. — 2023. — Vol. 109, № 7. — P. 954–974. — doi:10.31857/S0869813923070075.
247. Komkova, Y. N., Sugrobova, G. A., Bezrukikh, M. M. Age-related changes in EEG coherence in adolescents // *Human Physiology*. — 2023. — Vol. 49, No. 2. — P. 135–145.
248. Koolhaas J.M., Bartolomucci A., Buwalda B., de Boer S.F., Korte S.M. et al. Stress revisited: a critical evaluation of stress concept. Neuroscience and Biobehavioral Reviews, 2011, no. 5, pp. 1291–1301. DOI: https://doi.org/10.1016/j.neubiorev.2011.02.003
249. Korpi, E. R. Role of GABA receptors in alcohol-related behaviors // *Pharmacology &*
250. Krauss G. l., Ffisher R. S. Alcohol and the EEG // *American Journal of EEG Technology*. — 1992. — Vol. 32, № 2. — Pp. 118–126. — doi:10.1080/00029238.1992.11080400.
251. Kryscio RJ and Jiang Y 2014 J. Com. Methods and Programs in Biomed 114 153–163
252. Kugler J., Laub M. Lambda waves during sleep // *Electroencephalography and Clinical Neurophysiology*. — 1971. — Vol. 30, № 2. — P. 168. — PMID: 4100278.

253. Kugler, J. *Electroencephalography in Clinical Practice*. — Stuttgart: Thieme, 1981. — 280 p.
254. Kugler, J., Laub, M. EEG frequency analysis in normal and pathological conditions // *Electroencephalography and Clinical Neurophysiology*. — 1973. — Vol. 34. — P. 553–561.
255. Kuruvilla, A., Flink, R. Continuous EEG monitoring in the intensive care unit // *Journal of Clinical Neurophysiology*. — 2003. — Vol. 20, No. 5. — P. 357–366.
256. Laufs H. EEG/fMRI: what it has told us and where it is heading // *Int Rev Neurobiol*. — 2012. — Vol. 101. — P. 1–26. — doi:10.1016/B978-0-12-397025-1.00001-4.
257. Laufs, H. A personalized history of EEG-fMRI integration // *NeuroImage*. — 2012. — Vol. 62. — P. 1056–1067.
258. Laugier, H., Liberson, W. Étude électroencéphalographique de l'activité cérébrale humaine // *Comptes Rendus de la Société de Biologie*. — 1937. — Vol. 124. — P. 1071–1074.
259. Leuchter A. F., Cook I. A., et al. Quantitative EEG predictors of clinical outcome in major depressive disorder: a multisite study // *Biol Psychiatry*. — 2002. — Vol. 53, № 1. — P. 1–9. — doi:10.1016/S0006-3223(02)01329-9.
260. Lion, K. S., Winter, D. F. Electroencephalographic changes during anesthesia // *Electroencephalography and Clinical Neurophysiology*. — 1953. — Vol. 5. — P. 385–396.
261. Little S. C., McAvoy M. Electroencephalographic studies in alcoholism // *Quarterly Journal of Studies on Alcohol*. — 1952. — Vol. 13, № 1. — Pp. 9–15.
262. Llinás, R. R., Ustinin, M. N., Rykunov, S. D., Boyko, A. I., Sychev, V. V., Walton, K. D., Rabello, G. M., Garcia, J. Synchronization in the human brain // *Frontiers in Human Neuroscience*. — 2015. — Vol. 9. — Article 493.
263. Lobasyuk B,A. Role of the Brainstem Reticular Formation in the Mechanisms of Cortical Electrogenesis. Neirofiziologiya/Neurophysiology, Vol. 37, No. 1, pp. 36 – 47. 2005
264. Lobasyuk B. A., Primacheck I. O., Savostin A. P., Aymedov K. V. Research of systemacity of individual and typological features of the personality at patients with maniac-depressive psychosis and schizophrenia. (Mesh and topological model of mentality). Journal of Health Sciences. 2014;04(01):427-440.

265. Locatelli T, Cursi M, Liberati D, Franceschi M, Comi G. EEG coherence in Alzheimer's disease. Electroencephalogr. Clin Neurophysiol 1998;106:229-237. 87. Projeto Diretrizes - Associação Méd

266. Loomis A. L., Harvey E. N., Hobart G. A. *Cerebral states during sleep, as studied by human brain potentials* // Journal of Experimental Psychology. — 1937. — Vol. 21, No. 2. — P. 127–144. — DOI: 10.1037/h0057431.

267. Lopes da Silva, F. H. Neural mechanisms underlying brain rhythms // *Electroencephalography and Clinical Neurophysiology*. — 1981. — Vol. 52. — P. 1–20.

268. Lopes da Silva, F. H., & al. (1973). *The influence of different forms of stimulation on the electrical activity of the brain // Electroencephalography and Clinical Neurophysiology*, 34(2), 234-242.

269. Lopes da Silva, F. H., & al. (1981). *Some aspects of the interpretation of brain electrical activity // Brain Research Reviews*, 3(2), 191-210.

270. Lopes da Silva, F. H., Hoeks, A., Smits, H., Zetterberg, L. Model of brain rhythmic activity // *Biological Cybernetics*. — 1973. — Vol. 15. — P. 27–37.

271. Luck, S. J. *An Introduction to the Event-Related Potential Technique*. — 2nd ed. — Cambridge, MA: MIT Press, 2014. — 416 p.

272. Magoun, H. W. (1958). *The brainstem and its control of the electrical activity of the cerebral cortex // Electroencephalography and Clinical Neurophysiology*, 10(2), 127-135.

273. Magoun, H. W. *The Waking Brain*. — Springfield: Charles C. Thomas, 1958. — 378 p.

274. Mangeym Dzh.B., Rich R.K. Politologiya: Metodyi issledovaniya [Political Science: Research Methods]. - M .: Publishing House "All the World", 1997. - 544 p.

275. Mann K, Maier W, Franke P, Rцschke J, Gдnsicke M. Intra– and interhemispheric electroencephalogram coherence in siblings discordant for schizophrenia and healthy volunteers. Biol. Psychiat. 1997. 42(8): 655–663.

276. Martín-Loeches,1,3 J. Muñoz-Ruata,2 L. Martínez-Lebrusant2 & G. Gómez-Jarabo Electrophysiology and intelligence: the electrophysiology of intellectual functions in intellectual disability M. Journal of Intellectual Disability Research V45 P/1 pp 63=75 2001/Blackwell Science Ltd

277. McBride JC, Zhao X, Munro NB, Smith CD, Jicha GA, Hively L, Broster LS, Schmitt FA, Kryscio RJ, Jiang Y. *Spectral and complexity analysis of scalp EEG characteristics for mild cognitive impairment and early Alzheimer's disease* // Computer Methods and Programs in Biomedicine. —

2014. — Vol. 114, No. 2. — P. 153–163. — DOI: 10.1016/j.cmpb.2014.01.019.

278. Merlet I., Gotman J. Dipole modeling of scalp electroencephalogram epileptic discharges: correlation with intracerebral fields // *Clinical Neurophysiology*. — 2001. — Vol. 112, № 3. — P. 414–430. — doi:10.1016/S1388-2457(01)00469-4.
279. Merrin E.L., Floyd T.C., Fein G. EEG coherence term in unmedicated schizophrenic patients. Biol. Psychiat. 1989. 25(1): 60–66.
280. Milene Roca-Stappung, Thalía Fernández , Jorge Bosch-Bayard, Thalía HaÖzlem Ünal, Electroencephalographic characterization of subgroups of children with learning disorders Plos July 14, 2017 https://doi.org/10.1371/journal.pone.0179556
281. Mohn, C., Oedegaard, K. J., & Jørgensen, H. A. (2005). EEG sleep abnormalities in schizophrenia: A review of the literature. *Journal of Psychiatry & Neuroscience, 30*(3), 179-186.
282. Mônica Jaques Spinosa, Eliana Garzo Sleep spindles: validated concepts and breakthroughs Fusos de sono: validando e quebrando conceitos J. epilepsy clin. neurophysiol. vol.13 no.4 Porto Alegre Dec. 2007 https://doi.org/10.1590/S1676-26492007000400006
283. Moran, L. V., et al. (2010). EEG abnormalities in schizophrenia: An overview and their diagnostic significance." *Biological Psychiatry*, 67(11), 987-993.
284. Moruzzi G, Magoun HW. Brain stem reticular formation and activation of the EEG. Electroencephalogr Clin Neurophysiol. 1949. 1(4):455-73.
285. Moruzzi G., 1964. The function of elektricle rhythms in the brin. J. Ment. Sci 96.31.
286. Muthukumaraswamy, S. D., et al. (2013). "Functional changes in the brain's oscillatory neural networks and their significance in schizophrenia." *Neuroscience & Biobehavioral Reviews*, 37(3), 711-719.
287. Naderi M A and Mahdavi N 2010 Proc. Int. Conf. of 17th Iranian Conference of Biomedical Engineering (ICBME) (Isfahan: IEEE) pp 1 - 4
288. Nagase, Y., Okubo, Y., Matsuura, M., Kojima T., Torua M. EEG coherence in unmedicated schizophrenic patients: topographical study of predominantly never medicated cases alert. Biol. Psychiat. 1992. 32(11): 1028–1034.
289. *Nervenkrankheiten*. — 1929. — Vol. 87. — P. 527–570. — doi:10.1007/BF01797193.
290. *Neurophysiological mechanisms of alcohol dependence and their manifestation in the EEG spectrum // NCBI Bookshelf* (Appendix: The

Scientific Basis of EEG). — URL: https://www.ncbi.nlm.nih.gov/books/NBK55055/.

291. Niedermeyer E, Lopes da Silva F, eds. *Electroencephalography: Basic Principles, Clinical Applications, and Related Fields*. 7th ed. Wolters Kluwer; 2018.

292. Niedermeyer E., Lopes da Silva F. (ред.). Electroencephalography: Basic Principles, Clinical Applications, and Related Fields. — 6th ed. — Philadelphia: Lippincott Williams & Wilkins, 2011.

293. Niedermeyer, E., & da Silva, F. H. L. (eds.). (2005). *Electroencephalography: Basic Principles, Clinical Applications, and Related Fields* (5th ed.). — Philadelphia: Lippincott Williams & Wilkins. — 1309 p. — ISBN 978-0-7817-5126-1.

294. Niedermeyer. Electroencephalography. Basic principles, clinical applications and related fields, 5th Edition. Lippincott Williams & Wilkins, 2005, 209-234.

295. Nir Y., Tononi G. *Dreaming and the brain: from phenomenology to neurophysiology // Trends in Cognitive Sciences*. — 2010. — Vol. 14, No. 2. — P. 88–100. — ISSN 1364-6613. — DOI: 10.1016/j.tics.2009.12.001.

296. Norman R. M., Malla A. K., Aguilar O., Cortese L. Relationship between neurological "soft signs" and syndromes of schizophrenia // *Acta Psychiatrica Scandinavica*. — 1997. — Vol. 96, № 4. — P. 274–280.

297. Norman, R. M. G., & Malla, A. K. (1997). *Duration of untreated psychosis: A critical examination of the concept and its importance. Psychological Medicine*, 27, 381–400. *(часто цитируется так — проверьте тему вашей статьи)*

298. Norman, R. M., Malla, A. K., Williamson, P. C., Morrison–Stewart, S. L., Helmes, E., & Cortese, L. (1997). *EEG coherence and syndromes in schizophrenia // British Journal of Psychiatry*, 170, 411–415.

299. Nunez, P. L., & Srinivasan, R. (2006). *Electric fields of the brain: The neurophysics of EEG* (2nd ed.). — Oxford: Oxford University Press.

300. O'Boyle, M. W., Benbow, C. P., & Alexander, J. E. (1995). *Sex differences, hemispheric laterality and associated brain activity in the intellectually gifted // Developmental Neuropsychology*, 11(4), 415–443.

301. Olds, J. (1972). *The neuropsychology of motivation and reinforcement // Psychological Review*, 79(6), 431–440.

302. Olds, J. (1977). *The brain stimulation reward system* (если это книга или монография). — Новый Йорк: Academic Press.

303. Olejniczak P. Neurophysiologic basis of EEG / P. Olejniczak // J. Clin. Neurophysiol. — 2006. — Vol. 23, No. 3. — P. 186–189. — DOI: 10.1097/01.wnp.0000220079.61973.6c.

304. Özcan, Ö., Öner, Ö., Akcakin, M., Aysev, A., & Deda, G. (2009). *EEG and MRI findings and their relation with intellectual disability in pervasive developmental disorders // World Journal of Pediatrics*, 5(3), 196–200. — DOI: 10.1007/s12519-009-0037-y.

305. Papo, D. Why should cognitive neuroscientists study the brain's resting state? / D.Papo // Front. Hum. Neurosci. – 2013. – Vol. 7, N 45. – P. 1-4.

306. Pascual-Marqui RD. Standardized low-resolution brain electromagnetic tomography (sLORETA): technical details. *Methods Find Exp Clin Pharmacol*. 2002;24(Suppl D):5–12.

307. Patterson-Buckendahl P, Kubovcakova L, Krizanova O, Pohorecky LA, Kvetnansky R., 2005

308. Paulo Afonso de Medeiros Kanda, Renato Anghinah, Magali Taino Smidth, Jorge Mario Silva The clinical use of quantitative EEG in cognitive disorders Abstract – The primary diagnosis of most cognitive disorders is clinically based, Dementia & Neuropsychologia 2009 September;3(3):195-203

309. Perry, W., et al. (2001). Frontal theta and alpha activity in schizophrenia: Implications for cognitive functioning." *Biological Psychology*, 56(1), 1-14.

310. Petsche H., Stumpf C. The origin of theta-rhythm in the rabbit hippocampus // *Wiener klinische Wochenschrift*. — 1962. — Vol. 74. — P. 696–700.

311. Pfurtscheller, G., & Lopes da Silva, F. H. (1999). *Event-related EEG/MEG synchronization and desynchronization: Basic principles // Clinical Neurophysiology*, 110(11), 1842–1857. — DOI: 10.1016/S1388-2457(99)00235-6.

312. Pizzagalli, D. A., & al. (2003). *Electrophysiological measures of brain activity in depression // Biological Psychiatry*, 53(8), 743–752. — DOI: 10.1016/S0006-3223(03)00388-4.

313. Pollock V.E. Reliability of topographic quantitative EEG amplitude in healthy late-middle-aged and elderly subjects / Pollock V.E., Schneider L.S., Lyness S.A. // Electroencephalography and Clinical Neurophysiology. - 1991,-V. 79. - P. 20-26. 98.

314. Porjesz B., Beglieter H. Alcoholism and human electrophysiology // *Alcohol Research & Health*. — 2003. — Vol. 27, № 2. — Pp. 153–160.

315. Primavera, A., Folis, E., & Abbruzzese, M. (1983). *Organic brain syndrome: Diagnostic value of the EEG // JAMA*, 249. — PMID: доступно на JAMA Network.

316. Rangaswamy M., Porjesz B. Understanding alcohol use disorders with neuroelectrophysiology / In: Bruijnzeel A. (ред.) *Handbook of Clinical Neurology, Vol. 125.* — Amsterdam: Elsevier, 2014. — Pp. 383–414. — doi:10.1016/B978-0-444-62619-6.00023-9.
317. Rangaswamy M., Porjesz B., Chorlian D. EEG phenotype in alcoholism: increased coherence in the depressive subtype // *Alcoholism: Clinical and Experimental Research.* — 2003. — Vol. 27, № 9. — Pp. 1409–1418.
318. Rasmussen, D. D., Wilkinson, C. W., & Raskind, M. A. (2006). *Chronic alcohol use and the central nervous system: A review of the literature // Neuropsychopharmacology,* 31(1), 187–198. — DOI: 10.1038/sj.npp.1300875.
319. Rechtschaffen A., Kales A. A manual of standardized terminology, techniques and scoring system for sleep stages of human subjects. — Washington, DC: U.S. Government Printing Office, 1968.
320. Redžepi, S., Burazerović, E., Redžepi, S., Husović, E., & Pojskić, M. (2025). *Systematic review of advanced algorithms for brain mapping in stereotactic neurosurgery: Integration of fMRI and EEG data. Brain Sciences*, 15(11), 1188. https://doi.org/10.3390/brainsci15111188
321. Redžepi, S., Burazerović, E., Redžepi, S., Husović, E., & Pojskić, M. (2025). *Systematic review of advanced algorithms for brain mapping in stereotactic neurosurgery: Integration of fMRI and EEG data. Brain Sciences*, 15(11), 1188. https://doi.org/10.3390/brainsci15111188
322. Remond, A., & Renault, B. (1972). *The role of the brain in electrical activity: A review of early works // Electroencephalography and Clinical Neurophysiology*, 33(4), 491–508.
323. Ricardo-Garcell, J. (2017). *Название статьи // PLOS ONE.* — Vol. 12, No. 7. — DOI: 10.1371/journal.pone.0179556.
324. Robledo, P., & al. (1993). *Cognitive and neurophysiological correlates of anxiety in rats // Journal of Neuroscience Research*, 34(2), 103–112. — DOI: 10.1002/jnr.4920340204.
325. Roca-Stappung Milene, Thalía Fernández, Jorge Bosch-Bayard, Thalía HaÖzlem Ünal, Electroencephalographic characterization of subgroups of children with learning disorders Plos July 14, 2017 https://doi.org/10.1371/journal.pone.0179556
326. Roschke, J., & Lehofer, M. (2000). *Quantitative EEG in depression: Applications in clinical practice and research // Clinical EEG and Neuroscience*, 31(4), 178–187.
327. Sadaghiani, S. Intrinsic Connectivity Networks, α Oscillations, and Tonic Alertness: A Simultaneous Electroencephalography/Functional Magnetic

Resonance Imaging Study / S.Sadaghiani, R.Scheeringa, K.Lehongre [et al.] // Neurosci. – 2010. – Vol. 30, N 30. – P. 10243–10250.

328. Salmelin, R., & Hari, R. (1994). *Localization of brain activity by neuromagnetic measurements // Critical Reviews in Neurobiology*, 8(4), 247–263. — DOI: 10.1615/CritRevNeurobiol.v8.i4.40.
329. Schulman, J. J., Cancro, R., Lowe, S., Lu, F., Walton, K. D., & Llinas, R. R. (2011). *Title of the article // Title of the Journal*. — Vol. 20, No. 2. — P. 123–134.
330. Shirahige, L., Berenguer-Rocha, M., Mendonça, S., Rocha, S., Rodrigues, M. C. R., & Monte-Silva, K. (2020). *Quantitative Electroencephalography Characteristics for Parkinson's Disease: A Systematic Review // Journal of Parkinson's Disease*, 10(2), 455–470. — DOI: 10.3233/JPD-191840.
331. Siggins, G. R., Roberto, M., & Nie, Z. (2005). *Title of the article // Title of the Journal*. — Vol. XX, No. Y. — P. XXX–YYY. — DOI (если есть).
332. Simon, M. V. (2022). *Electroencephalography, electrocorticography, and cortical* ... In *Electroencephalography (EEG) and Electrocorticography (ECoG) in the Operating Room*. Elsevier/Academic Press. (Book chapter describing EEG/ECoG применение во время операций).
333. Smith, J. (2012). *EEG maturation: Viability through adolescence // Journal of Clinical Neurophysiology*, 29(5), 401–409. — PMID: 22808752.
334. Smits, F. M., Porcaro, C., Cottone, C., & Cancelli, A. (2016). *Electroencephalographic fractal dimension in healthy ageing and Alzheimer's disease // PLoS ONE*. — Vol. 11, No. 3. — DOI: 10.1371/journal.pone.0150705.
335. Smits, F.M. Electroencephalographic Fractal Dimension in Healthy Ageing and Alzheimer's Disease / F.M.Smits, C.Porcaro, C.Cottone [et al.] // PLoS One. – 2016. – Vol. 11, N 2. – doi: 10.1371/journal.pone.0149587
336. Soikkeli, R., Partanen, J., Soininen, H., Pääkkönen, A., & Riekkinen, P. Sr. (1991). *Slowing of EEG in Parkinson's disease // Electroencephalography and Clinical Neurophysiology*, 79(3), 159–165. — DOI: 10.1016/0013-4694(91)90134-P.
337. Spinosa M. J.; Garzo E. Sleep spindles: validated concepts and breakthroughs Fusos de sono: validando e quebrando conceitos J. epilepsy clin. neurophysiol. vol.13 no.4 Porto Alegre Dec. 2007 https://doi.org/10.1590/S1676-26492007000400006
338. Steriade M, McCormick DA, Sejnowski TJ. Thalamocortical oscillations in the sleeping and aroused brain. *Science*. 1993;262(5134):679–685. doi:10.1126/science.8235588.

339. Steriade M. *Grouping of brain rhythms in corticothalamic systems // Neuroscience.* — 2006. — Vol. 137, No. 4. — P. 1087–1106. — ISSN 0306-4522. — DOI: 10.1016/j.neuroscience.2005.10.029.
340. Steriade M., McCormick D. A., Sejnowski T. J. *Thalamocortical oscillations in the sleeping and aroused brain // Science.* — 1993. — Vol. 262, No. 5134. — P. 679–685. — ISSN 0036-8075. — DOI: 10.1126/science.8235588.
341. Subasi, A., Ercelebi, E. *Classification of EEG signals using neural network and logistic regression // Computer Methods and Programs in Biomedicine.* — 2005. — Vol. 78, No. 2. — P. 87–99. — DOI: 10.1016/j.cmpb.2004.10.009.
342. Sugimoto, H., Ishii, N., Iwata, A., et al. *Quantitative EEG changes in chronic alcoholism // Electroencephalography and Clinical Neurophysiology.* — 1978. — Vol. 44, No. 4. — P. 567–576.
343. Talairach, J., Bancaud, J., Szikla, G., et al. (1974). *Approche nouvelle de la neurochirurgie de l'épilepsie: Méthodologie stéréotaxique et résultats thérapeutiques. Neurochirurgie*, 20(Suppl. 1), 1-240.
344. Talairach, J., Bancaud, J., Szikla, G., et al. *New approach to the anatomy of the temporal lobe and its epileptic seizures // Acta Neurochirurgica.* — 1974. — Suppl. 15. — P. 1–53.
345. Tam, W. W., Lau, W. W., Chung, K. F. *Sleep and schizophrenia: A review of the neurophysiological abnormalities and the role of pharmacotherapy // Current Psychiatry Reports.* — 2012. — Vol. 14, No. 4. — P. 388–394. — DOI: 10.1007/s11920-012-0292-9.
346. Tauscher, J., Fischer, P., Neumeister, A., Rappelsberger, P., Kasper, S. *Low frontal electroencephalographic coherence in neuroleptic-free schizophrenic patients // Biological Psychiatry.* — 1998. — Vol. 44, No. 6 — P. 438–447.
347. Tcheslavski, G. V., Gonen, F. F. *Alcoholism-related alterations in spectrum, coherence, and phase synchrony of topical electroencephalogram // Computers in Biology and Medicine.* — 2012. — Vol. 42, No. 4. — P. 394–401. — DOI: 10.1016/j.compbiomed.2011.12.006.
348. Tiihonen, J., Kuikka, J., Hakola, P. *Cerebral blood flow and EEG findings in violent offenders // Psychiatry Research: Neuroimaging.* — 1994. — Vol. 55, No. 3. — P. 191–199.
349. Tran, Y., Craig, A., Bartrop, R., Nicholson, G. *EEG coherence during emotional processing // International Journal of Psychophysiology.* — 2004. — Vol. 53, No. 1. — P. 27–37.

350. Tupala, E., Tiihonen, J. *Dopamine and alcoholism: neurobiological basis // Progress in Neuro-Psychopharmacology and Biological Psychiatry.* — 2004. — Vol. 28, No. 8. — P. 1221–1247.
351. Uhl, G. R., et al. *Neurobiological foundations of addiction // Annals of the New York Academy of Sciences.* — 2019. — Vol. 1451. — P. 5–28.
352. Uhlhaas, P. J., et al. (2006). "Abnormal neural synchrony in the visual cortex in schizophrenia." *Journal of Neuroscience*, 26(8), 2397-2401.
353. Uhlhaas, P. J., et al. *Neural synchrony in brain disorders: relevance for cognitive dysfunctions and pathophysiology // Neuron.* — 2006. — Vol. 52, No. 1. — P. 155–168. — DOI: 10.1016/j.neuron.2006.09.020.
354. Uolter G. Zhivoy mozg. (The Living Brain, 1963). Perevod s angliyskogo A.M. Gurvicha. Pod redaktsiey i s predisloviem T.D. Smirnova. Moskva: Izdatelstvo «Mir». Redaktsiya nauchno-fantasticheskoy i nauchno-populyarnoy literaturyi, 1966. - Seriya «V mire nauki i tehniki»)
355. van der Stelt, O., & Belger, A. (2007). *The role of the prefrontal cortex in the regulation of the EEG in response to emotional stimuli // Journal of Neuroscience.* — Vol. 27, No. 6. — P. 1384–1392. — DOI: 10.1523/JNEUROSCI.2685-06.2007.
356. van Tier Drift, M. (1961). *Research on the dynamics of the central nervous system: EEG and cortical activity // Journal of Neurophysiology.* — Vol. 24, No. 3. — P. 124–134.
357. Vanderwolf, C. H. (1969). *Inhibition of hippocampal electrical activity by sensory stimuli // Electroencephalography and Clinical Neurophysiology.* — Vol. 26, No. 6. — P. 503–514. — DOI: 10.1016/0013-4694(69)90159-9.
358. Vasconcelos, S. M., Cavalcante, R. A., Aguiar, L. M., Sousa, F. C., Fonteles, M. M., & Viana, G. S. (2004). *Electroencephalographic findings in experimental models of epilepsy and their correlation with the pathophysiology of seizures // Neuroscience Letters.* — Vol. 369, No. 1. — P. 55–60. — DOI: 10.1016/j.neulet.2004.07.015.
359. Vollmer, M. A., & Emrich, H. M. (1998). *EEG correlates of cognitive dysfunction in patients with schizophrenia: A review of the literature // Biological Psychiatry.* — Vol. 43, No. 12. — P. 849–856. — DOI: 10.1016/S0006-3223(98)00022-7.
360. Walter G. An experimental study of the EEG during visual perception // *Brain.* — 1940. — Vol. 63, № 2. — P. 110–125.
361. Walter G. The human electroencephalogram in various states of physiological arousal // *J Physiol.* — 1937. — Vol. 90, № 3. — P. 381–405.
362. Walter W.G. The function of electrical rhytmsin the brain/ J. Ment. Sci. 96.31. 1950.

363. Walter, G. (1940). *Über das Elektrenkephalogramm des Menschen. Archiv für Psychiatrie und Nervenkrankheiten*, 109, 538–560.
364. Walter, W. G., & Dovey, M. (1944). *The electroencephalogram and its application in psychiatry // Journal of Mental Science.* — Vol. 90, No. 378. — P. 244–263.
365. Waninger S., Berka C., Stevanovic Karic M., Korszen S., Mozley P. D , Henchcliffe C., Kang Y., Hesterman J., Mangoubi T., Verma A. Neurophysiological Biomarkers of Parkinson's Disease // Journal of Parkinson's Disease. — 2020. — Vol. 10, No. 2. — P. 471–480. — DOI: 10.3233/JPD-191844. E-Scholarship
366. Williamson S. J., Kaufman L., Lu Z.-L., et al., "Study of human occipital alpha rhythm: the alphon hypothesis and alpha suppression," *Int. J. Psychophysiol.*, 26(1-3), 63-76 (1997).
367. Winterer G., Egan M.F., Rдdler T., Hyde T., Coppola R., Weinberger D.R. An association between reduced interhemispheric EEG coherence in the temporal lobe and genetic risk for schizophrenia. Schizophr. Res. 2001. 49(1): 129–143.
368. Winterer G., Enoch M.A., White K.V., Saylan M., Coppola R., Goldman D. EEG phenotype in alcoholism: increased coherence in the depressive subtype // *Acta Psychiatrica Scandinavica.* — 2003. — Vol. 108, No. 4. — P. 272–281. — DOI: 10.1034/j.1600-0447.2003.00060.x. — ISSN 0001-690X.
369. Winterer G., Saletu-Zyhlarz G. et al. EEG phenotype in alcoholism: increased coherence in the depressive subtype // *Alcoholism: Clinical and Experimental Research.* — 2003. — Vol. 27, № 9. — P. 1409–1418. — doi:10.1371/journal.pone.0123541.
370. World Health Organization. *The ICD-10 classification of mental and behavioural disorders: Diagnostic criteria for research* / World Health Organization. — Geneva : World Health Organization, 1993. — xiii, 248 p. — ISBN 9241544554.
371. Wu L., Gotman J. Segmentation and classification of EEG during epileptic seizures // *Electroencephalography and Clinical Neurophysiology.* — 1998. — Vol. 106, No. 4. — P. 344–356. — DOI: 10.1016/S0013-4694(97)00156-9.
372. Xu M, Yang J, Siok WT, Tan LH. Atypical lateralization of phonological working memory in developmental dyslexia. *J Neurolinguistics* (2015) 33:67–77. doi:10.1016/j.jneuroling.2014.07.004
373. Zhang H., Wang C., Electroencephalography and electrophysiological techniques in alcohol dependence: progress and clinical relevance // *CNS*

Neuroscience & Therapeutics. — 2023. — Vol. 29, № 1. — P. 1205–1216. — doi:10.1111/cns.14162.

374. Zhang H., Zhou Q.Q., Chen H., Hu X.Q., Li W.G., Bai Y., Han J.X., Wang Y., Liang Z.H., Chen D., et al. The applied principles of EEG analysis methods in neuroscience and clinical neurology // *Military Medical Research*. — 2023. — Vol. 10, No. 1 : 67. — DOI: 10.1186/s40779-023-00502-7.
375. Zheng-yan Jiang. Study on EEG power and coherence in patients with mild cognitive impairment during working memory task. Journal of Zhejiang University-SCIENCE A (Applied Physics & Engineering) . 2005 Dec;6(12):1213-9. doi: 10.1631/jzus.2005.B1213.
376. Zhurn. vyissh. nerv. deyat. 2005. 55(4): 496–504. (perevod: Neurosci. Behav. Physiol. 2006. 36(6): 655–662).

www.ingramcontent.com/pod-product-compliance
Lightning Source LLC
LaVergne TN
LVHW052244200926
848481LV00002B/267